THE LEAST WORST DEATH

Essays in Bioethics on the End of Life

MARGARET PABST BATTIN

New York   Oxford
OXFORD UNIVERSITY PRESS
1994

Oxford University Press

Oxford   New York   Toronto
Delhi   Bombay   Calcutta   Madras   Karachi
Kuala Lumpur   Singapore   Hong Kong   Tokyo
Nairobi   Dar es Salaam   Cape Town
Melbourne   Auckland   Madrid

and associated companies in
Berlin   Ibadan

Copyright © 1994 by Oxford University Press, Inc.

Published by Oxford University Press, Inc.
198 Madison Avenue, New York, New York 10016-4314

Oxford is a registered trademark of Oxford University Press

Library of Congress Cataloging-in-Publication Data
Battin, M. Pabst.
The least worst death : essays in bioethics on the end of life /
Margaret Pabst Battin.
p.   cm.   Includes index.
ISBN 0-19-508592-2; ISBN 0-19-508265-6 (pbk.)
1. Terminal care—Moral and ethical aspects. 2. Right to die.
3. Assisted suicide—Moral and ethical aspects. I. Title.
R726.B33   1994   179'.7—dc20   93-8276

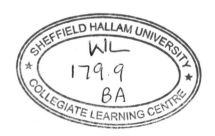

9 8 7 6 5 4 3
Printed in the United States of America
on acid-free paper

For Brooke Hopkins and Sarah Pabst Hogenauer,
for continuous enthusiasm and continuous challenge

Contents

THE LEAST WORST DEATH

Introduction: The Politics of Dying

How will we all die? This artless question may seem to be unanswerable—after all, how can we hope to see so far into our own personal futures? But it is our failure to confront this question directly, and to recognize that it has not only factual but normative components, that lies at the root of the issues addressed in this book. Of course, we cannot see our own personal futures in specific detail, but we can still know a great deal about how we are likely to die—it is a new picture, different from what it would have been only forty or fifty years ago. Furthermore, while we often think of dying as something that will eventually happen to us, we fail to see that our own deaths are a component of our lives about which we can make major, morally significant choices. Finally, even if we see that there are choices to be made, we fail to recognize that the choices that appear open to us are culturally limited in quite severe ways. *How will we all die?* This is not just a predictive empirical question; it is also a moral one.

The Political, Social, and Legal Background

Increasingly visible as topics of friction and contemporary social debate, the "right-to-die" issues—terminating medical care, withdrawing and withholding treatment, "pulling the plug," euthanasia, and assisted suicide—are rapidly becoming politicized. What fuels this increasing politicization is what we might call the *new epidemiology*, a basic change in the way we die, since with this change has come a rethinking of the purposes of medicine, an explosion of costs, and a savage challenge to traditional ideas about the ways we may die.

To see what massive but subtle transformations are taking place, consider two major twentieth-century mileposts in the public discussion of dying: the Existentialists' concerns about authenticity in life (especially their view that it is awareness of the everpresent possibility of death that first makes genuine authenticity possible), and Elizabeth Kübler-Ross's claim, put forward in *On Death and Dying*,[1] that it is permissible, indeed, desirable, to talk openly with dying patients about death. These mileposts have both contributed in important ways to the public discussion of issues in dying. But there is a substantial difference between them: what the Existentialists (especially Martin Heidegger, Karl Jaspers, Gabriel Marcel, Jean-Paul Sartre, and Albert Camus) were alert to is the possibility of unexpected death—the fact that death could happen tomorrow, today, or at any moment, though we tend to think of it as still far in the future and avoid any sense of death as a *present* possibility. Kübler-Ross, on the other hand, has in mind death that is foreseeable, indeed, death which is already in progress, in a situation in which the dying patient is beginning a series of predictable transitions through denial, anger, bargaining, depression, and a final detachment sometimes called "acceptance" on the way to death.

These two mileposts are marked by a small distance in time; most of the significant Existentialist writing appeared in the first half of the twentieth-century, up to about 1945; *On Death and Dying* appeared in the late 1960s. They are only a handful of decades apart. But they bridge a watershed transition in the new epidemiology: the Existentialists were writing largely before the discovery and dissemination of penicillin,[2] Kübler-Ross at the beginning of the major developments in what we now call life-prolonging terminal care technology: respirators, dialysis machines, artificial nutrition and hydration, and the sophisticated technology of the modern intensive-care unit. This is the leap from what is known as the third stage of the epidemiological transition to the fourth, as chapter 3, "Is There a Duty to Die?", explores in greater detail. Suddenly, penicillin and other "wonder drugs" could cure infections in injuries, childbirth, surgery, and many other situations; but they could also cure pneumonia and intercurrent infections in people with terminal illnesses, who before the development of these drugs and related technologies would have died not long after they had become bedridden. With this epidemiological transition, the dying patient would now face a much more lingering death, and pneumonia could no longer be regarded as "the old man's friend."

Thus, it should be no surprise that it is only in the last fifteen years or so that issues about sustained dying and death have become fully conspicuous. One of the earliest widespread public discussions of a specific case culminated in a state supreme court decision in 1976: this was the dispute over whether Karen Ann Quinlan could be disconnected from the respirator that had sustained her since she had fallen into a coma several years earlier, when she was in her early twenties. The New Jersey Supreme Court asserted that it had no doubt that if Karen could have regained consciousness for a moment and surveyed her own circumstances, she would have chosen to have the respirator disconnected; it ruled in favor of permitting her father to have this done.[3] Not only did this case involve the public in a broad and often virulent discussion of the issues in "pulling the plug," it also brought home the possibility that situations like Karen's could happen to anyone.

Fifteen years elapsed before the U.S. Supreme Court heard its first right-to-die case, that of another permanently comatose young woman, Nancy Cruzan. In 1990, the Court ruled that the state of Missouri could insist that Cruzan not be denied tube feedings and artificial hydration without clear and convincing evidence that that was what she would have wanted.[4] But in doing so, it gave substantial weight to a patient's own expression of his or her wishes, and did not foreclose the possibility of other states adopting less rigorous standards for determining such wishes than those of Missouri. Between *Quinlan* and *Cruzan,* a long series of cases in the courts of various states has explored, in a way open to public view, many other facets of the right-to-die issues.

Similarly, a series of publicly visible incidents has also attracted attention—sometimes supportive, sometimes appalled. They began with narrative accounts, often written by family members, of the deaths of loved ones: accounts of deaths from cancer, accounts of the long course of amyotrophic lateral sclerosis (ALS or Lou Gehrig's Disease), accounts of catastrophic burns, as in "Dax's Case."[5] They included accounts by nonparticipatory but horrified observers, as in the parents' story of heroic but futile treatment for their birth-defective newborn, *The Long Dying of Baby Andrew*.[6] They included doctors' accounts of their own practices in medicine, as, for example, Duff and Campbell's controversial account of withholding treatment from some newborns with spina bifida in an intensive-care unit (ICU).[7] And they also included stories of family members and physicians involved in more active roles in bringing about death. For example, Lael Tucker Wertenbacker's *Death of a Man* described her husband's dying of cancer and her own role in aiding his suicide; Jessamyn West, the noted Quaker author, described aiding her dying sister in the same way.[8] Betty Rollin portrayed helping her mother die.[9] By far the most influential of these, and with the most long-range effect, was *Jean's Way*, British journalist Derek Humphry's account of helping his wife, Jean, who was in the last stages of cancer, to drink a lethal potion.[10] There were further incidents: the 1977 suicide of Wallace Proctor, a seventy-five-year-old dermatologist with Parkinson's Disease whose friend, Morgan Sibbett, had consulted with the public prosecutor before aiding him;[11] the controversial 1979 suicide of artist Jo Roman, diagnosed with breast cancer, who composed a book and videotape describing her choice, and then invited her friends to a large party, after which she took her life;[12] and the double suicide of the distinguished former president of Union Theological Seminary, Henry P. Van Dusen, and his wife, Elizabeth, leaders in the ecumenical movement, whose joint suicide note read: "We still feel this is the best way and the right way to go."[13] In the early 1980s, Elizabeth Bouvia, severely handicapped by quadriplegia associated with advanced cerebral palsy, attempted to legally compel a California hospital to let her die of self-starvation while providing her with comfort care. In the early 1990s, a physician named Jack Kevorkian aroused enormous controversy by using his "suicide machine" to assist in the death of Janet Adkins, a middle-aged woman diagnosed with Alzheimer's, and then flaunting the Michigan legislature's attempts to stop him by assisting in a number of additional suicides. These accounts make very good press, and each exploited exhaustively the new medical prospects ordinary individuals would face in dying.

During the 1970s, and especially the 1980s, the media and entertainment industries were quick to make use of the compelling character of individual cases. Most popular among the resulting productions was "Whose Life Is It, Anyway?", a compelling drama asserting rights of self-determination for a young quadriplegic, which played on both the London and Broadway stages and also appeared in a film version.[14] This story also reflected new developments in medicine. At any much earlier period in medical history, before the development of penicillin and the antibiotics in general, someone born or rendered quadriplegic would have been a comparatively quick victim of such associated difficulties as pulmonary and bladder infections, as well as infections in pressure sores. The prospect of a whole life of complete immobility—which so caught audiences in its dilemma—would have been virtually nonexistent. Indeed, most of the controversial cases were ones that could not have occurred only a few decades earlier: not only would there have been no respirator to support Karen Ann Quinlan and no artificial nutrition or hydration for Nancy Cruzan, but there would have been no technology for supporting end-stage ALS, or catastrophic burns, or very serious birth defects in newborns, or even the sustained treatment of cancer.

"Whose Life Is It Anyway?" also captured another new element: the prospect of extensive "medicalization" of the predictable end of a person's life: a situation in which one's dying would be conducted largely in medical institutions. Much as childbirth had been transformed from a domestic occurrence usually taking place at home into a medical event usually taking place in a hospital, dying had also become far more highly medicalized. At the turn of the century, only a very small proportion of the population, mostly the poor, died in hospitals or institutions; today, about 85 percent of Americans do. This characteristically brought with it greater costs, greater disruption in the lives of family members, and a greater degree of isolation and disempowerment for the patient.

Concern about more active roles in dying also seemed to arise in a number of cases discussed originally within specific professional circles. The 1988 case published in the *Journal of the American Medical Association,* ambiguously entitled "It's Over, Debbie,"[15] described a sleepy resident giving a lethal injection in the middle of the night to a young woman dying of ovarian cancer; this highly problematic case seemed to electrify the medical community, and the public prosecutor made an intense (but unsuccessful) effort to identify the physician who had done it. But just a year or so later, Dr. Timothy Quill published a straightforwardly autobiographical account of his role in providing lethal drugs for a leukemia patient, Diane, who declined therapy though it offered her about a 25 percent chance of survival, and chose to die at home by her own hand.[16] Quite unlike the hostile response to Dr. Kevorkian's assistance in suicide and to the "Debbie" case, Dr. Quill's account was received with much greater sympathy. A New York grand jury refused to indict Dr. Quill, and the New York State Board for Professional Medical Conduct ruled that no charge of misconduct was warranted. The Debbie and Diane cases were originally published in medical journals for an audience of physicians, but they, too, became subject of considerable public discussion, as physicians themselves began to rethink their own rules vis-à-vis their patients' deaths.

During these decades, new legislation and public policies also came into being. California's Natural Death Act of 1976 seemed to be a breakthrough: by protecting physicians from action for failure to treat, it had the effect of empowering patients to stipulate, before they became unable to make their own choices at the end of life, what treatment they would—or, more to the point, would not—want to have. By 1983, ten other states had developed their own versions of this law; by 1993, forty-seven states—all but New York, Massachusetts, and Michigan—had "living will" laws. But there was some disenchantment with the rather anemic power of living wills: they seemed to have no teeth (providing only for professional "censure" of the physician who ignored the patient's wish to be allowed to die), and they took effect only after the patient was certified to be terminally ill and where further medical treatment would not succeed in prolonging life very much. However, states had also begun to modify existing statutes or to adopt new ones to provide a durable power of attorney for health care; by 1993, forty-eight states—all but Alaska and Alabama—had some statutory mechanism for appointing a surrogate, so that a person could select someone—a friend, relative, or anyone he or she trusted—to make medical decisions for him or her authorizing the withholding or withdrawing of life-sustaining treatment if he or she were no longer able to do so. In November 1991, the state of Washington's ballot contained a measure that would have legalized physician-assisted suicide and voluntary active euthanasia; so did California's ballot in 1992. While initially expected to pass, both lost by the fairly close margin of 54 to 46 percent. In the wake of defeat, a new group was formed in Washington: Compassion in Dying, based in Seattle, which announced its willingness to assist with the suicides of terminally ill patients in extreme suffering who make such a request. In 1993, it made public the fact that it had performed its first actual case of assisted suicide.

The responsibility for much of the increased awareness of right-to-die issues fell to a number of different groups. Hospice, begun in England by Dame Cicely Saunders, had originally challenged standard medical practice for its ineffectiveness in pain control for the dying: Hospice pioneered techniques of controlling pain before it is felt, rather than treating it afterwards, and became a major force in protecting the terminally ill from uncontrolled pain and unwanted treatment. Formed as a union of Concern for Dying, an organization promoting education about rights to refuse treatment, and the Society for the Right to Die, a group specifically advocating legal change to protect such rights, the broad group Choice in Dying emerged in 1990 to address both educational and legislative efforts. Meanwhile, Derek Humphry, who had moved to the United States from England after the publication of *Jean's Way*, had formed the Hemlock Society, a group advocating the legalization of both physician-assisted suicide and voluntary active euthanasia. It was Hemlock and its lobbying arm that had drafted and sponsored the proposed legislation in Washington and California to legalize assisted suicide and voluntary active euthanasia. Hemlock, which developed a vigorous network of nearly one hundred local members' groups, had grown extraordinarily rapidly, reaching some 50,000 members by the early 1990s, and achieved very broad visibility with the publication in 1991 of Humphry's *Final Exit*, a how-to book providing explicit information about the dosages of drugs required for "self-deliverance."[17] *Final Exit* sold more than 540,000 copies within a year and a half of publication and hit the top of the *New York Times* how-to bestseller list. The message to the medical establishment was clear: the public intended to wrest the control of dying from the physician and from medical institutions, and return it directly to the patient.

The United States was by no means the only country in which such ferment was taking place. Many other countries already had voluntary euthanasia societies and vocal individual advocates for legal change. Britain's Voluntary Euthanasia Society, renamed EXIT, had been providing drug dosage information to its members for years, sometimes directly, sometimes through its Scottish affiliate. The Dutch had established a set of guidelines under which voluntary active euthanasia, though technically illegal, would not be prosecuted; these guidelines gradually emerged in a series of court cases, both in the lower courts and in the supreme court. Meanwhile, in Germany, where assisting a suicide is not illegal, provided the person is competent and acting voluntarily, there is a large private (though controversial) organization devoted to providing assistance with suicide for the terminally ill. Late in 1993, Canada's Supreme Court heard the Rodriguez case, in which a forty-three-year-old woman with ALS directly challenged Canada's law against assisted suicide. She lost, but by a narrow 5–4 margin. The right-to-die movement has become very active in a number of countries; by 1993, such diverse countries as Japan, India, Israel, Colombia, Sweden, Australia, Belgium, South Africa, and France had right-to-die organizations that are members of the World Federation of Right-to-Die Societies.

Meanwhile, right-to-life groups were beginning to take notice of these developments. Although originally involved primarily in the public debate over abortion, by the late 1980s the right-to-life groups were beginning to focus on right-to-die issues as well, and there were several quite vocal anti-euthanasia societies. Public debate seemed to be aligned along the same general axis as the abortion issue, even though the issues are disanalogous in one central feature: in assisted suicide and voluntary active euthanasia, the death in question is a voluntary one and there is no other life at stake, whereas in abortion this is what is at issue. Right-to-life groups, together with the Catholic church, were primarily responsible for the defeat of Initiative 119 and Proposition 161. Right-to-life books and movies, often concerned with the obstacles faced by people with severe disabilities and their courage in overcoming them, have become more available. So too have explorations of the depth of prejudice—not only others' but their own—faced by persons with disabilities, as recounted in Joseph Shapiro's *No Pity*.[18] It is the disabled whom right-to-life organizations fear would be most at risk if euthanasia or assisted suicide were legal.

In this political contest, many were surprised by role of Hospice, which joined the right-to-life groups and the Catholic church to defeat the aid-in-dying initiatives. What surprised observers, despite the fact that Hospice had long been developing a philosophy in this direction, was its seeming transformation from a group that advocated patient autonomy into a group that appeared to be opposing it.[19] Hospice argued against the initiatives on what were essentially slippery-slope grounds, intimating that patients would be pressured into choices of death, but because Hospice could not claim that it was universally successful in controlling pain, this argument appeared to some to be suspiciously self-serving. The political contest will continue: Hemlock has announced plans to reintroduce legislation regarding voluntary active euthanasia and physician-assisted suicide in Oregon and Washington in 1994 and California in 1996, while at the same time some states in which assisted suicide has not been prohibited by statute have introduced "anti-Kevorkian" measures to make it so.

Thus, the situation is growing increasingly volatile. Indeed, I think the right-to-die issue, including the three topics of this book, withholding and withdrawing treatment, assisted suicide, and active euthanasia, will become *the* major social issue of the next decade—that is, the focus of the most volatile public controversy—replacing abortion in that role. This is not to say that such social concerns as child abuse, world hunger, drugs, racism, ethnic violence, prison conditions, and the like will not also be major causes of concern, and certainly not that they are less important nor that they do not also generate deep dissent. Yet, I do think that right-to-die issues involve disagreement at a deeper level, concerned as they are about the role one may or may not take in matters so directly affecting one's own being as whether one lives or dies.

As is emphasized repeatedly throughout this book, the epidemiology of how we die is changing, and an individual's chances of dying in certain highly predictable ways are increasing. In the technologically advanced nations, only about 10 percent of deaths are completely unexpected, including accident, homicide, and suicide, and around 70 to 80 percent of deaths are the result of degenerative diseases marked by a long downhill decline. It is no doubt true that right-to-die issues concerning old, terminally ill people are unlikely to exercise a youth-oriented culture in the same way that the envisioned destruction of unborn babies produces visceral responses in the abortion debate—at least until individuals watch a parent, a sibling, a child, or another close family member or friend die, especially of a protracted deteriorative illness in a highly medicalized situation. It is personal experience of this sort—which increasingly involves painful decisions to terminate treatment, overwhelming cost pressures, and devastating nursing-care choices—that galvanizes individuals on one side or another of a major public issue. It is true that in our youth-oriented, seemingly death-proof culture we do not like to think about dying—certainly not about our own deaths, and certainly not much in advance—but politicization occurs when we are forced by circumstances to see what is involved in the ways we now usually die. Thus, it is ultimately a personal issue: that is, right-to-die issues are issues about our own *personal futures.* As we discover this, public ferment over right-to-die issues is likely to increase and to involve disagreement at a deeper level. It is the aim of this book to explore these deeper disagreements.

It is important to see how contingent an issue this is. Our new concerns with the ways we die are, I think, largely a product of our new epidemiology, the fact that we now typically die late in life of deteriorative disease. But this could change: global environmental damage could cause our life expectancies to drop dramatically, or extraordinary developments in medicine or genetic technology could cause them to rise equally dramatically. Or, more likely, gains in life expectancies may inch upward, but our technological situation may remain more or less the same. If there is dramatic change, either up or down, the ethical dilemmas that confront us will also change; but the likelihood is that those which confront us now are dilemmas we shall be facing for some time to come.

Institutional Pressures

This chronicle of specific events, court cases, groups, and the other features of which the recent history of dispute over right-to-die issues consists, can be described, I think, in terms of pressure and ferment within at least three major institutions: law, medicine, and religion.

Ferment within the Law

In the long series of cases occurring in the fifteen years between *Quinlan* and *Cruzan*, a series that included, among many others, *Saikewicz, Spring, Eichner, Barber, Bartling, Conroy, Brophy, Bouvia,* and the trio *Farrell, Peter,* and *Jobes,* state courts have developed a rich texture of decisions about withholding and withdrawing treatment from patients who can no longer, or never could, indicate their wishes.[20] *Saikewicz,* for example, involved withholding chemotherapy from a sixty-year-old man with an IQ of 10 and a mental age of about two years and eight months. *Spring* concerned terminating dialysis treatments for a seventy-eight-year-old man with profound dementia. *Brophy* involved the withdrawal of artificial nutrition from a forty-nine-year-old former firefighter and emergency medical technician who had said of a man he'd helped pull from a burning truck but who suffered a great deal before dying several months later, "If I'm ever like that, just shoot me, pull the plug."[21] These court decisions have been rendered at the same time as state legislatures have been enacting so-called "natural death" laws, providing the structures of living wills and durable powers of attorney for health care to enable patients to direct their care after they are no longer competent. In general, the courts have been willing to respect clearly expressed antecedent patient declarations, even when they involve withholding or withdrawing care after the patient is no longer competent, in a way that will result in death.[22] And the courts have long recognized, since the 1914 *Schloendorff* case, that the competent patient may refuse any treatment he or she wishes. But what they have not addressed, or addressed in only the most tangential way, are first-party choices by the competent patient for more active forms of intervention in the dying process. Virtually all the major court cases have been cases about withholding or withdrawing treatment from somebody else—*second-party cases*—and only a handful—*Bouvia, Rhodas,* and a few others—have been about first-party refusal of treatment in a way that results in death. And none has directly concerned the issue of patient requests for active termination of their own lives, either in assisted suicide or voluntary active euthanasia, though there have been a few voices, for example, Justice Compton's concurring opinion in *Bouvia* and Justice Scalia's in *Cruzan,* that have spoken to the larger issue. Writing of Elizabeth Bouvia's request to be allowed to starve herself to death while receiving comfort and care in a California hospital rather than continue a life severely handicapped by cerebral palsy, Justice Compton said that Bouvia had an "absolute right" to effectuate her decision, and that the state and the medical profession should "assist her to die with ease and dignity."[23] In *Cruzan,* Justice Scalia seemed almost to equate refusal of treatment with suicide, and rejected any claim that suicide was a right.[24]

Yet it is here that the major issue lies. It can be understood as a basic constitutional conflict, one that U.S. law has never addressed squarely.[25] On the one hand, the U.S. Constitution protects the right of self-determination in many significant matters of personal choice, including choices involving the treatment of one's own body; although these have sometimes been described as issues of privacy, the

Supreme Court is now tending to treat them as issues of self-determination or liberty. Such protected personal choices include those that may result in death, such as refusing a blood transfusion on religious grounds or refusing medical treatment for personal reasons. On the other hand, the courts have also appeared to recognize state interests in preventing suicide: this is one of the four virtually universally cited state interests in these areas, namely: (1) the preservation of life, (2) the protection of the interests of innocent third parties, (3) the prevention of suicide, and (4) safeguarding the integrity of the medical profession.[26] But no rationale is cited for the state's interest in preventing suicide, and hence there is no way of discerning what the state's interest might be, if any, in preventing suicide in medical cases of terminal illness that are at issue here.

The law itself is in a state of active flux. In all but two or three states, it is not a crime to commit or attempt to commit suicide,[27] though in no state is it a crime to intervene to prevent a suicide. Suicide had earlier been treated as a felony in many U.S. jurisdictions and remained so in England and Wales until 1961; decriminalization was intended to permit the treatment of mentally ill suicide attempters without criminal onus. In recent times, only slightly more than half of the U.S. states have had statutes explicitly criminalizing assisted suicide; yet in the wake of the Kevorkian case Michigan and several other states—Illinois, Indiana, and Tennessee—have passed new statutes, making a total (as of this writing, October 1993) of thirty-two.[28] Twelve more states and the District of Columbia have adopted English common law, making assisted suicide a criminal matter. Two states (Iowa and Virginia) prohibit assisted suicide on the basis of case law, and one (Louisiana) protects citizens from euthanasia under constitutional law. Three states (North Carolina, Utah, and Wyoming) do not have explicit statutes, do not recognize common law, and have no holding or court case in the matter. Yet observers in some states which appear to have statutory prohibitions of assisted suicide have challenged these interpretations—as Compassion in Dying has done in the state of Washington. The ACLU has entered the Michigan case, arguing that a statute passed specifically to stop Kevorkian is unconstitutional and that it undermines patients' rights to decide when and how they die. Furthermore, three states—Maine, New Hampshire, and Vermont—are all considering legislation which would legalize physician-assisted suicide, and ballot measures are expected during the next several years in Oregon, Washington, and California. And some observers point out that common-law prohibitions of suicide are historically rooted in medieval ecclesiastical conceptions of suicide as a sin, and thus to be challenged on grounds of separation of church and state. Thus the current legal situation is extraordinarily fluid, with some state legislatures reacting to events by passing "anti-Kevorkian" laws while others consider legalization of assistance or physician-assistance in suicide, and critics pointing out the unresolved constitutional issue of the state's interest in preventing suicide and the scope of individual liberties. As attorney Alan Sullivan puts it:

> In a culture that places freedom of choice among the most important of all protected values, the state has no plausible interest in preventing suicide by competent people. Rather, the state's "compelling interest" is in protecting choice, in insuring that persons making critical decisions within the ambit of the right to

privacy are not coerced, are mentally competent, and are sufficiently informed to decide for themselves. The state should intervene to prevent suicide where the individual lacks the capacity or the competence to make a choice in the matter. The state should not intervene merely because the incipient suicide's decision appears foolish or because it is regarded as morally wrong.[29]

This view may be contrasted with the position taken by Justice Scalia in his vehement concurring opinion in *Cruzan,* in which he rejected the claim that aid in dying could be a right, and appealed to the traditional claim that suicide is *always* wrong. Many viewed this opinion as tangential to the issue in *Cruzan,* if not altogether irrelevant, and not only did no other justices join it, none of them, whether in the majority or minority, gave any sense that they saw the issue in this way. Nevertheless, Scalia's opinion was treated as unusually farsighted by other observers: Scalia, some claimed, was seeing what the deeper issue not just in *Cruzan,* but in all right-to-die cases, really is.

Thus, it would seem there is remarkable tension concerning this central point of law. The question can be understood as a fundamental civil liberties issue: What role may the individual play in his or her own death? To what degree does the state have an interest in controlling the character of a person's death? Thus, the issue turns to challenge the alleged state's interest in preventing suicide: Does the state always have an interest in preventing suicide, or just when the person's choice is impaired? If, as I expect, right-to-die issues do eclipse abortion as the focus of social ferment in the next decade, it is a decision on basic issues in suicide that will serve the same pivotal legal and political function as *Roe v. Wade,* and will no doubt generate the same turbulent public discussion.

It is also crucial to note the differences between the positions on these issues that characterize U.S. law and those of various other nations. Consider, for instance, the differences between the United States, the Netherlands, and Germany (a trio that will often be discussed in this volume): three advanced, industrial nations, with roughly similar demographic patterns of life expectancy and population age, equally sophisticated medical establishments, common roots in the European Enlightenment, and legal environments similar in many (though by no means all) respects. All of these nations have entered the fourth stage of the epidemiological transition, when the majority of their populations will die late in life of degenerative rather than parasitic or infectious diseases, and all now have the medical capacity to prolong the ending of life considerably. But whereas U.S. law has recognized only a patient's right to refuse unwanted treatment, so that Americans are forced in principle to rely only on withholding or withdrawing treatment in their approach to death, Dutch law (as described in detail in chapter 6, "A Dozen Caveats for the Discussion of Euthanasia in the Netherlands") has come, in a delicately balanced way, to recognize choices of euthanasia as well, and German law (described in chapter 12, "Assisted Suicide: Can We Learn from Germany?") permits assistance in suicide, provided that the person who wishes to die is competent and acts voluntarily. Thus, under their respective bodies of law, both Dutch and German patients facing the end of life have choices not legally open to Americans, and hence, one may wish to claim, an environment for dying in which the state is less constricting and in which a fuller range of civil liberties exist.

Ferment in Health Financing and Health Policy

If the situation in U.S. law seems unsettled, that in American health financing and health policy must appear tempestuous. Cost issues have become acute, and they increasingly challenge the very structure of contemporary medicine. Currently reaching around 14 percent of the gross domestic product (GDP), U.S. expenditures on health care are the highest per capita in the world, but they do not provide health care for all citizens or residents and they do not produce the highest level of health status. On the contrary, the United States ranks well behind most industrialized nations in many indicators of health status. This is associated with the fact that the United States has had only a partial national health system, comprised of distinct programs such as Medicare and Medicaid, and those of the Veterans Administration (VA), the Indian Health Service, and CHAMPUS, which provides care for the elderly, the poor, veterans, Native Americans, and military and government employees, but not for others. The majority of the population has depended on health insurance obtained through their employers, and at the time of this writing some thirty-seven million Americans—mostly employed, primarily by small firms unable or unwilling to provide health insurance—still have no coverage at all. A similar number have coverage that is grossly inadequate. The Clinton administration's efforts to develop a national health plan is in response to broad public concern about the state of U.S. medicine, and whatever form it takes, it will have substantial impact on the way we die.

In the current tempest, blame is leveled at many parties: at physicians for charging huge fees, at hospitals for inflating charges by cost-shifting, at developers of high-tech medical devices for inviting overuse, at lawyers for malpractice litigation, at medical suppliers for inflating costs, at insurance companies for poor capital investment and for screening out the ill, at administrative functions for consuming, it is sometimes estimated, as much as a quarter of total health care costs, and, not least, at patients for their failures to adopt healthier life-styles. But blame is very often also leveled indirectly at those groups of patients with whom this book is primarily concerned: those for whom "death and dying" issues are most pressing—the terminally ill and the elderly. An estimate originally based on Medicare expenditures, now employed across the board in discussions of health policy and financing, holds that care for those within the last six months of life consumes some 30 percent of the total health care budget. To be sure, those within the last six months of life include newborns with serious defects who do not survive and accident, homicide, and suicide victims who receive some treatment before they succumb, but by far the largest group are those reaching late life: older individuals in the process of dying, usually slowly and usually in hospitals or nursing homes, of essentially degenerative diseases that typically exhibit an extended downhill course. As several of the chapters in this book discuss in greater detail, some 70 to 80 percent of persons can now expect to die of diseases or conditions that may lead to death in this protracted way: this is the new epidemiological circumstance, new in the developed nations in this century and still not achieved in many developing ones, that gives rise to the issues discussed in this book.

But dying later in life of deteriorative rather than acute diseases, at the conclusion of a long downhill course, is expensive, and hence many of the cost-control proposals focus on those groups of patients with whom we are especially concerned here. Thus, we see proposals for age-rationing (for example, those by Daniel Callahan and Norman Daniels are discussed in chapter 3, "Is There a Duty to Die?"), and sometimes, proposals for time-to-death rationing intednded to limit terminal care. There are also cloaked cost-control proposals: indeed, as I suggest in chapter 8, "Voluntary Euthanasia and the Risks of Abuse," I believe the 1991 Patient Self-Determination Act (PSDA) to be an example—even though there is not a word either in the act itself or in its legislative history to suggest that its motive is cost control. After all, it is easily and predictably misunderstood to require execution of an advance directive, and since advance directives are almost always used to decline rather than request care, the PSDA will most likely have the effect of reducing end-of-life health care costs.[30] Pressures for cost control are certain to become still more severe in coming years, regardless of what structural changes medicine does or does not undergo.

But cost-control pressures readily fuel fears of abuse: they insert considerations of money into the relationship between physician and patient, and in effect give other entities—insurers, HMOs, hospitals, government—veto power over the way in which the physician treats the patient. The degree of mistrust is increasing, and the traditional professional posture of medicine—that the physician's primary concern is the welfare of the patient—is under severe threat. Physicians fear being forced to practice within inappropriate limits; patients fear being written off. These effects of turbulence in financing and health policy—the fears of abuse they generate, and with this, the slippery-slope arguments they stimulate—are a central concern of this book.

Ferment in Religion

As the people of the state of Washington prepared to go to the polls in November 1991 to vote on Initiative 119, they were confronted with a remarkable degree of involvement by religious groups. Urging voters to reject the measure was the Catholic church, the source of most of the substantial funding raised by opponents of the bill to defeat it, as well as virtually all fundamentalist groups. But on the other side, urging passage, were, among others, a regional group of the Methodist church, the United Church of Christ, and the Unitarian/Universalists, together with a coalition of ministers from a very wide range of denominations.

Although the positions and activities of religious groups are not always accorded central importance in our reflections on social issues, I think it is crucial not to underestimate their influence here—influence not only on their own members, but on members of other groups and on those with no religious affiliation at all. This is not merely the view that religion has always influenced politics and will no doubt continue to do so; it is the view that there is something distinctive about right-to-die issues that should lead us to expect that religion will play a much more important role. After all, it is primarily religion, including both religious belief and the religious institutions that foster this belief, that interprets for a culture what the significance of death is and, hence, what one's attitude toward dying and role in one's own death ought to be. To what I think is a substantial degree, both medicine and the law tend to operate within the conceptual frameworks and assumptions about dying originally marked out by religion, even where they appear to be wholly secular enterprises.

The ferment within religion in the United States at root is due, as I discuss in some detail in several of these chapters, to a set of background circumstances related to the epidemiological point made previously. Traditional Christian thought connects death with sin; death is the penalty for original sin. Death is also associated with redemption and a beatific afterlife: it is the point at which one is judged for salvation. In traditional thought, the believer's appropriate posture should be acceptance of the penalty, repentance of sin, willing acceptance of suffering, and devout hope of grace for admission into heaven. This is a *passivist* posture, as I argue toward the end of chapter 4, "Dying in 559 Beds": one is to accept the death meted out to oneself and the suffering that may accompany it. That is, for many traditionalists, what it is to believing and devout. But these beliefs were developing during historical periods when the principal causes of death were parasitic and infectious diseases, occurring in pandemic or epidemic conditions and associated with such circumstances as malnutrition, trauma, and childbirth. Infection frequently dispatched accident victims (and wounded soldiers) who survived the initial trauma. Death was often sudden and unexpected, and except for sepsis in childbirth, could occur at any chronological age. Furthermore, medical care was of very little efficacy in changing the course of these diseases: it could comfort and perhaps ease the transition, but it could not prevent death. Today, of course, at least in the advanced nations, deaths from parasitic and infectious diseases are comparatively few and, except for AIDS and trauma, we now die of degenerative conditions instead. The background religious beliefs of Western culture developed under very different epidemiological conditions, and what is provoking the new ferment—and will continue to do so—is the perception, however inchoate, that these religious beliefs and their associated practices are simply no longer very well suited to the much more extended, much more predictable ways we now die.

Philosophic Issues in the Background

Right-to-die issues are becoming increasingly politicized, it is true; but they also raise more complex philosophic issues, discussed in various contexts and used in various ways in the right-to-die debates. These philosophic issues also permeate this volume. I'd like to call attention to what I think are the three most basic issues, and provide some clues about where to see them in action in the chapters of this book.

Killing versus Letting Die

Exhaustively discussed in the academic literature, the distinction between killing and letting die is central to all discussion here. Is there really a difference, an important difference, between these two? To be sure, the very organization of this volume seems to trade on this distinction: it begins with a set of selections on withholding and withdrawing treatment—or, in less disguised terminology, allowing the patient to die—and moves on to two sections involving different forms of killing: killing by the physician and killing by the patient—respectively, euthanasia and suicide. It seems easy to identify the conceptual distinction between the two: killing involves intervening in ongoing physiological processes that would otherwise have been adequate to support life, whereas letting die involves not intervening to aid physiological processes that have become inadequate to support life. But there are a number of ambiguous cases: on the one hand, removing a respirator may seem to be letting the patient die, because his or her lung function has become inadequate to support life; on the other hand, it may seem to be killing, because removing the respirator intervenes in the physiological process of air exchange in the lungs, which so far has actually been supporting life. Clearly, although it may in general be intuitively simple to distinguish between killing and letting die, in many of the kinds of cases of interest here the distinction is not quite as straightforward as it may seem.

There is, as one might imagine, an immense literature devoted to the analysis of this complex philosophical problem.[31] It is a crucial issue, since on it rides the success of any rule-based system, whether moral, legal, religious, or otherwise, that rests on assertions about the categorical impermissibility of certain cases of killing, but also maintains that certain cases of letting die are permissible. No doubt, the most loudly proclaimed categorical assertion currently invoked in right-to-die discussions is Mark Siegler's table-thumping *"Doctors must not kill!"*[32] But categorical assertions are also to be found, for example, in the Hippocratic Oath. The oath stipulates "I shall not give a deadly drug, not even if asked," a clear prohibition of the then-current practice among mainstream Greek physicians of providing a euthanatic drug on request to patients they could not cure. The American Medical Association's 1973 policy statement that the physician is always morally prohibited from killing patients but is not morally bound to preserve life in all cases[33] also involves the same categorical assertion—that is, that even if the physician may sometimes allow a patient to die, the physician must never kill.

But to grant, despite gray cases, that there is "a difference" between killing and letting die that is adequate to support categorical assertions against killing is only to grant a conceptual point; it is not yet to grant that there is or must be a moral difference, or that a moral difference must run in a certain way. This point was raised most vividly by James Rachels's tiny but famous article, "Active and Passive Euthanasia," which appeared in the *New England Journal of Medicine* almost two decades ago.[34] Rachels challenged the conventional conception of the moral difference between killing and letting die by posing the following now-famous case: Smith and Jones, let us imagine, will each inherit a considerable fortune from their respective six-year-old cousins, should the cousins die. One evening, while his cousin is taking his bath, Smith sneaks into the bathroom and drowns him. Meanwhile, Jones is also planning to drown his own cousin, who is also taking a bath, but as Jones sneaks into the bathroom the child hits his head and slips under the water, and Jones does nothing to save him. Now both children are dead. Smith has killed his cousin; Jones has merely allowed his cousin to die.

Clearly there is a conceptual and causal difference in what the two men did—one pushed the child's head under the water, the other sat back and watched—but even so, Rachels argues, we ought not grant that there is any *moral* difference. They both acted despicably, and it is no excuse for Smith to say that he didn't kill his cousin, he "merely" let his cousin die.

Not so, argued Richard Trammell, in a nearly equally famous reply.[35] Discerning the difference between Jones' killing and Smith's letting die is like trying to taste the difference between two fine wines when they are mixed with green persimmon juice: there *is* a difference between the wines, but in these overpowering circumstances we cannot see what it is. Just so with the drowned cousins: because the behavior of both men is so repugnant, it has a ''sledgehammer'' or ''masking'' effect, and we cannot see the difference in what they did.

This of course, is an attempt to try to preserve the categorical injunction against killing: the view that killing is always intrinsically wrong, or, if the categorical view does not prohibit killing in warfare, capital punishment, or self-defense, then that killing is always wrong in medicine. But this view is readily challenged by moral experience, which suggests that in some cases killing is right: for example, the coup de grace granted a mortally wounded, dying soldier who cannot be saved on the battlefield, abortion in order to save the life of the mother, or selective termination of a multiple pregnancy when without it none of the fetuses would survive. Of course, whether there are any noncontroversially permissible examples of killing in medicine is just what is at issue.

Beyond question, the most influential strategy to try to preserve the categorical injunction against killing in the face of such challenges is traditional Catholicism's principle of double effect. According to this principle, one may perform an action with a bad effect—for instance, the death of a person—provided one foresees but does not intend that bad effect; one must be doing the act to achieve a different, good effect (hence the name, ''double'' effect). More rigorously stated, the principle of double effect requires that four conditions be met: (1) the action must not be intrinsically wrong; (2) the agent must intend only the good effect, not the bad one; (3) the bad effect must not be the means of achieving the good effect; and (4) the good effect must be ''proportional'' to the bad one, that is, outweigh it.[36] Thus, to use an example widely discussed in Catholic moral theology, a surgeon may remove a cancerous uterus in order to save the life of the mother, though this will also bring about the death of a fetus developing there, provided the surgeon's intention is to save the mother: the surgeon foresees, but does not intend, that the procedure will also kill the fetus. The case is said to meet all four of the conditions: removing the cancerous uterus is good, or at least morally neutral; the surgeon intends only to save the mother; killing the fetus is not the means of saving the mother; and saving the mother's life outweighs saving that of the fetus, which in the circumstances could not survive in any case.

But even if it seems plausibly applied here, the principle has been used in some very strained ways in the Catholic tradition. For example, a Jesuit writing in 1936, attempting to explain the view that Christian virgins seeking to escape violation during the Roman persecutions could not be said to be guilty of suicide when they flung themselves from rooftops as the soldiers approached (as Eusebius, Jerome, and Ambrose had said they were not), claimed that they merely ''wished the jump, and put up with the fall.''[37] But this is remarkably stretched, and it is simply implausible to claim that someone who knows with certainty that a specific, central effect will result, namely, her own death at the bottom of the fall, can be said not to intend it when she leaps; she knows what she is doing—what she must do to escape violation—and intends to do it. Such examples raise the more general difficulty of distinguishing ''intended'' from ''unintended'' effects, and constitute a serious challenge to the principle. Of course, it may be true that the parent who gives a child medicine to cure an illness does not intend the bad taste it causes in the child's mouth, but this is more a comment on the magnitude, not the moral status, of the foreseeable effects. To claim that a doctor can give a patient a massive overdose and foresee, without intending, the patient's death serves more as a *reductio ad absurdum* than a confirmation of the principle, more like "wishing the jump and putting up with the fall" than giving the child the bad-tasting medicine.

A second stategy for trying to distinguish permissible from impermissible kinds of acts at the end of life, also inherited from the Catholic tradition, seeks to distinguish between *ordinary* and *extraordinary* means of sustaining life; it holds that although it is always obligatory to provide ordinary means of treatment and care, it is permissible to withhold or withdraw extraordinary ones. Thus, this additional principle supplements the principle of double effect by showing which forms of letting die are permissible and which are not in medical situations. But it has not proved very workable in many of the hard cases: Is a respirator ordinary or extraordinary treatment? (Answer: sometimes one, sometimes the other.) Is artificial nutrition and hydration ordinary or extraordinary? (same answer) and so on. This account has proved no more persuasive than that of the principle of double effect in drawing tenable distinctions, and reveals itself as an essentially heuristic device for trying to draw a moral distinction by means of a conceptual one.

Quite current in contemporary medical ideology concerning end-of-life issues is a secular variant of the principle of double effect, one that comes without the sophistication of the traditional four-point Catholic version. This secular variant seems to hold simply that there is no moral disapprobation to be attached to doing something the effect of which one does not intend. So, for example, it is very often claimed that it is permissible for a physician to administer heavy doses of morphine to a terminally ill patient close to death, knowing that the morphine will depress respiration and make that death occur earlier, provided the physician's intention is to relieve suffering, not to cause the death. There is rarely discussion, in this ideology, of whether the agent also intends the death as well as the relief of suffering, whether the death is intended to relieve the suffering, or whether the goodness of the good effect is proportional to the badness of the bad, that is, outweighs it. That using morphine in this way is all right seems, rather, to be a view widespread in terminal care, but rarely carefully challenged. Yet, depending on how the elements of such cases are described, it may seem that they violate several of the conditions of the principle of double effect—indeed, all but the last. It can easily be argued that what the physician is doing in giving the patient the very heavy dose of morphine is killing the patient (though the physician would resist this label); that it is impossible for the physician to "foresee" but not intend that the patient will die as a result of the dose (especially when far larger doses are used than are actually required to produce sedation sufficient to control pain); and that bringing about the patient's death is used as a way of controlling the pain—now the pain can no longer occur. But in actual contemporary medical practice the principle of double effect is hardly formally recognized; what actually happens, it is surely more accurate to say, is that medical culture has developed a prevailing mythology that giving high doses of morphine at the end is not killing (even though the patient dies as a result) and hence not subject to moral (or legal) censure. Even in the Netherlands, which legally tolerates voluntary active euthanasia—for example, by lethal injection—both of the recent empirical studies (the Remmelink Commission report and that by van der Wal, both described in chapter 6), draw a conceptual distinction between euthanasia and the use of opiates at doses sufficient to bring about an earlier death. Only 1.8 percent of deaths annually in the Netherlands are the result of euthanasia, but 17.5 percent of deaths occur in connection with the use of heavy doses of opiates.

Thus, we must recognize that the distinction between killing and letting die does not succeed in carrying the moral weight often placed on it. Even if it were always possible to draw clear conceptual lines between the two, the conceptual distinction almost always brings along with it an unjustified moral distinction in the bargain. For example, to describe a procedure as "mercy killing" invites the inference that because it involves killing it is wrong; this is to take the moral baggage along with the conceptual distinction, though the inference does not follow. To claim that it is permissible to let newborn infants die, if their defects are so severe that they cannot survive, but not to kill them, is also to beg the question; one cannot assume that in such cases killing is worse than letting die. Rather, each such issue needs to be argued on its own merits, and the conceptual distinction between killing and letting die cannot do all the work instead.

Nor does it help to try to see the killing/letting die distinction as simply one instance of the more general *act/omission* or *active/passive* distinction. To be sure, by looking at other examples we can see how fragile a basis such distinctions provide for categorical moral claims. Consider one in a positive context: the distinction between *teaching* and *letting learn*. There are clearly conceptual differences here, for example, between teaching the young child (say, by explaining to him or her) that the stove is hot, and letting the child learn by touching it; but even granting the conceptual distinction, we can still argue at length about which is the "better" (less painful? more effective? quickest?) and more morally defensible method of inculcating this knowledge. In some cases teaching is the only option: you cannot simply "let" someone learn, say, the theory of relativity. And, in some cases teaching rather than letting learn is the only morally defensible course: you could teach a parachutist to pull the ripcord or let him or her learn (the hard way), but only one of these is defensible. On the other hand, many cases are the other way around. Thus, the more general distinction does not really help. Killing and letting die are much like teaching and letting learn: acts and omissions, doings and lettings, of which each must be examined more closely for its moral features. To discover differences between active and passive causal roles still does not answer the moral issues. In short, we cannot sweep these moral problems under the rug with categorical conceptual claims.

Nevertheless, the killing/letting die distinction is not without its uses, especially as it makes possible a more general challenge to the assumption that killing is worse than letting die. I think this challenge is especially important as we approach the distributive issues posed under the question of justice. The root question soon to be publicly raised (though probably not to be formulated in this way, since this phraseology evokes associations with the thrift-euthanasia of the early Nazi program) is this: given the enormous expense of medical care and the fact that in some situations continuing life seems to be of no benefit to the patient at all, is letting die worse than killing, or the other way around? Both result in the death of the patient, but letting die can consume huge amounts of resources; killing minimizes expense. This discussion, I repeat, is unlikely to be conducted in these terms, but it is already operative in practice: we give large doses of morphine, we disconnect respirators, we discontinue artificial nutrition and hydration, under the tacit assumption that to let these patients die at a longer, slower rate would be not only cruel, but a tremendous waste of resources. The *Wanglie* case, in which physicians sued to remove a respirator from a permanently comatose elderly woman, claiming it was of no benefit to her, over the objections of her husband who insisted that she wanted her life preserved even if she would never recover to a conscious state, is a foreshadowing of this, and whether we interpret the removal of a respirator as killing or as merely letting die, it is a case that clearly raises what I think will be central issues in the future.[38] After all, the *Wanglie* case was seen in these two different ways by the different parties involved: the family saw disconnecting Mrs. Wanglie's respirator as killing her, while the doctors clearly viewed it, though they did not use quite this language, as a routine, normal case of letting a hopelessly ill, unsalvageable patient die.

Virtually all the essays in this book presuppose, or make use of, the distinction between killing and letting die, and they all refrain from supposing that killing is worse than letting die. Chapter 1, the title piece, discusses ways the physician can attempt to accommodate a patient's desire for "natural death" without either active euthanasia or assisted suicide: it does not reject either of these, but simply assumes that for those patients and physicians who do see a moral distinction and who do take direct killing to be wrong, there are still ways to pursue strategies of "letting die" to maximize choice and minimize the risk of suffering. Chapter 3, "Is There a Duty to Die?" directly explores the distinction between killing and letting die; it argues that policies developed to satisfy the demands of distributive justice cannot rationally be restricted to letting die, especially letting die as a result of disenfranchisement in a rationing scheme.

Chapter 7, "Fiction as Forecast: Euthanasia in Alzheimer's Disease?" explores the distinction between killing and letting die by employing a first-person, quasifictional strategy to see what the experienced difference between being killed and being allowed to die may be to an advanced Alzheimer's patient. This chapter too challenges the conventional assumption that killing is always worse than letting die. Finally, the accounts of euthanasia in the Netherlands and assisted-suicide practices in Germany also rest on this distinction, portraying two very different societies that do not see the fit between the conceptual and the moral issues in quite the same way Americans do.

The Slippery Slope

The second of the three principal philosophical issues permeating this volume, that concerning the soundness of the slippery slope argument, is taken extremely seriously here. As I argue in chapter 8, "Voluntary Euthanasia and the Risks of

Abuse," both those opposing and those favoring the expansion of right-to-die practices to include active euthanasia and assisted suicide ought to attend to this argument with care, since there are claims of potential abuse going both ways: the abuse
that may occur if direct killing practices are permitted, and the abuse that may
(already) occur if they are not.

The slippery slope argument occurs under a variety of names and in a variety of
forms, including those that appeal to direct causation and those that appeal to
precedents, to psychological and sociological changes, and to a variety of other
mechanisms. They are all used to resist the acceptance, performance, or legalization
of specific practices, and they all predict a slide down the slippery slope if these
practices are not resisted. Of course, as is pointed out in chapter 5, "Euthanasia: The
Fundamental Issues," each of these metaphorical names for the argument—
"slippery slope," "camel's nose under the tent," "edge of the wedge," and so
on—carries with it a concealed assumption about causal force: in the "slippery
slope" version, it is gravity that pulls you down; in the "camel's nose" version, it is
the camel's curiosity or appetite that propels it further into the tent; and in the "edge
of the wedge" version, it is assumed that someone or something will strike the
wedge, for if not, the wedge constitutes no further risk. Since their cute metaphorical
names alone cannot grant them logical validity, adequate evaluation of slippery
slope arguments must involve identifying and ascertaining the actual causal force
assumed to be at work.

Alternative versions point not to causal forces unleashed by the practice in
question but to precedents set by them, in view of which other causal forces will
work to start the slide down the slope. Favorites here are claims about the greed or
evil of human nature, about the natural abusiveness of human institutions, or the lure
of money. Most realistic among these, I've argued in several places (see chapters 4
and 8), are the tensions in medicine set up by pressures for cost control. But the root
difficulty of this, like any other consequentialist argument (as slippery slope arguments are), is that of making secure predictive claims. Indeed, the argument form
has not been in particularly good philosophic repute in recent years, not only because
the predictive claims on which it trades are difficult to formulate and support in any
rigorous way, but because it is so frequently used in such uncritical ways by those
who oppose various forms of social change.

Of course, not all slippery slope arguments trade on simple empirical claims.
Here's an example of one that trades on legal precedent independently of claims
about human nature, human institutions, or money. It has been rather widely employed in the right-to-die literature:

> . . . recognition of a true right to die [that is, a right to commit suicide, with or
> without assistance] would revolutionize much of the legal system, having serious
> impacts in the areas, for example, of constitutional law, torts, mental health law,
> and criminal law . . .
>   . . . a right to commit suicide could not be limited to dying, terminal patients.
> Under the equal-protection clause of the Fourteenth Amendment to the U.S. Consti-
> tution, legislative classifications that restrict constitutional rights are subject to strict
> scrutiny and will be struck down unless narrowly tailored to further a compelling
> government interest . . . there appears no reason why the right to die should

apply only to terminally ill people or any other limited class of individuals. In the context of a right to refuse treatment, such limitations have not withstood judicial review [references to *Bouvia* and *Conroy*]. Therefore the "young woman tragically disappointed in love, the middle-aged man who has lost his family and whose career has been destroyed, the depressed teen, and the . . . severely disabled [person]" would share equally in the right to kill themselves.

    . . . the right to die would apply not only to adults, but also to mature minors . . .

    . . . a right to choose death for oneself would also probably extend to incompetent individuals . . . Therefore infants, those with mental illness, retarded people, confused or senile elderly individuals, and other incompetent people would be entitled to have someone else enforce their right to die.

    . . . counselors [would be required] to advise a client that he or she has a right to die and that the means are available to effectuate that decision.

    . . . police and firefighters who rescue potential suicides would risk provoking a federal civil rights action for the deprivation of the right to die . . .

    . . . the state could not justify a blanket authorization of civil commitment for mentally ill persons dangerous to themselves . . .

    . . . A right to kill oneself would at least partially invalidate or require judicial reconstruction of all current homicide and assisted-suicide laws . . . consent of the slain would be a defense to homicide, and laws forbidding homicide would be unenforceable as applied to the killing of willing victims. Substituted judgment doctrine, where adopted, would extend this exception to minor and other imcompetent victims "substitute-judged" to desire death.

    . . . recognition of a right to die would virtually demolish whatever minimal state interest remained in preserving human life. In the face of a right to die, the state would be largely powerless to do anything other than safeguard the integrity of the decision whether to live or die. Consequently, a substantial body of law premised upon a governmental interest in protecting human life—health and safety regulations, for example—would suffer the loss of its primary justification, and thus face drastic limitation.[39]

This argument displays at least four of the most common errors of slippery slope reasoning. First, it fails to identify clearly what the feared outcome is—the bottom point of the slide. The feared outcome is alluded to in the claim that "whatever minimal state interest remained in preserving human life" could have been demolished: but what, exactly, are the new circumstances feared? A society of universal suicide? A Hobbesian war of all against all, with anyone able to impose death on anyone else? A new Nazism, in which "unfit" individuals are declared candidates for euthanasia and suicide on the basis of "substituted judgment"? The argument points to an intolerable outcome that will result if a "full right to die," including rights to voluntary active euthanasia and assisted suicide, are recognized, but although this intolerable outcome is used as the basis for not recognizing these rights, it is nowhere clearly described.

Second, and related, this slippery slope argument, like many others, fails to identify the causal force presumed to fuel the slide from the current situation to the predicted bad outcome. An implicit reference to human greed or the pressure of economic circumstances could conceivably be discovered here, but it is by no means articulate. Third, the argument does not demonstrate the badness of the outcome. To be sure, this is in part because the bad outcome is not clearly identified, but if the bad outcome is simply that any individual would be recognized to have the right to die while the "integrity of the decision whether to live or die" were safeguarded, it is by no means clear that this would be a bad thing; after all, this would still preclude virtually the entire range of suicides with which we are now familiar, including all those by people who were depressed, disturbed, or otherwise mentally ill, as well as those coerced or manipulated in any way. Finally, the argument also fails to take account of the current state of affairs and its relationship to the predicted bad outcome. Suicide is not now against the law; right-to-die decisions effected by refusal of treatment are now in principle respected; and assisted suicide is not a statutory violation in nearly half the states. What is the bad outcome this slippery slope argument foresees, and would it indeed be worse?

Of course, a slippery slope argument can be much more effective than this one, if it is stated clearly, exhaustively, and with as much conscientiously assembled evidence as possible to back up the predictive claims it makes. Even where slippery slope arguments do not meet these standards of rigor, however, I think it is important to try to take account of the often inchoate intuitions expressed there, and to try to anticipate, if possible, the kinds of predictive arguments that might be made against the right-to-die policies proposed. That is why this volume contains so many essays that in one way or another address forms of slippery slope arguments, not only explicitly, as in chapter 5 and chapter 8, but generally in chapters 4, 7, and 10. These chapters all point to various kinds of pressures, including individual, institutional, and societal ones, that might occur to push a culture from humane practices to morally repugnant ones.

However, taking account of these pressures in a serious way produces another effect, one that in this volume may appear to be vacillation. Indeed, it has sometimes resulted in essays that may look as though they must have come from a different pen: for example, chapters 10 and 14. These two essays are actually a matched set, written at about the same time, reflecting two complementary sets of concerns about the same issue. (My only gripe has been that one of these essays is regularly quoted by right-to-life advocates, the other only by those favoring the right to die.) Some of the chapters in this book seem to defend the recognition of rights to both voluntary active euthanasia and physician-assisted suicide; others seem much more wary of active euthanasia, and argue instead that assisted suicide is to be preferred as a matter of social policy. This seeming vacillation is a direct result of taking the slippery slope argument seriously, but responding at both theoretical and practical levels. I argue that both voluntary active euthanasia and assisted suicide can be defended on moral grounds; but, as I acknowledge in comparing the United States with the Netherlands, I worry that the circumstances of the contemporary United States, with its currently chaotic, inequitable health-care system, its comparatively inflexible legal system, its increasing racism, its discontinuous relationships between doctors and patients, and its tremendous financial pressures in medicine, may make recognizing the practice of physician-performed euthanasia more problematic than recognizing physician-assisted suicide. After all, assisted suicide gives the patient one final measure of control because, in the end, death is brought about by the patient, not the physician. This is not to say that physician-performed euthanasia is wrong, but rather that it may be riskier *for us* here and now. At the same time, I think it should be legalized, in part because I think greater visibility makes possible greater protection from abuse. I remain deeply ambivalent about this issue, and it is for this reason that in these various essays I've spent so much time reflecting on the nature of these risks and whether there are ways to prevent abuse. Thus, what appears to be vacillation is rather, I think, the product of switching one's view from an ideal-world perspective to the messier, flawed, often blatantly unjust aspects of the real world, and also the product of shifting perceptions about just how messy the real world actually is. As I argue at length in chapter 8, I think there are theoretically adequate, practical ways of preventing abuse—but that does not keep me from worry.

Autonomy

At the deepest level of these three background philosophical issues is the troubling issue of autonomy. Thanks to the virtual canonization of this concept as one of the four major principles of bioethics—autonomy, beneficence, nonmaleficence, and justice[40]—the concept of autonomy is vastly overworked and remarkably variously understood. It is, nevertheless, intuitively accessible: put in less mystifying language, it is the capacity for self-determination, or for making basic-level human choice, free from both exterior compulsion and internal impairment. The autonomous person acts freely; the person of diminished autonomy cannot, either because of some external pressure or because of some loss in internal capacities for deliberation, reflection, intention, or comprehension of the matters involved in choice.

It has been widely assumed in contemporary bioethics—and the pieces in this collection are no different in this regard—that the answers to the two principal questions usually asked about autonomy: *"Is autonomy possible?"* and *"Is autonomous choice always to be respected?"* are both *yes*. Indeed, both answers were defended by Immanuel Kant.[41] Translated into the currency of modern medicine, these questions just mean that the competent patient can, and ought to be accorded the right to, determine what is to be done to him or her, even if—as in the cases I am concerned with here—it means he or she will die. This principle of autonomy is the basis for the legal right of informed consent.

The traditional counterobjection to the autonomist view is the position known as *paternalism:* the view that it is sometimes appropriate to interfere in a person's liberty for his or her own good. Chapter 2 is quite directly concerned with related issues in paternalism, though not perhaps by this name. "The Eclipse of Altruism" argues that by deferring decision-making in end-of-life situations until a point at which the patient is no longer competent, the very possibility of altruistic choice by the patient—that is, choice running counter to his or her own interests—is precluded. In effect, caregivers and institutions thus override the possibility of choice, ensuring that decisions will be made, though only later, for that person's own good. This posture, which favors deciding by others over deciding for oneself, thus has a paternalistic effect. Chapter 7, which explores the issue of euthanasia in Alzheimer's disease, also looks at various views of autonomy, including the issue of what constitutes a person and whether antecedent autonomous choices should govern persons who have radically changed.

Although paternalism in medicine is far from extinct, there is a much more serious challenge to the prevailing assumption that autonomy is to be regarded as one of the four basic moral principles to be observed in bioethics. This is the claim that autonomy isn't really possible at all. Individual choice, both about superficial everyday matters and about deeper personal preferences and life plans, is, on this view, so thoroughly conditioned and shaped by its cultural situation that it is no longer meaningful to speak of autonomy in any full-blooded sense. People are best understood as communally structured and coded, not as truly discrete individuals. It is naive, on this view, to speak of the individual as "self-legislating"; although he or she can make personal choices that appear different from those of others, this marks only superficial difference, and the individual is really not independent from the linguistic and social structures in which he or she is situated. This point has been argued heavily within cultural studies and literary theory in recent years and is coming only slowly to bioethics; but it is a point with real bite: the autonomist view, that individuals ought to be able to make their own, personal choices about how to die, reinforced in such doctrines as informed consent, is under substantial challenge. This view argues that personal choice is a sham: liberal notions of autonomy and individuality are misleading, and personal choice is merely the product of larger communal understandings of such matters as what death is, what is the purpose of life, what obligations one has to one's fellows, and so on. One can try to go against the grain, but for the most part one cannot even see which way the grain is running or understand that it could run in a different direction. In a word, individuals are not really *individuals,* and are not capable of deeply independent choice.

None of the essays included here adopts the vocabulary current in contemporary cultural studies, but many of them are directly concerned with these issues. Taking as its focus the issues of distributive justice, chapter 3, "Is There a Duty to Die?" addresses background cultural assumptions about active versus passive ways of coming to the end of life, and in doing so it explores the possibility that there could develop a notion of a "time to die," the product of radical cultural change. Chapter 4, "Dying in 559 Beds," treats of standardization as a threat to autonomy, citing Rilke's continuing preoccupation with precisely the kind of situated perspective that constitutes the challenge. Chapter 10, "Manipulated Suicide," points out that these much deeper cultural commonalities can and do change. Indeed, if our eyes are sharp enough to see them and we are able to shed some of our own encompassing cultural assumptions, we notice that deeper cultural commonalities also vary in cultures that seem otherwise very much alike; this is what both chapter 6 and chapter 12, "A Dozen Caveats Concerning the Discussion of Euthanasia in the Netherlands" and "Assisted Suicide: Can We Learn from Germany?" explore. These concerns also explain this volume's sustained interests in cross-cultural issues, not only by attempting to shed some rather constricting American cultural assumptions in scrutinizing euthanasia practices in the Netherlands as well as some equally limiting constrictions of the English language in looking at the terminology of suicide in Germany, but by looking at historical cultural transitions as well, particularly the differences between Stoic and Christian views of the individual's appropriate posture in approaching death.

This challenge to traditional autonomist views may also explain some of my continuing ambivalence about the slippery slope arguments against euthanasia and suicide. As I have argued in several places, it seems to me that the best barrier against the slide down the slippery slope is the reinforcement of individual choice; but individual choice may only be possible in a superficial way within the larger scope of cultural and linguistic constraints. Nevertheless, while at a theoretical level true autonomy may be rare or virtually impossible, I do not regard this as a counsel of despair: I believe that social policy and the law must act as if autonomy were both possible and desirable. Hence, social issues are discussed here in the language of rights, and health policy is said to have an obligation to preserve and enhance autonomous choice. I also contend that it is possible to imagine cultural evolution in a direction in which individual choice is encouraged not only at a superficial level but also at a deeper one. A number of these essays have as their objective making a plausible case for this view.

These background philosophical issues—the distinction between killing and letting die, the soundness of the slippery slope argument, and the nature and possibility of autonomy, are just three that are raised here. There are many other concerns directly or tangentially addressed in this volume—for example, the nature of justice, the appropriate scope and nature of health policy, the character of religious belief—but rather than address them in this introduction, it is best, I think, to turn to the essays themselves.

The essays in this book were written between 1977–78 (when the National Endowment for the Humanities generously supported me with a year-long Fellowship for Independent Study and Research) and 1992—a long chronicle of continuous ruminating on a set of closely related issues. I've also been helped by support from the Utah Endowment for the Humanities and the University of Utah Research Committee. Several are the product of research travel in the Netherlands and Germany. Many of these essays have been retitled; some are amalgamated out of other, smaller pieces, and there are some deletions to try to minimize overlap. I have not tried to obscure the major ambivalence of this body of work by revising pieces to preserve the appearance of consistency; I've preferred to leave the two principal areas of ambivalence exposed to view—whether the slippery slope argument is really persuasive against legalizing voluntary active euthanasia in the United States, as distinct from assisted suicide, and whether autonomy is really possible in any full sense at all—as evidence that I continue to think these problems are real and difficult, and that it is better to leave threads dangling than to knot them off into quick, easy solutions. I've been thinking about these issues for fifteen or twenty years so far; I expect I'll be ambivalent about these issues for some time to come.

This is, in the end, an optimist's book: it sees that the ways in which we go about dying are often not very good, but imagines modifications of our assumptions and practices in which they could be very much better. It is also a pessimist's book: it sees the dangers involved. In the end, it works for a realist vision: dying can hardly be regarded as good, but we may hope for less bad deaths, especially if we are alert to the ways in which they could be still very much worse.

Notes

1. Elizabeth Kübler-Ross, *On Death and Dying* (New York: Macmillan, 1969).

2. Penicillin was discovered in 1940, but initially was made available only to combat soldiers; it became widely available to the public after the war. The antimicrobials had been developed in the 1930s.

3. *Matter of Quinlan*, 355 A. 2d 647 (1976). The respirator was removed, but because Karen Ann had been weaned from it in advance, she did not die; she remained in a coma for another ten years before she died.

4. *Cruzan v. Director, Missouri Department of Health*, 497 U.S. 261 (1990).

5. Videotape of Dax Cowart's treatment, "Please Let Me Die," is available from the Department of Psychiatry, University of Texas Medical Branch, Galveston, Texas; a film version of his story called "Dax's Case."

6. Robert and Peggy Stinson, *The Long Dying of Baby Andrew* (Boston: Little Brown, 1983).

7. Raymond S. Duff and A. G. M. Campbell, "Moral and Ethical Dilemmas in the Special-Care Nursery," *New England Journal of Medicine* 289 (1073): 890–94.

8. Lael Tucker Wertenbacker, *Death of a Man* (Boston: Beacon Press, 1974): Jessamyn West, *The Woman Said Yes* (New York: Harcourt Brace Jovanovich, 1976).

9. Betty Rollin, *Last Wish* (New York: Linden Press/Simon & Schuster, 1985).

10. Derek Humphry, with Ann Wickett, *Jean's Way* (London, Melbourne, New York: Quartet Books, 1978).

11. See *The New York Times*, December 11, 1977, and Berkeley Rice, "Death by Design: A Case in Point," *Psychology Today*, January 1978, p. 1.

12. *The New York Times*, June 17, 1979.

13. *The New York Times*, February 26, 1975, p. 1. He was seventy-seven and had had a disabling stroke; she was eighty and had serious arthritis.

14. Brian Clark, *Whose Life Is It, Anyway?* (New York: Dodd Mead, 1978); film version, starring Richard Dreyfuss and John Cassavetes, New York: MGM/UA Entertainment Co., 1982.

15. "It's Over, Debbie," *Journal of the American Medical Association* 259 (Jan. 8, 1988): 272.

16. Timothy E. Quill, "Death and Dignity: A Case of Individualized Decision Making," *The New England Journal of Medicine* 324 (1991): 691; see also his *Death and Dignity: Making Choices and Taking Charge* (New York: W. W. Norton, 1993).

17. Derek Humphry, *Final Exit: The Practicalities of Self-deliverance and Assisted Suicide for the Dying* (Eugene, Oregon: The Hemlock Society, 1991; pbk. edn., New York: Dell, 1992).

18. Joseph Shapiro, *No Pity: People with Disabilities Forging a New Civil Rights Movement* (New York: Times Books, 1993).

19. Courtney Campbell, "Dying Well: Hospice Confronts Physician-Assisted Suicide," *Biolaw* 11:4 (April 1993), 29–36.

20. For citations to these cases and for accounts and/or texts of them, see for example, Barry R. Furrow, Sandra H. Johnson, Timothy S. Jost, and Robert L. Schwartz, *Health Law: Cases, Materials, and Problems* (St. Paul, Minn.: West Publishing Co., 1987).

21. Brief accounts of these cases are readily accessible in Thomas L. Beauchamp and James F. Childress, *Principles of Biomedical Ethics*, 3rd ed. (New York: Oxford University Press, 1989).

22. Actually, the courts have been more ready to respect expressions of a patient's wishes when the patient is male, and more ready to consider the patient's best interests when the

patient is female. See Steven Miles and Alison August, "Courts, Gender, and the Right to Die." *Law, Medicine, and Health Care* 18 (Spring–Summer 1990): 85–95.

23. 179 Cal. App. 3d 1127, 225 Cal. Rptr. 297 (1986).

24. 497 U.S. 261 (1990) at 295.

25. See Alan Sullivan, "A Constitutional Right to Suicide," in *Suicide: The Philosophical Issues,* ed. M. Pabst Battin and David J. Mayo (New York: St. Martin's, 1980), 229–253. Although Sullivan's analysis was published over a decade ago, Yale Kamisar has recently called it "one of the best arguments for a constitutional right to suicide" ("Are Laws Against Assisted Suicide Unconstitutional?" *Hastings Center Report* 23 (May–June 1993): 32–41.

26. Cited, for example, in *Bartling,* 163 Cal. App. 186 (1984); *Conroy,* 98 N.J. 321 (1985), and *Bouvia,* 179 Cal. App. 3d 1127 (1986), to name but a few.

27. More precisely, no state or federal statute punishes an individual who commits or attempts suicide, though a few still retain the common-law classification of suicide as a crime. Maria T. CeloCruz, "Aid-in-Dying: Shoud We Decriminalize Physician-Assisted Suicide and Physician-Committed Euthanasia?" *American Journal of Law & Medicine* 18 (1992): 369–396, specifically p. 377, incl. n. 60.

28. Information provided by Choice in Dying, 200 Varig Street, New York, NY 10014.

29. Sullivan, "A Constitutional Right," 244.

30. The PSDA requires hospitals, nursing homes, and other health-care institutions that accept Medicare or Medicaid funds to ask all patients whether they have a living will, durable power of attorney, or other advance directives. It does not require the patients to have one. But the likelihood of misunderstanding on the part of both patients and hospital employees is substantial, and since advance directives are typically used to decline treatment rather than request it, the effect is likely to be a cost-saving one. See Jay A. Jacobson et al., "Patient Awareness, Understanding, and Use of Advance Directives," *Western Journal of Medicine,* 1993, in press.

31. For example, see the collection edited by Bonnie Steinbock, *Killing and Letting Die* (Englewood Cliffs, NJ: Prentice-Hall, 1980).

32. Siegler is not the only physician who argues this way. See the editorial, "Doctors Must Not Kill," *Journal of the American Medical Association* 259 (April 8, 1988): 2139–40, signed by Willard Gaylin, M.D., Leon R. Kass, M.D., Edmund D. Pellegrino, M.D., and Mark Siegler, M.D.

33. Beauchamp and Childress, *Principles of Biomedical Ethics,* 135.

34. James Rachels, "Active and Passive Euthanasia," *New England Journal of Medicine* 292 (1975): 78–80.

35. Richard L. Trammell, "Saving Life and Taking Life," *Journal of Philosophy* 72 (1975): 131–137.

36. An accessible discussion of the principle of double effect can be found in Beauchamp and Childress, *Principles of Biomedical Ethics,* 127–134.

37. Henry Davis, S.J., *Moral and Pastoral Theology,* vol. 2 (London: Sheed and Ward, 1936) 116.

38. See Marcia Angell, "The Case of Helga Wanglie," *New England Journal of Medicine* 325 (1991): 511.

39. Walter M. Weber, J.D., "What Right to Die?" (letter to the editor) *Suicide and Life-Threatening Behavior* 18 (Summer 1988): 182. For an extended treatment of some of the same themes, see Thomas J. Marzen et al., "Suicide: a Constitutional Right?" *Duquesne Law Review* 24 (1985): 102ff.

40. This set of four principles is to be attributed to Beauchamp and Childress's *Principles*

of Biomedical Ethics, a text that has been extraordinarily influential in shaping contemporary bioethics.

41. See especially Kant's *Groundwork of the Metaphysics of Morals,* as well as his *Lectures on Ethics, The Metaphysical Principles of Virtue* and *The Critique of Practical Reason.* A lucid discussion can be found in Warner A. Wick's introduction to Immanuel Kant, *Ethical Philosophy* (Indianapolis: Hackett Publishing Co., 1983), pp. xxff.

I

Withdrawing and Withholding Treatment

1

The Least Worst Death

In recent years right-to-die movements have brought into the public consciousness something most physicians have long known: that in some hopeless medical conditions, heroic efforts to extend life may no longer be humane, and the physician must be prepared to allow the patient to die. Physician responses to patients' requests for "natural death" or "death with dignity" have been, in general, sensitive and compassionate. But the successes of the right-to-die movement have had a bitterly ironic result: institutional and legal protections for "natural death" have, in some cases, actually made it more painful to die.

In the United States, there is just one legally protected mechanism for achieving natural death: refusal of medical treatment. It is available to both competent and incompetent patients. The competent patient is legally entitled to refuse medical treatment of any sort on any personal or religious grounds, except perhaps where the interests of minor children are involved. A number of court cases, including *Quinlan, Saikewicz, Spring,* and *Eichner,*[1] have established precedent in the treatment of an incompetent patient for a proxy refusal by a family member or guardian. In addition, eleven [in 1983; by 1993, forty-seven] states now have specific legislation protecting the physician from legal action for failure to render treatment when a competent patient has executed a directive to be followed after he or she is no longer competent. A durable power of attorney, executed by the competent patient in favor of a trusted relative or friend, is [as of 1993] also used in forty-eight states to determine treatment choices after incompetence occurs.

An Earlier but Not Easier Death

In the face of irreversible, terminal illness, a patient may wish to die sooner but "naturally," without artificial prolongation of any kind. By doing so, the patient may believe he or she is choosing a death that is, as a contributor to the *New England Journal of Medicine* has put it, "comfortable, decent, and peaceful";[2] "natural death," the patient may assume, means a death that is easier than a medically prolonged one.[3] That is why he or she is willing to undergo death earlier and that is

From *The Hastings Center Report* 13:2 (April 1983): 13–16. Copyright © 1983 by the Hastings Center. Reprinted by permission of the publisher.

why, he or she assumes, natural death is legally protected. But the patient may conceive of "natural death" as more than pain-free, and may assume that it will allow time for reviewing life and saying farewell to family and loved ones, for last rites or final words, for passing on hopes, wisdom, confessions, and blessings to the next generation. These ideas are, of course, heavily stereotyped; they are the product of literary and cultural traditions associated with conventional deathbed scenes, reinforced by movies, books, news stories, religious models, and just plain wishful thinking. Even the very term "natural" may have stereotyped connotations for the patient: something close to nature, uncontrived, and appropriate. As a result of these notions, the patient often takes "natural death" to be a painless, conscious, dignified, culminative slipping-away.

Now consider what sorts of death actually occur under the rubric of "natural death." A patient suffers a cardiac arrest and is not resuscitated. Result: sudden unconsciousness, without pain, and death within a number of seconds. Or a patient has an infection that is not treated. Result: the unrestrained multiplication of micro-organisms, the production of toxins, interference with organ function, hypotension, and death. On the way there may be fever, delirium, rigor or shaking, and light-headedness; death usually takes one or two days, depending on the organism involved. If the kidneys fail and dialysis or transplant is not undertaken, the patient is generally more conscious, but experiences nausea, vomiting, gastrointestinal hemorrhage (evident in vomiting blood), inability to concentrate, neuromuscular irritability or twitching, and eventually convulsions. Dying may take from days to weeks, unless such circumstances as high potassium levels intervene. Refusal of amputation, although painless, is characterized by fever, chills, and foul-smelling tissues. Hypotension, characteristic of dehydration and many other states, is not painful but also not pleasant: the patient cannot sit up or get out of bed, has a dry mouth and thick tongue, and may find it difficult to talk. An untreated respiratory death involves conscious air hunger. This means gasping, an increased breathing rate, a panicked feeling of inability to get air in or out. Respiratory deaths may take only minutes; on the other hand, they may last for hours. If the patient refuses intravenous fluids, he or she may become dehydrated. If he or she refuses surgery for cancer, an organ may rupture. Refusal of treatment does not simply bring about death in a vacuum, so to speak; death always occurs from some specific cause.

Many patients who are dying in these ways are either comatose or heavily sedated. Such deaths do not allow for a period of conscious reflection at the end of life, nor do they permit farewell-saying, last rites, final words, or other features of the stereotypically "dignified" death.

Even less likely to match the patient's conception of natural death are those cases in which the patient is still conscious and competent, but meets a death that is quite different than the one bargained for. Consider the bowel cancer patient with widespread metastases and a very poor prognosis who—perhaps partly out of consideration for the emotional and financial resources of the family—refuses surgery to reduce or bypass the tumor. How, exactly, will he or she die? This patient is clearly within his or her legal rights in refusing surgery, but the physician knows what the outcome is very likely to be: obstruction of the intestinal tract will occur, the bowel wall will perforate, the abdomen will become distended, there will be intractible vomiting (perhaps with a fecal character to the emesis), and the tumor will erode into adjacent areas, causing increased pain, hemorrhage, and sepsis. Narcotic sedation and companion drugs may be partially effective in controlling pain, nausea, and vomiting, but this patient will *not* get the kind of death he or she bargained for. Yet, the patient was willing to shorten life, to use the single legally protected mechanism—refusal of treatment—to achieve that "natural" death. Small wonder that many physicians are skeptical of the "gains" made by the popular movements supporting the right to die.

When the Right to Die Goes Wrong

Several distinct factors can contribute to the backfiring of right-to-die choices. First, and perhaps the most obvious, patients may misjudge their situations in refusing treatment or in executing a natural-death directive; refusal may be precipitous and ill informed, based more on fear than on a settled desire to die. Second, the physician's response to the patient's request for "death with dignity" may be insensitive, rigid, or even punitive (though in my experience most physicians respond with compassion and wisdom). Legal constraints may also make natural death more difficult than might be hoped: safeguards often render natural death requests and directives cumbersome to execute, and in any case, in a litigation-conscious society, the physician will often take the most cautious route.

But most important in the backfiring of some right-to-die choices is the underlying ambiguity in the very concept of "natural death." Patients tend to think of the character of the experience they expect to undergo—a death that is "comfortable, decent, peaceful"—but all the law protects is the refusal of medical procedures. Even lawmakers sometimes confuse the two. In their first version, the California and Kansas natural death laws claimed to protect what they romantically described as "the natural process of dying." North Carolina's statute says it protects the right to a "peaceful and natural" death. But because these laws actually protect only refusal of treatment, they can hardly guarantee a peaceful, easy death. Thus, we see a widening gulf between the intent of the law to protect the patient's final desires, and the outcomes if the law is actually followed. The physician is caught in between: he or she recognizes the patient's right to die peacefully, naturally, and with whatever dignity is possible, but foresees the unfortunate results that may come about when the patient exercises this right as the law permits.

Of course, if the symptoms or pain become unbearable the patient may change his or her mind. The patient who earlier wished not to be "hooked up on tubes" now begins to experience difficulty in breathing or swallowing, and finds that a tracheotomy will relieve this distress. The bowel cancer patient experiences severe discomfort from obstruction, and gives permission for decompression or palliative surgery after all. In some cases, the family may engineer the change of heart because they find dying too hard to watch. Health-care personnel may view these reversals with satisfaction: "See," they may say, "he really wants to live after all." But such reversals cannot always be interpreted as a triumph of the will to live; they may also be an indication that refusing treatment makes dying too hard.

Options for an Easier Death

How can the physician honor the dying patient's wish for a peaceful, conscious, and culminative death? There is more than one option.

Such a death can come about whenever the patient is conscious and pain-free; he or she can reflect and, if family, clergy, or friends are summoned at the time, will be able to communicate as he or she wishes. Given these conditions, death can be brought on in various direct ways. For instance, the physician can administer a lethal quantity of an appropriate drug. Or the patient on severe dietary restrictions can violate the diet; the kidney-failure patient, for instance, for whom high potassium levels are fatal, can simply overeat on avocados. These ways of producing death are, of course, active euthanasia, or assisted or unassisted suicide. For many patients, such a death would count as "natural" and would satisfy the expectations under which they had chosen to die rather than to continue an intolerable existence. But for many patients (and for many physicians as well) a death that involves deliberate killing is morally wrong. Such a patient could never assent to an actively caused death, and even though it might be physically calm, it could hardly be emotionally or psychologically peaceful. This is not to say that active euthanasia or assisted suicide are morally wrong, but rather that the force of some patients' moral views about them precludes using such practices to achieve the kind of death they want. Furthermore, many physicians are unwilling to shoulder the legal risk such practices may seem to involve.

But active killing aside, the physician can do much to grant the dying patient the humane death he or she has chosen by using the sole legally protected mechanism that safeguards the right to die: refusal of treatment. This mechanism need not always backfire. For in almost any terminal condition, death can occur in various ways, and there are many possible outcomes of the patient's present condition. The patient who is dying of emphysema could die of respiratory failure, but could also die of cardiac arrest or untreated pulmonary infection. The patient who is suffering from bowel cancer could die of peritonitis following rupture of the bowel, but could also die of dehydration, of pulmonary infection, of acid-base imbalance, of electrolyte deficiency, or of an arrhythmia.

As the poet Rilke observes, we have a tendency to associate a certain sort of end with a specific disease; it is the "official death" for that sort of illness. But there are many other ways of dying than the official death, and the physician can take advantage of these. Infection and cancer, for instance, are old friends; there is increased frequency of infection in the immuno-compromised host. Other secondary conditions, like dehydration or metabolic derangement, may set in. Of course, certain conditions typically occur a little earlier, others a little later, in the ordinary course of a terminal disease, and some are a matter of chance. The crucial point is that certain conditions will produce a death that is more comfortable, more decent, more predictable, and more permitting of conscious and peaceful experience than others. Some are better, if the patient has to die at all, and some are worse. Which mode of death claims the patient depends in part on circumstance and in part on the physician's response to conditions that occur. What the patient who rejects active euthanasia or assisted suicide may realistically hope for is this: the least worst death among those that could naturally occur. Not all unavoidable surrenders need involve rout; in the face of inevitable death, the physician becomes strategist, the deviser of plans for how to meet death most favorably.

He or she does so, of course, at the request of the patient (or if the patient is not competent, at the request of the patient's guardian, designee, or kin). Patient autonomy is crucial in the notion of natural death. The physician could, of course, produce death by simply failing to offer a particular treatment to the patient. But to fail to *offer* treatment that might prolong life, at least when this does not compromise limited or very expensive resources to which other patients have claims, would violate the most fundamental principles of medical practice; some patients do not want "natural death," regardless of the physical suffering or dependency that prolongation of life may entail.

A scenario in which natural death is accomplished by the patient's selective refusal of treatment has one major advantage over active euthanasia and assisted suicide: refusal of treatment is clearly permitted and protected by law. Unfortunately, however, most patients do not have the specialized medical knowledge to use this self-protective mechanism intelligently. Few are aware that some kinds of refusal of treatment will better serve their desires for a "natural death" than others. And few patients realize that refusal of treatment can be selective. Although many patients with life-threatening illness are receiving multiple kinds of therapy, from surgery to nutritional support, most assume that it is only the major procedures (like surgery) that can be refused. (This misconception is perhaps perpetuated by the standard practice of obtaining specific consent for major procedures, like surgery, but not for minor, ongoing ones.) Then, too, patients may be unable to distinguish therapeutic from palliative procedures. And they may not understand the interaction between one therapy and another. In short, most patients do not have enough medical knowledge to foresee the consequences of refusing treatment on a selective basis; it is this that the physician must supply.

It is already morally and legally recognized that informed consent to a procedure involves explicit disclosure, both about the risks and outcomes of the proposed procedure and about the risks and outcomes of alternative possible procedures. Some courts, as in *Quackenbush,*[4] have also recognized the patient's right to explicit disclosure about the outcomes of refusing the proposed treatment. But though it is crucial in making a genuinely informed decision, the patient's right to information about the risks and outcomes of alternative kinds of refusal has not yet been recognized. So, for instance, in order to make a genuinely informed choice, the bowel cancer patient with concomitant infection will need to know about the outcomes of each of the principal options: accepting both bowel surgery and antibiotics, accepting antibiotics but not surgery, accepting surgery but not antibiotics, or accepting neither. The case may, of course, be more complex, but the principle remains: to recognize the patient's right to autonomous choice in matters concerning the treatment of his or her own body, the physician must provide information about all the legal options open to him or her, not just information sufficient to choose between accepting or rejecting a single proposed procedure.

One caveat: It sometimes occurs that physicians disclose the dismal probable consequences of refusing treatment in order to coerce patients into accepting the treatment they propose. This may be particularly common in surgery that will result in ostomy of the bowel. The patient is given a graphic description of the impending abdominal catastrophe—impaction, rupture, distention, hemorrhage, sepsis, and death. He or she thus consents readily to the surgery proposed. The paternalistic physician may find this maneuver appropriate, particularly because ostomy surgery is often refused out of vanity, depression, or on fatalistic grounds. But the physician who frightens a patient into accepting a procedure by describing the awful consequences of refusal is not honoring the patient's right to informed, autonomous choice; he or she has not described the various choices the patient could make, but only the worst.

Supplying the knowledge a patient needs in order to choose the least worst death need not require enormous amounts of additional energy or time on the part of the physician; it can be incorporated into the usual informed consent disclosures. If the patient is unable to accommodate the medical details, or instructs the physician to do what he or she thinks is best, the physician may use his or her own judgment in ordering and refraining from ordering treatment. If the patient clearly prefers to accept less life in hopes of an easy death, the physician should act in a way that will allow the least worst death to occur. In principle, however, the competent patient, and the proxy deciders for an incompetent patient, are entitled to explicit disclosure about all the alternatives for medical care. Physicians in burn units are already experienced in telling patients with very severe burns, where survival is unprecedented, what the outcome is likely to be if aggressive treatment is undertaken or if it is not—death in both cases, but under quite different conditions. Their expertise in these delicate matters might be most useful here. Informed refusal is just as much the patient's right as informed consent.

The role of the physician as strategist of natural death may be even more crucial in longer-term degenerative illnesses, where both physician and patient have far more advance warning that the patient's condition will deteriorate, and far more opportunity to work together in determining the conditions of the ultimate death. Of course, the first interest of both physician and patient will be strategies for maximizing the good life left. Nevertheless, many patients with long-term, eventually terminal illnesses, like multiple sclerosis, Huntington's chorea, diabetes, or chronic renal failure, may educate themselves considerably about the expected courses of their illnesses, and may display a good deal of anxiety about the end stages. This is particularly true in hereditary conditions where the patient may have watched a parent or relative die of the disease. But it is precisely in these conditions that the physician's opportunity may be greatest for humane guidance in the unavoidable matter of dying. He or she can help the patient to understand what the long-term options are in refusing treatment while competent, or help him or her to execute a natural death directive or durable power of attorney that spells out the particulars of treatment refusal after incompetence sets in.

Of course, some diseases are complex, and not easy to explain. Patients are not always capable of listening very well, especially to unattractive possibilities concerning their own ends. Physicians are sometimes reluctant to acknowledge that their efforts to sustain life will eventually fail, or believe that providing such information may undermine the patient's hope. And some conditions offer little to choose from among an unappetizing range of deaths: the least worst isn't much less awful than the worst. But the very fact that the patient's demise is still far in the future makes it possible for the physician to describe various scenarios of how that death could occur, and at the same time give the *patient* control over which of them will actually happen. Not all patients will choose the same strategies of ending, nor is there any reason that they should. What may count as the least worst death to one person may be the most feared form of death to another. The physician may be able to increase the patient's psychological comfort immensely by giving him or her a way of meeting an unavoidable death on his or her own terms.

In both acute and long-term terminal illnesses, the key to good strategy is flexibility in considering *all* the possibilities at hand. These alternatives need not include active euthanasia or suicide measures of any kind, direct or indirect. To take advantage of the best of the naturally occurring alternatives is not to cause the patient's death, which will happen anyway, but to guide him or her away from the usual, frequently worst, end.

In the current enthusiasm for natural death it is not patient autonomy that dismays physicians. What does dismay them is the way in which respect for patient autonomy can lead to cruel results. The cure for that dismay lies in the realization that the physician can contribute to the *genuine* honoring of the patient's autonomy and rights, assuring him or her of "natural death" in the way in which the patient understands it, and still remain within the confines of good medical practice and the law.

Notes

I'd like to thank Howard Wilcox, M.D., and, at a later date, Jay Jacobson, M.D., for contributions to this paper.

1. *In re Quinlan*, 355 A. 2d 647 (N.J. 1976); *Superintendent of Belchertown v. Saikewicz*, 370 N.E. 2d 417 (Mass. 1977); *In re Spring*, Mass. App., 399 N.E. 2d 493; *In re Eichner*, 420 N.E. 2d at 72 (1981).

2. S. S. Spencer, "'Code' or 'No Code': A Nonlegal Opinion," *New England Journal of Medicine*, 300 (1979): 138–140.

3. See Dallas M. High's analysis of various senses of the term "natural death" in ordinary language, in "Is 'Natural Death' an Illusion?" *Hastings Center Report* (August 1978): 37–42.

4. *In re Quackenbush*, 156 N.J. Super. 282, 353 A. 2d 785 (1978).

2

The Eclipse of Altruism:
The Moral Costs of Deciding for Others

Lay decision-making on behalf of a patient—by family, guardians, and nonmedical professionals such as judges—may be superior in certain respects to that of medical professionals, since it may be both more sensitive to the patient's preferences and rights and less rigid in imposing an artificial conception of his or her medical needs. But whatever its virtues, lay decision-making shares with professional decision-making a disturbing common feature: both tend to obscure the possibility of other-regarding, altruistic choice and behavior on the part of the patient. Whether this is to be regarded as a virtue, however, or as a serious moral abuse, will have considerable bearing on the kinds of decision-making to be permitted and encouraged in medicine.

Treatment choices made on behalf of a patient vary widely as a function of two principal factors: the differing competencies and fields of expertise of the decision-makers, and the differing influences and pressures characteristically placed upon them. But they all properly share one central moral characteristic: if made in a morally correct way, they must all have the patient's interests at heart. (This characteristic may be said to be rooted in an obligation of beneficence, reflected in the Hippocratic Oath's requirement to act "for the sake of the patient.") Whatever the practical differences of decisions by professionals and laypersons, they ought not be *morally* diverse: they will all conform, if made correctly, to the canon that it is the interests of the patient that are to be served.

Although perhaps less straightforward in its application, this moral obligation also holds for medical professionals and laypersons who occupy policy-making positions governing medical research and experimentation, from federal officials to local members of institutional review boards. Though they must take into account the needs and research goals of medical science, they are morally required to give the interests of the subject or potential subject priority over those of anyone else, including both the experimenters and any future patients who might benefit from the research.

From *The Journal of Medicine and Philosophy* 10 (1985): 19–44. Originally titled "Non-Patient Decision-Making in Medicine: The Eclipse of Altruism." Copyright © 1985 by *The Journal of Medicine and Philosophy*. Reprinted by permission of the publisher.

The fundamental obligation of the decision-maker to keep the interests of the patient at heart operates not only in cases where the patient is incompetent or has ceded his or her decision-making authority, but in contexts involving competent patients as well. Although it is most frequently articulated where the fiduciary character of the professional-patient relationship is recognized, this moral obligation operates wherever a second party influences, shapes, or controls the patient's decision, whether by suggestion, provision of information, giving of advice, or by any other means, both in therapeutic and experimental cases. In practice, it is also often taken to apply even where the patient clearly asserts a contrary choice of his or her own; though this raises the much disputed issue of paternalism, claims are often made that the professional or layperson ought to cooperate only with those of the patient's decisions that are actually in the patient's interests, and ought to ignore, discourage, or actively intervene in self-harming choices a patient makes. Only when there are compelling reasons for doing so are the interests of other persons, organizations, or causes to take precedence over the decision-maker's primary obligation to the patient.

Paradoxically, it is this very dedication to the patient's interests that raises serious issues about the moral costs of second-party, non-patient decision-making in medicine. Exclusive commitment to patient interests by both professional and lay second-party decision-makers tends to limit the kinds of choice the patient can make, and in particular tends to preclude the possibility of altruism. Because altruism may be of considerable moral significance, one ought not be too cavalier about a system that seems to simply preclude it.

The Patient's Choices: Self-Interest and Altruism

Most patients, it is reasonable to assume, will make most medical decisions, or will consent to decisions that have been made for them, in ways that they take to serve their own self-interests, usually understood to coincide with their own well-being. Of course, some patients harbor unusual beliefs about what serves their interests, and some patients are not rational in choosing the most effective means to promote their interests, but in general most patients attempt to make rationally self-interested choices. Thus, since their choices are intended to serve their own interests, the decisions of patients, although they are perhaps the quintessential laypersons in medicine, coincide in principle with the choices both professional and lay second-party, non-patient decision-makers would be required to reach for them.

However, while non-patient decision-makers are morally required to act in the patient's interests, the patient is not. All that is morally required of the patient's decision is that it harm no one else, directly or indirectly; if it meets this condition and is made in an unimpaired way, the principle of autonomy requires that it be honored. Thus, because altruistic choices are intended to benefit others and consequently are not in general excluded under the harm principle, they too, like the self-interested choices a patient may ordinarily make, are to be respected under the principle of autonomy. Of course, in some patients the proportion of altruistic commitments may be vanishingly small, and in some what appears to be altruism is self-interest in disguise, but if—as shall be assumed here—there is any possibility of altruism at all, it presents disturbing issues in medicine.

Altruistic choices vary in at least three ways. First, they vary in respect of the immediacy of the object of the other-regarding interests, from commitments to one's nearest family, immediate clan, party, political unit, nation, or religious group, to abstract institutions or ideas, or to remote groups with which one is not identified and which are independent of oneself, or to a deity, or to the world as a whole. Second, altruistic commitments may range from the completely personal to the wholly impersonal: one's attention may be directed to other individual persons (for instance, those who are members of one's family, clan, or nation), or toward the interests of the group or abstract institution without specific reference to its members. Third, altruistic motivation and behavior may vary in strength, from forms that are quite mild to extremely robust varieties, depending on the degree to which the other-regarding interests coexist or conflict with interests of one's own.[1]

In the weaker cases, egoism and altruism are not incompatible.[2] Altruism may be understood as "merely a willingness to act in consideration of the interests of other persons, without the need of ulterior motives,"[3] as Thomas Nagel describes it; this need not involve sacrifice of one's own interests at all. Altruism of intermediate strength can be described, as it is by Serge-Christophe Kolm, as that in which "the person takes himself to be a person of the same general importance as anyone else and acts accordingly"; Kolm's example is St. Martin, who does not give his coat away to the shivering pauper, but divides it in two.[4] In the most robust cases of altruism (those that Nagel calls "abject self-sacrifice"), egoism and altruism are incompatible: the agent's interests are completely subordinated to the interests of the other.

Altruistic choices by patients, subjects, and consumers of health-care services can occur at all levels of medicine and health-related activity. For example, although perhaps most health-preserving life-style choices (e.g., to exercise, quit smoking, or reduce the animal fats in one's diet) are made in a self-interested way (e.g., to increase one's own attractiveness or to prolong one's own life), similar choices could also be made on altruistic grounds, such as to promote the welfare of one's spouse, to serve as a model for one's community, or to avoid becoming a burden upon the society as a whole. (Whether altruistically motivated life-style choices can always be accurately distinguished in practice from self-interested ones, either by an external observer or by the agent, is quite another question.) Choices at other levels within medicine can also be self-interested or altruistically motivated; for example, the husband who undergoes a vasectomy may do so to increase his own control over reproduction, or, on the other hand, to spare his wife the riskier methods of female birth control. The patient who participates in an experimental drug or surgical study may do so in hopes of cure, or in order to contribute to the advance of medical science. Such actions may, of course, be based in both self-interested and altruistic reasons, but they become both morally significant and problematic in medicine when other-regarding concerns outweigh self-interested ones.

Particularly significant and problematic are the altruistic choices a severely ill or dying patient may make. His nonmedical decisions can range over all the aspects of his life over which he retains control—for instance, the disposition of his property, the bestowing of his affection or advice, the assertion of his political power or cultural influence, and so forth—but his *medical* options are quite limited in scope. He can choose to accept one among whatever forms of aggressive treatment are offered him; he can choose merely palliative care; he can choose to remove himself from medical treatment altogether, or even to directly end his life. Generally speaking, his central choice is for or against attempting to prolong his life. But because this choice has consequences not only for himself but for his family, associates, caregivers, heirs, and other patients, his decisions about his own living and dying can be made in altruistic as well as self-interested ways.

A patient's altruistic choices in the matter of dying may be immediate, personal, and comparatively mild; so, for instance, a person hoping to spare her family the burdens of extended terminal care might forgo treatment in such a way that death intervenes before a lengthy coma can set in. (In altruism of this weak sort, although the benefit to her family may be great, the sacrifice to the patient herself is small or nil: all that she loses is an indefinite period of unconscious existence.) Of course, the terminal patient might equally altruistically choose to stay alive: she does it not so much to gain something for herself (since what she gains may be only pain), but, for instance, to serve her family's desire to keep her alive or to postpone their grief. (This, too, is immediate, personal altruism, but because the sacrifice is greater, of a more robust sort). Patients might choose to stay alive to complete tasks of importance to others (as did Freud), fulfill contracts, or keep promises (like Regulus), or they might choose to die to spare loved ones the psychological as well as financial burdens of care. Patients might choose to stay alive for political causes, or to die for them instead; patients might make similarly altruistic commitments to nations or religious groups or abstract principles as well. Choosing to die is not itself inherently altruistic, nor is prolonging one's life always self-interested; one can choose to die for oneself or for others, or choose continuing life in the same diverse ways.

Medicine and the Eclipse of Altruism

Despite the various possibilities of altruism, the institution of medicine appears to respect overt expressions of it only in quite restricted forms. Altruism is typically permitted among patients and research subjects only when it is either strongly personal, quite immediate, or very mild; in most cases, it must be all three. The most frequent examples are familial, such as the parent who makes a minor sacrifice (say, postponing nonurgent surgery) to help his or her child. More robust acts of altruism (say, donating a kidney) are typically permitted only if they are personal and immediate. Nonimmediate personal altruism is regarded with some suspicion: as Robert Steinbrook hints,[5] altruistic acts are more readily accepted between family members than strangers (as is evident in policies and practices discouraging organ transplants from unrelated living donors even when there is a reasonable chance of medical success), and even "altruism" within the family is often treated with suspicion. Nonimmediate, nonpersonal altruism, such as that in national, ideological, or universal forms, is tolerated in medicine only if it is very very mild: one may volunteer for a low-risk experimental study, for instance, or donate a pint of blood, but more robust acts of self-sacrifice, such as probably fatal experimentation and donation of unpaired vital organs, are not allowed.

One way to account for such situations involves postulating that the institution of medicine itself affects the expression of altruism. This yields the working hypothesis, to be adopted here, that under the moral principles widely accepted as governing its practice, medicine tends (except in the limited cases already noted) to inhibit, suppress, or altogether preclude altruism on the part of the patient. Under this assumption, two kinds of structures may appear to produce this eclipse.

Formal Policies Precluding Altruism

Medicine has certain policies, evident for instance in professional codes, research regulations, hospital policies, and malpractice law, which may preclude altruism. Some prohibit the physician from performing elective nontherapeutic procedures that cause serious harm to the patient, regardless of how sincere and well-informed the patient is in requesting them: the surgeon may not perform a procedure, for instance, in which the patient donates her only remaining kidney, even to her own child. Others prohibit the physician or researcher from performing experimental procedures that are not potentially therapeutic but pose serious risk to the subject or patient, even with adequately informed, voluntary consent. Of course, such policies are designed to prevent coercion of patients or subjects by researchers and caregivers, and to protect patients and subjects from the consequences of their own misjudgments and irrational choices. But they may also prevent the expression of any altruistic desires the patient may have had, at least where these desires are robust enough to involve conflict between the interests of others and the patient's own.

The possibility that medical policy precludes altruism may be of particularly great significance in prison settings, where protections of prisoner-subjects against coercive environments are at their strongest. It cannot, of course, be assumed that these policies in fact preclude altruism; altruism may be at its lowest ebb among those who commit crimes. But the contrary cannot be assumed either, since at least on theories that stress the repentance value of punishment, one might expect that altruistic motivation could be quite strong. Before the implantation of the Jarvik-7 artificial heart in Barney Clark, for instance, the surgical team at Utah received over a dozen offers from death-row prisoners to volunteer for the procedure.[6] Of course, an underlying desire to be spared from execution or to manipulate the justice system may be suspected in many of these cases; nevertheless, there is no basis for *assuming* that no such cases could be genuine.

Such offers are by no means limited to prisoners or to others who may seem to have little to lose. For instance, a sixty-one-year-old woman from Las Vegas wrote to the same heart team, explaining that she was in perfectly good health, that she had no dependents, and that she had lived a full and satisfying life. Now, she said, she would like to do something for science by volunteering for the artificial heart. Perhaps the woman was crazy, or simply eager for the publicity that would accompany implantation of the heart, although her letter gave no indication that this was so. She knew about the risks and restrictions that implantation of the heart would involve, and that if she did not die during the procedure, she would face permanent tethering to the air-drive mechanism. But she also believed that she, as a healthy subject, would be a much more informative candidate for testing the heart than the already extremely ill patients on whom it would otherwise be tried. Her offer cannot be merely discarded by assuming that it could not have been genuine; it may have been self-seeking, in some odd, pathological way, but then again it may have been the product of an altruism of the most robust and universal sort.

Informal Practices Precluding Altruism

Medicine may also preclude altruism not as a matter of policy but of practice. Because this phenomenon involves a much more subtle process, it is less likely to be explicitly defended than formally developed policies. Yet its effects may be still more far-reaching. It should be particularly conspicuous, if it occurs, in decisions about death.

Some decisions about death are dictated by the patient's direct request, or by his antecedent request in a living will or similar declaration. Some are reached by courts or guardians after the patient is legally incompetent or can no longer register his preferences at all. But by far the largest (and morally most difficult) group of decisions about death are made by the physician, together, perhaps, with the patient's family or other lay and professional consultants, as the patient's illness overwhelms him and he begins to sink: death now seems probable but perhaps not fully certain, and the choice concerns whether to let it occur or attempt to stave it off.

As has already been said, the patient can make choices to accelerate death or to prolong life in either self-interested or altruistic ways; under the principle of autonomy, these choices are to be respected, provided that they satisfy the harm principle and are made without impairment. However, as has also been said, decisions made by second-party professional and lay decision-makers on behalf of a patient must, under the principle of beneficence, be made with the interests of the patient in mind. Thus, what is significant about decisions about dying is that, in the vast majority of cases, they are made in circumstances in which the conditions for moral adequacy undergo a shift. At the start of a patient's decline (assuming that she is still lucid and competent), autonomy is the appropriate principle to observe; at the conclusion of this decline, when her competency is threatened and her ability to formulate and articulate desires perhaps severely impaired, those making decisions on her behalf must observe the principle of beneficence. Of course, in that gray, declining range where most decisions about dying are made, competency may be intermittent, varying with drug schedules, pain, fear, depression, intimidation in a hospital setting, isolation, and the many other psychological factors of serious illness that can erode a person's capacity to make and defend choices of her own. But intermittent competency is also often treated as evidence that the principle of autonomy is no longer appropriate to observe, and that the conscientious caregiver must attend to the patient's interests, not follow her wishes—if they have not been previously declared—during the remainder of her decline.

The moral tensions in decisions about dying, which increase as the appropriate principle of decision-making begins to shift from autonomy to beneficence, may be exacerbated by two additional features of decision-making about dying. These features are ubiquitous in medical practice, and may at first seem to be both innocuous and medically justified. Nevertheless, their moral consequences may be profound.

First, decisions about dying are rarely explicitly discussed in advance, and though open conversation about death is now in fashion, specific treatment decisions about death are not typically made until a crisis or change in status occurs. This is true even for patients who have signed living wills or durable powers of attorney; although in these cases a general strategy concerning death may have been outlined, the specific details of treatment and the withdrawal of treatment typically are not. It is still almost always the physician, perhaps in conjunction with the patient's family, who decides at what moment the plug should be pulled or who determines what count as the "heroic" measures that should or should not be introduced.

Second, because decisions about death are typically decisions about whether to give up or persevere against the odds, they are typically made as late as possible in the game: since no advantage seems to be gained by making an expeditious choice, postponement of the decision is naturally favored. This is true even if the decision is to continue to fight: after all, the physician has (presumably) been fighting for the patient all along, and nothing is lost by postponing the decision about whether to continue to do so or not.

It is as a consequence of these two features that decisions about death typically concern patients in debilitated, fluctuating states, for whom the decline is already comparatively advanced. Not all deaths occur in this way or involve an extended decline, of course, but those which involve *decisions* about death—whether to accelerate or delay it—typically do. Except for those few cases where the patient articulates his or her desires in detail well in advance and establishes a reliable mechanism for effectuating them, decisions about death are almost always made by others, after the patient is already largely gone.

An additional factor in dying, also compounded by delay, likewise affects the moral criteria for decision-making. As a dying patient declines, the nature of his interests may change. Aesthetic, social, and intellectual interests may subside; biological and psychological ones assume a much larger role. These may center upon the maximization of comfort and the minimization of pain, and include specific interests such as adequate nourishment, affectionate care, maintenance in a nonthreatening setting, and so on.[7] In general, the more advanced the patient's decline, the more limited his interests; toward the end they may be reduced almost entirely to seeking comfort and avoiding pain. Continuing life may not always be in a patient's interests, although it normally is—even for someone in a terminal decline. In some cases, however, it may serve a person's interests to have his death occur in an earlier, better controlled, pain-free way. This is not to deny that a person cannot have "pre-posthumous" and posthumous interests, whether approaching death or already dead, in such things as the welfare of his family, the success of his projects, or the triumph of his political cause, but these are not the sorts of interests *medicine* serves. Beneficence in medicine serves the patient's interests, but restricts its concerns to those interests that are fundamentally biological and psychological in scope.

This shift in interests has its consequences in the moral sphere. As the patient's decline continues and her discomfort becomes more acute, the nature of her choices is likely to shift: she becomes more likely to seek respite from her condition in satisfaction of her immediate physical interests, like avoiding pain, and less likely to cling to her altruistic ideals. Altruistic choices—at least, the robust and interesting ones—do involve sacrifice of one's own interests, but it is very difficult to make such choices when one is already suffering erosion of them. Altruism is sufficiency-motivated, so to speak: it is the kind of choice a person can make in advance of difficult circumstances, but which becomes much more difficult when actually in those circumstances. Even milder cases of altruism, where serving the interests of others does not run counter to interests of the patient's own, may grow less likely when choice is postponed until medical circumstances worsen; this is because suffering itself tends to produce a self-centeredness more pronounced than in ordinary life. As the patient's awareness of her own anguish or pain intensifies, she begins to focus almost entirely on the relief of this distress, and involvement with other persons, institutions, or causes recedes. Thus, because concern for the interests of others wanes as the patient's own needs and sufferings grow, the practice of postponing decisions about death will, in effect, tend to preclude reaching or reaffirming altruistic decisions at all.

Of course, it might be objected that if altruism fades as the patient's own needs and sufferings grow, this simply shows that antecedent altruistic choices fail to be adequately informed: the altruist's sacrifice turns out to be worse than she expected, and when she discovers how bad it is, she reverses her choice. But this is not a sufficient reason for discouraging or prohibiting altruistic choice in the first place—even if such choice might later be reversed. Altruism, at least in its more robust forms, always involves self-sacrifice, that is, the choice of a course of action that one expects to damage one's own interests but favor the interests of others. There is no requirement that one enjoy the damage when it later occurs, nor is the fact that one will not enjoy the damage when it does occur adequate reason for curtailing or overriding the original choice. I may, for instance, decide to contribute unusually handsomely to CARE, knowing I will wince when I see the sum removed from my pay, or volunteer to visit a crotchety old uncle even though I know I will fail to enjoy myself when I am there. But that I regret the deduction or the tedious visit when they occur is not reason for preventing my prior self-sacrificial choice: I *knew* I was choosing courses of action that would make me unhappy, and taking this into account, as well as the interests of others, was part of my choice. Paternalist considerations may underwrite intervention when the agent miscalculates the size of the sacrifice to be made, but not where the choice is knowingly made.

Of course, not all second-party decisions in medicine naturally favor delay. For instance, the kinds of decisions typically made by judges and courts stress attention to the patient's rights, and these rights may be better protected if asserted clearly and unambiguously early in the game—say, while the patient is still competent enough to state his own views or to assert his own moral or religious beliefs. Similarly, certain kinds of decisions made by family members on behalf of a patient (for instance, to support her request for procedures like dialysis or organ transplants thought to require a supportive family setting) favor expeditious making: the sooner the family indicates to the medical team its willingness to undertake care of the patient, the stronger the patient's chance of access to care is likely to be. Nevertheless, many professional and lay decisions in medicine, particularly those about dying, do naturally favor delay, and it is this delay that, according to the working hypothesis adopted here, tends to inhibit or preclude the possibility of altruism on the part of the patient.

Even if decision-making is postponed until a crisis or change in status occurs, the patient may retain sufficient capacity to give or withhold consent for treatment. Nevertheless, this right of ratification will not protect any residual altruistic commitments he may have had. Because under the principle of beneficence the physician or other decision-maker is obligated to reach only a decision that serves the patient's interests, she will not (if she acts in a morally appropriate way) reach a decision in which the patient sacrifices himself for others. Consequently, the patient will not be presented with an altruistic decision to ratify. In some cases the patient may be able to accomplish altruistic purposes by refusing to consent to a decision made in his interests, but he cannot act on his altruistic commitments in any more direct way. A patient might also hope to achieve his altruistic aims by allowing decision-makers to favor the interests of, say, his family, other patients, or society, and then simply acquiescing in these decisions.[8] But relying on such circumstances is hardly a foolproof procedure for accomplishing the altruistic ends one believes important, since the decision-maker may violate the patient's interests for some quite different end. More important, such a tactic would set an undesirable precedent in inviting decision-makers whose primary moral obligation is to the patient to fail to satisfy it, without protest on the part of the patient or perhaps anyone else. Finally, though gaining respect is not part of the true altruist's motivation in making his self-sacrificial choices, to rely on the moral failures of second-party decision-makers, rather than to assert one's own altruistic choices directly, would preclude observers from according respect where respect is clearly due. If altruistic choices are to be made in medicine at all, respect can be granted them only if they are made openly and forthrightly, not covertly as the by-product of others' moral faults.

The working hypothesis adopted here suggests that the institution of medicine itself, in a variety of policies and practices, tends to preclude altruistic commitment and choice. Of course, it may be the case that no individuals would volunteer for high-risk experimentation or self-sacrificial donations, even if such altruistic choices were allowed. It may also be the case that dying patients would always make self-interested, nonaltruistic choices, even if they were to make their decisions well in advance and to avoid postponement until crisis occurs. If some patients' decisions were other-regarding, it might be that most would favor the interests of others only very mildly, in ways not inconsistent with interests of their own. Perhaps only very, very few dying persons would make self-sacrificial decisions that might be described as robustly altruistic, and perhaps there would be none at all—not because altruism is impossible, but because in both experimental and therapeutic medical situations it simply does not occur. But notice that there is virtually no evidence available which bears on such claims, for the factors that would preclude these choices are already in place. Thus, the working hypothesis can neither be confirmed nor rejected; consequently, it is not possible to establish that any altruistic choices are actually prevented at all. Yet this does not settle the moral issues raised.

Perhaps the mechanisms of restrictive policy, delay, and displacement onto second-party decision-makers are necessary in order to prevent the abuse of vulnerable persons; this would be a very strong reason for curtailing altruistic practices both in therapeutic and experimental situations, if indeed they occur. But the possibility of abuse cannot count as a sufficient reason for precluding altruism unless it is impossible to protect against abuse without such restrictions, and unless nothing of still greater value would be lost. The argument from the possibility of abuse for limiting altruism can form only a secondary, later stage in the general assessment of professional and lay decison-making in medicine; the issue of whether altruism is morally desirable at all is independent of, and prior to, such further questions.

The Value of Altruism

In discussions of social institutions such as voluntary blood donation systems, altruism is frequently described as a precious social resource, a phenomenon to be protected and reinforced.[9] Altruistic donation, it is said, makes possible low-cost blood supplies, free from contaminants, which can be provided with little waste to the very wide range of patients who have need of blood; this is an important social good. The altruism involved is comparatively mild: inasmuch as the procedure is virtually painless and risk-free, the sacrifice that the donor makes to the unknown recipient is extremely small. Yet even mild altruism is a fragile thing, it is argued, and such a tradition must be protected against the encroachments of a paid-donor system. More robust altruism, if it could be sustained and encouraged, would provide still more important social goods, and very robust, self-sacrificial altruism—such as organ donation and volunteering for high-risk experimentation—could provide extremely valuable social goods that, without violations of individual rights, could be obtained in no other way.

Altruism may seem particularly precious as a social resource when it not merely confers gratuitous benefits upon someone else, but when it prevents serious harms to other persons or contributes to greater justice in the distribution of goods. Because the altruist recognizes the interests of others in addition to her own, she may be particularly perceptive in noticing that the interests of others are not served, and hence in noticing harms and injustice. Both small acts of altruism—say, yielding one's place in an emergency-care line—and more robust ones may not only have significant consequences in preventing harms to the beneficiary, but may rectify substantial injustices in access to health care. Even indirect altruistic donations, such as the savings of resources that might result from a patient's refusal of treatment, might redress serious inequities in the health-care system, particularly if such donations were directed to otherwise disadvantaged persons or groups. If what the altruist does is to relinquish her claims to resources, this choice, in a system with vast inequities in health-care access, may contribute to greater justice among the remaining claimants, particularly if it is based on an accurate perception of others' needs and if it is accompanied by measures ensuring that the desired redistribution will take place. Since, at least in many cases, it is the altruist herself who both identifies the need of the other and moves to correct that need, the potential effects of wide-scale altruism in medicine might be extremely profound.

Yet altruism ought not be valued for these reasons alone. If so, in effect it is to value the benefits of altruistic self-sacrifice to recipients, and to ignore or downplay the costs to donors; altruism is seen merely instrumentally, as a means of preventing harms or achieving a desired distribution of goods. But this is a remarkably callous view. It fails to recognize that protection from harms for some or a more just distribution of goods is achieved at the expense of others, namely, the altruists themselves. Nor does such a view acknowledge the distinctive moral feature of these costs, namely, that they are voluntarily sustained. To treat altruism as a "precious social resource" is to countenance a sacrifice without morally acknowledging either the fact or the unique features of it.

This attitude is particularly callous where altruistic sacrifices made by many individuals on a society-wide scale have pronounced effects on the distribution of resources within that society. Suppose, for instance, terminally ill patients were routinely to relinquish their claims on resources by declining treatment and accelerating their own deaths, not just for self-interested reasons such as avoiding pain or dependency but to conserve these resources and ease the burdens for others.[10] The aggregate effects of widespread individual choices of this sort might be significant indeed, and if redistribution of the savings to other claimants within the health-care system were actually to occur, it might do much to correct a variety of injustices within this system. This is an outcome much to be prized. But to value these choices *because* they effectively redistribute goods, even where they in fact contribute to greater justice, is to miss what is morally central in altruism. This callousness is exacerbated if altruism is encouraged through legislation, social policy, or other means that may diminish but not eliminate the voluntariness of the choice, since they diminish the morally distinctive feature of altruism and instead simply manipulate the goodwill of altruistic persons for other persons' sakes.

"Encouraged" altruism is particularly disturbing when it is encouraged by the expected beneficiary of the act. Homegrown cases of the "do it for me" variety are familiar enough, and, indeed, have their analogues in medicine; equally familiar are group, clan, tribe, and nation-focused forms of "altruism" fomented and encouraged by the group, clan, tribe or nation that stands to benefit. These groups demand self-sacrifice and loyalty, sometimes even to the point of death; in effect, they use these persons, by preying on their capacity for genuinely altruistic action, to advance their own interests. This not only abuses the potential altruist by misinforming, manipulating, and coercing him, but it distorts the central feature of altruism itself by valuing it for its social consequences alone.

Alternatively, altruism might be valued for one, or both, of the kinds of distinctive psychological consequences it brings. Acts of altruism can produce satisfactions for the agent, even if these satisfactions are not the basis of the altruistic motivation, and they can be substantial even in the face of sizeable material or physical losses. Then, too, altruism might be valued for its psychological consequences for the beneficiary: receiving altruistic aid from a friend, as distinguished from aid simply required by duty, not only improves the recipient's situation but enhances her self-esteem, by letting her know that someone cares about her: thus, altruistic help provides psychological benefits dutiful help does not.[11] Such evaluations of altruism, however, may prove to be a two-edged sword: the psychological consequences of altruistic action are not always good. Some self-sacrifice is pathological, and the harms it incurs bring further damage to the agent. Altruism may also harm its intended beneficiaries, since the altruist may misjudge what will serve their interests and impose upon them the altruist's own, foreign conception of the good. (Indeed, the worst vices of altruism may be located here.[12]) Even where the altruistic act produces its intended, beneficial results, it may also engender upon the part of the beneficiary quite damaging feelings of guilt for having been the subject of someone else's sacrifice. This is particularly frequent in altruistic choices about dying, where the patient makes a grave, irreversible choice for others' sakes: they may well feel responsible for her death.

Finally, institutionalized altruism, even if it remains voluntary, may bring devastating consequences in its wake. A recent writer in the *New Zealand Medical Journal* claims that altruism is "the secret of man's inhumanity to man," and cites practices from widow-burning to military self-sacrifice to support his claim.[13] Although this author's conception of altruism may be comparatively loose, his examples do challenge the claim that altruism is a "precious social resource."

Consequentialist views of altruism, such as those considered here, fail to capture what is of crucial moral significance about altruism itself. But there is a second, nonconsequentialist sense in which altruism might be considered a "precious social resource"; here, it might be considered an intrinsically good condition or activity of human beings, and for this reason, something to be protected, promoted, and revered. Altruism might be characterized as a virtue, a kind of moral heroism, the goodness of which resides in the individual's capacity to will the benefit of someone other than himself. What would be praiseworthy would be the altruist's underlying value system, particularly reflected in the relative priority he assigns to his own interests and those of others. If he is a moderate, Kantian altruist of the sort envisioned by Kolm, he equates others' interests with his own: "the person takes himself to be a person of the same general importance as anyone else." If he is a more robust altruist, he puts others' interests first and his own in second place; when the two conflict, he prefers theirs to his. Either or both of these priorities, it might be argued, is worthy of moral praise.

Nevertheless, the altruist's priorities may not be morally defensible ones. Norman Gillespie proposes the example of the altruist who sees that I have dropped my umbrella on the New York subway tracks, and successfully jumps down in front of an arriving train to retrieve it for me: this act, although altruistic, perhaps, is foolish or ridiculous, not morally good.[14] This altruist risks too much for the benefits others receive. Even in more plausible, ordinary cases, one might more generally argue, altruism is not heroism but a kind of self-deprecation, in which the individual counts herself as unworthy or valueless in comparison to those whose interests she serves. The altruist's underlying priorities are not symptomatic of moral strength, on this view, but of weakness; and although self-abnegation may be genuinely voluntary and genuinely other-regarding, and although it may have extremely beneficial outcomes for other parties, it is, nevertheless, not praiseworthy if it is rooted in abject feelings of personal worthlessness or despair. The altruist lacks, in short, a fundamental kind of self-respect. This may be true of even the most noble-seeming self-sacrificer. His act is, so to speak, morally pathological: it is a candidate for "treatment" and for both paternalistic and moralistic intervention, but it is not an act deserving moral praise.

But is there not at least one respect in which the altruist is deserving of moral praise? Nagel, for instance, holds that the altruist succeeds at a difficult cognitive task at which the egoist fails; it is this, one might argue, that is a praiseworthy achievement. The altruist *sees* the needs of others, in a way that egoists do not, and hence responds to them.[15] Indeed, developing the capacity for altruistic perception and action might be taken as an index of advanced moral capacities, in which the individual abandons sheer self-interest for the higher levels of concern for other persons and for the human community as a whole; and it is particularly praiseworthy when it is a moral *achievement,* not merely the product of ordinary moral growth. On this view, altruism would indeed be a candidate for moral commendation, since it represents actualization of the highest potential of the moral agent in acting in the world.

The issues posed by this sort of intentionalist assessment of altruism may be particularly pressing in medical situations of the sort under discussion here. What is the morally appropriate response, for instance, to a dying patient's request that treatment be discontinued "so I won't become a burden"—to consider this a mark of moral heroism, or to treat it as the symptom of the patient's moral failure to count herself a worthy competitor among those with claims to resources? What about offers to submit to risky experimentation "for the good of science," like that of the woman from Las Vegas who volunteered for the artificial heart? This requires a more careful analysis of altruism, in which the good-making feature, if there is any such, is clearly identified. It might be located in moral perception itself, though this may raise more questions than it answers. Or altruism might be recognized as morally heroic only when based upon relatively sturdy feelings of self-worth, so that in sacrificing oneself for others one sacrifices something of value; on this interpretation, it is the sacrifice itself that is the good-making feature, worthy of praise. On this view, very mild altruism, involving little sacrifice of the agent's interests, will be of little value; very robust altruism, great, and the residual moral problems will focus on whether a sacrifice can be disproportionately large for the benefit conveyed: was the future Sakyamuni, whom Buddhist legend says fed himself to a starving tiger, a saint or a fool? Then again, it might be said that intensity of devotion to the interests of others is the primary morally relevant feature; on this view, the altruist most strongly committed to others is most worthy of praise, whether or not she holds herself in much esteem. On this view, both mild and robust altruism may be of great value, though both may be valueless, too. Here, the principal remaining moral problems will concern evaluating the person whose devotion to others is not fully voluntary but involves a kind of obsession or fixation: does what is viewed as pathology by nonaltruists preclude moral praise? Whichever way this issue is resolved, to sort morally heroic cases of altruism from unpraiseworthy or debased ones would in practice no doubt be difficult to do, and would often be obscured by the temptation to value altruism for its consequences alone. Yet this does not provide a basis for any assumption that the possibility—and importance—of altruism can simply be dismissed. In the end, the precise moral assessment of the value of altruism will be a function of the moral theories employed to evaluate the specific actions in which it occurs—whether utilitarian and consequentialist, principle-based and nonconsequentialist, or some variant of virtue ethics. But *all* of the principal moral views, excepting egoism, presuppose the possibility of altruism in the sense of taking the interests of others into account in making choices of one's own: indeed, for all except egoism, it is this capacity that is essential to moral choice.[16] *Moral* choice cannot occur when one perceives no differences between others' interests and one's own, or among the varying interests of those whom one's choices might affect.

Protecting the Possibility of Altruism

If the possibility of moral choice is to be preserved, then specific changes are indicated concerning decision-making in medicine. To offset the effects of those structures by which medicine may tend to inhibit or preclude altruism, it is possible to formulate policies and practices that, if the working hypothesis employed here is correct, would tend to protect or promote it. There are two general areas within which this can occur.

First, patient-protective regulations in experimental situations could be revised. Rather than restrict the kinds of choices the patient may make by prohibiting dangerous nontherapeutic research, revised regulations would instead focus on developing more stringent methods for controlling coercion and manipulation of the subject by the researchers. (Whether such regulations could be effectively designed is a quite different issue.) Thus, the choice of whether or not to submit to dangerous experimentation would remain the subject's choice, not a choice made in advance for him or her by policymakers at the federal level or in local review boards. Under such regulations, the possibility of altruism would remain open—even nonimmediate, impersonal, ideological altruism of a very robust sort. Such regulations would not prevent the Las Vegas woman from volunteering for the artificial heart, provided that she understood the extraordinary risks and that she was not coerced, and it would permit many similar such cases. (Apparently offers like hers are not uncommon in medical research.[17]) It is possible that such a revision of the regulations could have quite wide impact, though of course it is also possible that if there were any possibility that such offers might be accepted, most would be hastily withdrawn.[18]

Second, the possibility of altruism in ordinary medical decision-making might be promoted and protected by placing increasing emphasis on the importance of patient-made decisions. Assignment of primary decision-making responsibilities to either medical professionals or laypersons on behalf of patients would be discouraged, except in cases where the patient is irreversibly incompetent and no alternatives remain. Particularly in decisions about dying, postponement favors reliance on physician and lay second-party, nonpatient decisions, thus predetermining the basis upon which such decisions are appropriately made. But this pattern can be blocked by retrieving responsibility for such decisions from the physician or other second party, and holding the *patient* morally obligated to make the central decisions about his or her own death. This is not to say that the patient is morally obligated to make altruistic decisions, but rather that he or she is obligated to make decisions that involve moral choice: though he or she may not be obligated to practice altruism, he or she must keep its possibility open. However, if the patient is to preserve the possibility of altruism in his or her own decision-making, he or she must make the central decisions about his or her own death at a time when it can be done in an informed, unimpaired way. Thus, he or she cannot accede to medicine's naturally favored tendencies to postpone this choice until the last possible moment. Consequently, the patient must make those choices about dying well in advance, much as he or she now makes a property will, insofar as that patient can foresee the kinds of medical eventualities that could arise.[19] Furthermore, the patient must take whatever steps are necessary to ensure that when the time comes, the physician or other decision-maker, professional or lay, will *follow his or her desires, not act in his or her interests*—that is, respect the principle of autonomy and not that of beneficence—in making specific decisions about his or her care, unless the patient explicitly reverses his or her choice. Consequently, the patient must make such choices before the condition is very far progressed, before he or she begins to succumb to pain, weakness, depression, or fear, and in particular before that self-centeredness so characteristic of the final stages of acute and terminal illness sets irrevocably in.

These are not mere prudential maxims; they harbor a fundamental moral obligation. Yet there is nothing mysterious about this obligation; it is only the obligation to see that the decisions surrounding one's dying are made *morally,* that is, that the interests of others as well as oneself are taken into account. This, of course, is just the same as the obligation one has concerning other major (and minor) decisions in one's life: one has an obligation to see that they, too, are made in a morally satisfactory way. This is *not* to say that one ought to submerge or sacrifice one's own interests to those of others, and indeed, it may be the case that in a good many sorts of decisions in medicine, as in other areas, one ought to favor interests of one's own, even at the expense of others. It is not to presuppose that egoistic choices are of less intrinsic value than altruistic ones, either in dying or elsewhere, at least until an account of the value of altruism is complete. It is not to say that acceding or deferring to choices made on one's behalf cannot sometimes serve as mechanisms of effecting one's own choices, and that these can have moral value as well. But it is to say that one ought to recognize that situations such as these invite moral *choice,* not abject moral passivity. Moral choice-making, in any circumstance, at any time, requires at a minimum the recognition that there are others with interests different from and perhaps competing with one's own, and that one must recognize and acknowledge them if one is to act morally at all.

Perhaps this can be put in a slightly different way. What the patient ought not do is allow him- or herself to succumb to a system in which all the morally relevant choices will be made for him or her, at least without recognizing what this involves. He or she must recognize in advance that when professionals or laypersons are deciding for him or her they are obliged to decide (if they do so morally correctly) in a way that serves the patient's interests. To allow the medical system to do the decision-making for you is morally tantamount to making all your own choices in a self-interested way. Yet this is what we often do. Perhaps we can speak of a kind of "learned helplessness" in the moral domain: because we recognize, however dimly, that our institutions will do our moral choice-making for us once we are within their care, we behave as if we had no antecedent control over these moral choices at all. We may even invite ourselves to think that being ill absolves one of moral responsibility altogether, especially in decisions about death. But this is to fail to notice that the very assumption that the ill person is excused from moral choice-making is itself a self-serving one. A long, expensive dying can wreak havoc on one's spouse, family, or communal group, and one facing dying (as we all shall) should recognize this; collectively, avoiding such deaths could ease enormous burdens on one's society as a whole. On the other hand, a heroic stand against an inexorable and painful death can serve as a model of heroism, courage, and solace for one's spouse, family, communal group, or even institutions and societies on the largest scale; one facing dying should recognize this, too. This is not to say whether one must choose for or against delaying or accelerating dying. Nor is it to say that one ought to volunteer for potentially dangerous research. Nor, again, is it to say that one ought to make altruistic choices at all. But it is to say that one ought not protect oneself from making moral choices altogether by acceding to practices and policies under which they will be made for you in a predetermined way, unless they coincide with your considered choice.

In recognizing such an obligation, it is crucial to understand upon whom it falls. The making of moral choices cannot be imposed upon patients for whom it is already too late, and it would invite manipulation to advertise the possibility of altruism to those whose declining condition and fluctuating competency make them easy targets for abuse. Thus, it is not so much present patients upon whom the obligation falls, but future ones: namely, those of us whose decline and dying has not yet begun. Such an obligation would, of course, be mooted if one's death were to occur in some sudden, accidental way, but this does not relieve us of the obligation now. To retrieve the primary responsibility for decision-making in medicine from both professional and lay nonpatient second parties, however competent and trustworthy they may be, is, so to speak, the only *morally* responsible thing to do.

Recognition in policy and practice of the importance of preserving the possibility of altruism would, no doubt, bring losses due to miscalculation and abuse. It is true that an altruistically motivated patient's or subject's decision may be, medically speaking, a mistake; but it is a "mistake" only if the criterion of correctness is coherence with self-interests. And it is true that the potential altruist can be manipulated or coerced, but one is most manipulated and coerced in a system in which one is denied any genuine moral choice at all. Thus, just one thing is clear: until the issue of the moral status of altruism itself is resolved, we ought not uncritically perpetuate policies and practices in medical decision-making that preclude its possibility altogether. To do so is to deprive the patient of the possibility of retaining his or her status as a moral agent, and to make him or her a "patient" in not only a medical but a moral sense as well. Among the indignities that medicine is capable of inflicting, this may be among the most profound.

Notes

I wish to thank Saul Moroff, Ron Bayer, and Joanne Lynn for comments on an earlier version of this paper, and Bruce Landesman, Leslie Francis, Don Garrett, Peter Windt, and Diana Ackerman for attention to more recent versions.

1. The term "altruism" is variously used to cover motivation and behavior varying along all three scales. Mild altruism that is also personal and usually, though not necessarily, immediate we often call "benevolence" or "generosity," perhaps also "kindness," "thoughtfulness," "considerateness," or "goodness." We use the term "charity" (at least in a contemporary, secular sense) to denote other-regarding behavior that is either personal or impersonal but is typically directed to persons or groups not immediately associated with oneself. The social science terms "caring behavior" and "helping behavior" appear to denote mild altruism, where attention to the interests of others does not conflict with interests of one's own (indeed, one may make a profession of doing so). "Unselfishness," "self-disinterestedness," and "self-indifferentness" are sometimes used to emphasize the self-effacing nature of other-regarding behavior without specifying its object; these terms also tend to suggest an other-regardingness that is impersonal and comparatively weak. In contrast, the term "self-sacrifice" is generally reserved for quite robust forms of other-regarding behavior, whatever the object and whatever its degree of personalness or impersonalness; indeed, the term "altruism" itself is very frequently used in this way. Other-regarding behavior may also vary in purity, from those forms that are undivided in their attention to the interests of others to those that are wholly infected by ulterior motives, especially by desires to manipulate and control, but we tend to withhold most of the above terms from cases of the latter sort. We also tend to withhold most of these terms from other-regarding acts required by duty (for instance, supporting one's children), but not from acts considered supererogatory, typically the more robust ones. By and large, the terminology for forms of other-regarding behavior appears to vary primarily with robustness, that is, the degree to which these forms of behavior involve the sacrifice of interests of one's own; it also exhibits an ambiguity between terms denoting acts that are intended to benefit others and those that succeed in doing so, though this ambiguity does not appear to be systematic. In general, the grammar of these terms is by no means tidy, and we shall here adopt the terms "altruism" and "other-regarding behavior" to cover them all.

2. Indeed, see Richard Norman, "Self and Others: The Inadequacy of Utilitarianism," *Canadian Journal of Philosophy,* supp. vol. 5, *New Essays on John Stuart Mill and Utilitarianism* (1979): 182 and *passim,* for an argument that the dichotomy between egoism and altruism is false.

3. Thomas Nagel, *The Possibility of Altruism* (Oxford: The Clarendon Press, 1970), 79; earlier in his text, Nagel defines altruism as "any behavior motivated by the belief that someone else will benefit or avoid harm by it" (footnote, p. 16).

4. Serge-Christophe Kolm, "Altruism and Efficiency," *Ethics* 94 (1983): 62.

5. Robert Steinbrook, "Unrelated Volunteers as Bone Marrow Donors," *The Hastings Center Report* 10 (1980): 13.

6. William DeVries, M.D., the surgeon in the Utah artificial heart case, personal communication, for this and the next case.

7. In some cases of profound incompetence, such as anencephaly and brain death, the patient may not have interests at all, except perhaps certain posthumous ones; the criteria for decision-making may be very different here.

8. This devious suggestion is Diana Ackerman's, though she does not endorse this approach.

9. See, for example, Ronald M. Green, "Altruism in Health Care," in *Beneficence and*

Health Care, E. E. Shelp, ed. (Dordrecht: D. Reidel, 1982), 239–254, and much of the discussion surrounding R. M. Titmuss's *The Gift Relationship* (London: George Allen and Unwin, 1970), on blood donation systems. Titmuss also claims to see intrinsic value in the altruistic sentiments engendered in a voluntary blood donation system, above and beyond their value as mechanisms for providing important social goods.

10. Mary Rose Barrington, "Apologia for Suicide," in *Euthanasia and the Right to Death,* A. B. Downing, ed. (London: Peter Owen, 1969), reprinted in M. Pabst Battin and David Mayo, eds., *Suicide: The Philosophical Issues* (New York: St. Martin's Press, 1980). Barrington argues that the elderly should consider this both a benefit and an obligation.

11. This point is discussed at length in Lawrence A. Blum's very interesting volume *Friendship, Altruism, and Morality* (London: Routledge and Kegan Paul, 1980), especially Chapter 7.

12. See C. Dyck, "The Vices of Altruism," *Ethics* 81 (1971): 241–252.

13. See William Weddel, "Are Ethics Necessary in Medical Care?" *New Zealand Medical Journal* 94 (1981): 186.

14. Norman Gillespie, Review of *Friendship, Altruism, and Morality* by Lawrence A. Blum, *Ethics* 93 (1983): 597.

15. Indeed, Thomas Nagel claims that the possibility of altruism is rooted in the capacity of an individual to recognize not just the needs but the reality of other persons, in a way that out-and-out egoists apparently cannot: "Altruism itself depends on a recognition of the reality of other persons, and on the equivalent capacity to regard oneself as merely one individual among many." *The Possibility of Altruism,* 3.

16. See Bernard Williams, "Egoism and Altruism," in *Problems of the Self: Philosophical Papers 1956–1972* (Cambridge: Cambridge University Press, 1973), 205–265.

17. Renée Fox, comments at a symposium on the artificial heart, Alta, Utah, October 1983.

18. In "Attitudes toward Clinical Trials among Patients and the Public," *Journal of the American Medical Association* 248 (1982): 968–970, authors Barrie Cassileth, Edward J. Lusk, David S. Miller, and Shelley Hurwitz report that a study of cancer and cardiology patients and members of the general public showed that although 71 percent believed that patients should serve as research subjects and that 69 percent gave "benefit to society or others, or an increase in medical knowledge" as their reason for this belief, this altruistic stance seemed to fade when patients were confronted with the possibility of their own participation: only 23 percent said they themselves would participate in medical research to contribute to scientific knowledge, whereas over half (52 percent) said their main reason for participating would be "to help me get the best medical care."

19. Only about one death in ten is entirely unforeseen, and the progression of most illnesses is fairly predictable. See "The Least Worst Death," chapter 1 in this volume.

3

Is There a Duty to Die?
Age Rationing and the Just
Distribution of Health Care

In the fifth century B.C., Euripides addressed "those who patiently endure long illnesses" as follows:

> I hate the men who would prolong their lives
> By foods and drinks and charms of magic art
> Perverting nature's course to keep off death
> They ought, when they no longer serve the land
> To quit this life, and clear the way for youth.[1]

These lines express a view again stirring controversy: that those of the elderly who are irreversibly ill, whose lives can be continued only with substantial medical support, ought not be given treatment; instead, their lives should be brought to an end. It should be recognized, as one contemporary political figure is said to have put it, that they have a "duty to die."[2]

Although this controversy achieves a new urgency as pressures for containment of health-care costs escalate, the notion is hardly new that there is a time for the ill elderly to die, a time at which they are obligated to bring their lives to an end or allow others to do so. A number of conspicuous voices in the historical tradition have advanced such a notion, variously recommending denial of treatment, euthanasia, or socially assisted "rational" suicide as a means of bringing it about. Plato, for instance, said that the chronically ill or disabled patient ought to refuse medical treatment and, if he cannot return to work, simply die.[3] In Thomas More's *Utopia*, the priests and magistrates are to urge the person who suffers a painful incurable illness "to make the decision not to nourish such a painful disease any longer" and to "deliver himself from the scourge and imprisonment of living or let others release him."[4] Nietzsche claimed that the physician should administer a "fresh dose of disgust," rather than a prescription, to the sick man who "continues to vegetate in a state of cowardly dependence upon doctors" and who thus becomes a "parasite" on society; it is "indecent," he said, "to go on living."[5]

From *Ethics* 97:2 (1987): 317–340. Originally titled "Age Rationing and the Just Distribution of Health Care: Is There a Duty to Die?" Copyright © 1987 by the University of Chicago Press. Reprinted by permission of the publisher.

Not only have individual thinkers recommended such practices, but a variety of primitive and historical societies appear to have engaged in them. Although the anthropological data may not be fully reliable, there seems to be evidence of a variety of senicide practices, variously involving abandonment, direct killing, or socially enforced suicide. The Eskimo, for instance, are reported to have practiced suicide in old age "not merely to be rid of a life that is no longer a pleasure, but also to relieve their nearest relations of the trouble they give them."[6] The early Japanese are said to have taken their elderly to a mountaintop to die.[7] Various migratory American Indian tribes abandoned their infirm members by the side of the trail. The Greeks on the island of Ceos, at least while it was under siege, required persons reaching the age of sixty-five to commit suicide. Except within the school headed by Hippocrates, Greek physicians apparently made euthanasia or assistance in suicide available to those whose illnesses they could not cure, and there is some evidence that hemlock was developed for this purpose.[8] Greek and Roman Stoics—most notably Seneca—recommended suicide as the responsible act of the wise man, who ought not assign overly great importance to mere life itself but, rather, achieve the disengagement and wisdom required to end his own life at the appropriate time. Of course, not all of these practices have been humane, either in their initial intent or in their final outcome. Although the early Nazi euthanasia program known as T4, which actively terminated the lives of chronically ill, debilitated, or retarded Aryans, was advertised as a benefit to these persons as well as to the state, it became the training ground for concentration camp personnel.[9] But although practices that range from recommending refusal of medical treatment to encouraging suicide to deliberate, involuntary killing may seem to differ sharply in their ethical characteristics, there is nevertheless an important, central similarity: they are all the practices of societies which communicate to their members that when they reach advanced old age or become irreversibly ill, it is time to die, and that they have an obligation to acquiesce or cooperate in bringing this about. The question to be explored here, in the light of current issues concerning distributive justice in health care, is whether there is any moral warrant at all to this underlying view and, if so, precisely what consequences this would have for the health care of the aged.

The Economics of Health Care for the Aged

In contemporary society, a discomforting set of economic facts brings this issue into prominence. Health-care use by the aged constitutes a major component of medical spending and exacerbates that scarcity of medical resources which generates distributive dilemmas in the first place. People reaching old age, and especialy those entering extreme old age, are people for whom late-life dependency has, or may become, a reality, for whom medical-care expenses are likely to escalate, and for whom needs for custodial and nursing care will increase. Three out of four deaths of persons of all ages in the United States occur as a result of degenerative diseases, and the proportion is much higher in old age;[10] the multiple infirmities and extended downhill course characteristic of these diseases greatly elevate the need for medical care. People over sixty-five use medical services at 3.5 times the rate of those below sixty-five.[11] In 1981, the 11 percent of the population over sixty-five used 39.3 percent of short-stay hospital days, and the 4.4 percent over seventy-five used 20.7 percent.[12] There are now about six million octogenarians, and the federal government provides an estimated $51 billion in transfers and services to them.[13] People eighty years of age or older consume, on average, 77 percent more medical benefits than those between sixty-five and seventy-nine.[14] Nursing home residents number about 1.5 million, of whom 90 percent are sixty-five or over, at an average cost of $20,000 per year.[15] Although only 4.7 percent of persons sixty-five or over are in nursing homes, rates rise with age. About 1 percent of persons sixty-five to seventy-four are in nursing homes; of those seventy-five to eighty-four, 7 percent, and of those eighty-five and over, about 20 percent are in nursing homes on any given day.[16] Even so, institutionalized persons represent a comparatively small fraction of the elderly suffering chronic illnesses and disabilities, and it is estimated that for every nursing home resident, there are two other people with equivalent disabilities in the community.[17] One estimate suggests that 70 percent of the elderly who need care rely on relatives to provide it.[18] Even if a person maintains functional independence into old age, the risk of becoming frail for a prolonged period is still high: one study found that for independent persons between sixty-five and sixty-nine, total life expectancy was 16.5 years, but "active life expectancy," or the portion of the remaining years that were characterized by independence, was only 10 years, and the remaining 6.5 years were characterized by major functional impairment. Furthermore, this risk increases with age: persons who were independent at eighty-five were likely to spend 60 percent of their remaining 7.3 years requiring assistance.[19] Expenditures are particularly large for those who are about to die. For instance, for Medicare enrollees in 1976, the average reimbursement for those in their last year of life was 6.2 times as large as for those who survived at least two years, and although those who died constituted only 5.9 percent of Medicare enrollees, they accounted for 27.9 percent of program expenditures.[20] Although this figure is not confined to deaths among the elderly, a 1983 survey of cancer deaths conducted for Blue Cross/Blue Shield predicted that the average American who died of cancer in that year would incur more than $22,000 of illness-related expenses during the final year of life.[21]

Clearly, contemporary analogues of the practices of the historical and primitive societies just mentioned, ranging from refusal or denial of treatment to outright senicide and societally mandated suicide, would have pronounced impact upon the health-care resources available for other persons in society. It is this that gives rise to the quite painful distributive question to be examined here. If scarcity precludes granting all persons within society all the care they need for all medical conditions that might arise, some persons or some conditions must be reduced or excluded from care. But if so, it is often held, those excluded should be the elderly ill: after all, the medical conditions from which they suffer are often extraordinarily expensive to treat; the prognosis, as age increases, is increasingly poor; and in any case, they have already lived full life spans and had claim to a fair share of societal resources. It is this view, or constellation of views, which seems to underlie and motivate practices suggesting that there is a time for the elderly to die.

Justice and Age Rationing

If societal resources are insufficient to provide all the health care all persons in all medical conditions need, some sort of limiting distributive practice will of necessity emerge. Several writers have argued recently that rather than let the market control the distribution of health care, a rationally defended rationing policy can be developed under accepted principles of justice, and that this policy will justify rationing by age: old people should be the first to be excluded from medical care. However, assuming the underlying formal principle of justice to require that like cases and groups be treated alike, it is by no means initially clear that plausible material principles of justice will differentiate the elderly from other claimants for care. For instance, if an individual's claim to care were taken to be a function of the contributions society may expect as a return on its investment in him or her, this might seem to support age rationing, disfavoring those no longer capable of making contributions; but, of course, the elderly have already made contributions, contributions that in fact are more secure than the still potential contributions of the young. Alternatively, it might be argued that the elderly have greater claims to care in virtue of their greater vulnerability, in virtue of the respect owed elders, or in virtue of the intrinsic value of old age. This sort of discussion, characteristic of many analyses of distributive justice, involves identifying the possible desert bases of claims to health care—the grounds on which health care is said to be deserved—and then considering whether the elderly can satisfy these conditions as well as other age groups. If they can (which I think likely), policies that restrict the access of the elderly to health care must be seen as the product of simple age bias.

But an influential conceptual observation has been made by Norman Daniels.[22] Most analyses of distributive justice, Daniels observes, assume that the elderly constitute one among a variety of age groups, including infants, adolescents, and the middle-aged, all of which compete for scarce resources in health care. But this, in Daniels's view, is misleading; the elderly should be viewed as the same persons at a later stage of their lives. The mistake lies in considering distributive problems as problems in allocating resources among competing groups and among competing individuals, when they are more correctly understood as problems of allocating resources throughout the duration of lives. Given this conceptual shift, Daniels then employs Rawlsian strategies to determine just allocations of care. He considers what distributive policies prudential savers—the rational, self-interest-maximizing parties of the Rawlsian original position—would adopt if, unable to know their own medical conditions, genetic predispositions, physical susceptibilities, environmental situations, health maintenance habits, or ages, they must decide in advance on a spending plan, budgeting a fixed amount of medical care across their whole lives. He quite plausibly conjectures that prudential savers, behind the veil of ignorance in this original position, would choose, where scarcity obtains, to allocate a greater amount of resources to care and treatment required for conditions that occur earlier in life, from infancy through middle age, but not to underwrite treatment that would prolong life beyond its normal span. By freeing resources that might otherwise have been devoted to prolonging the lives of the elderly for use instead in the treatment of diseases that cause death or opportunity-restricting disability earlier in life, such a policy would maximize one's chances of getting a reasonable amount of life within the normal species-typical, age-relative opportunity range. (Presumably, such a policy would not allocate extensive care to severely defective neonates, cata-strophically and irreversibly damaged accident victims, or other persons whose medical prognoses are so dismal that the prospect of achieving even remotely normal species-typical age-relative opportunity is extremely poor. Thus, savings resulting from rationing care to the elderly would not be entirely consumed in treating the worst-off newborns or others in similarly hopeless circumstances, and the "black hole" problem would be avoided.) If this is a policy upon which prudential savers would agree, Daniels holds, it will show that—at least under scarcity conditions against a background of just institutions—age rationing is morally warranted for making allocations of health care.

But this leaves unanswered a crucial issue of application. If, in a situation of scarcity, a rationally defended rationing policy for health-care resources is more just than market control, and if the most just form of rationing for health care is rationing by age, this still does not determine what policies and practices for putting age rationing into effect are themselves just. Arguments for rationing are always morally incomplete without attention to the crucial details of precisely how such policies are to be given effect, because intolerable features of such policies may force recon-sideration of the rationing strategy from the start. Thus, employing Daniels's Rawl-sian strategy, it is necessary to consider what age rationing policies rational self-interest maximizers in the original position would accept.

Independent of whatever merits it may have as an application of the Rawlsian conception of justice, Daniels's strategy is intuitively attractive for assessing the moral justifiability of age rationing in health care. This is because those of us who are considering this issue—who would be prepared to develop policy requirements on the basis of these considerations and who would be governed by whatever policies might be devised—are effectively behind the "veil of ignorance" with respect to the specific events of our own aging and death. Although Rawls claims that we can enter the original position any time simply by reasoning for principles of justice in accordance with the appropriate restrictions on not taking into account one's own specific interests,[23] such self-restriction is hardly necessary: when consid-ering issues of justice with respect to aging and death, we are already there. Of course, it is true that most persons who are reasonably familiar with background medical and genetic information and who have some knowledge of their own ances-try, previous health history, and health maintenance habits are not completely igno-rant of the probable circumstances of their own aging and death. Yet they are able to eliminate with certainty only a very few types and causes of death (e.g., specific hereditary diseases for which one is not at risk) and to assign rough probabilities to the likelihood of contracting the major killer diseases; even those with early symp-toms of a disease syndrome cannot be sure that some other fatal event will not intervene. What they are not able to do is prospectively identify with certainty the actual cause of their own deaths or the precise events of a future terminal course. By and large, persons still in a position to consider the issue of health-care age rationing for the elderly and to develop policy responses do not yet know when or how they will age and die. But we are all in this position, and we find ourselves obliged to evaluate policies and applications of age rationing practices without knowing how they will affect our own interests when the time comes. Yet, despite the fact that we thus replicate the Rawlsian original position quite naturally, our reluctance to look squarely at death and its often unpleasant circumstances may undermine both the rationality and the justice of the death-related policies we adopt.

If the Rawls/Daniels strategy is employed, then, possible practices and policies for effecting age rationing, including denial or refusal of treatment, senicide, euthanasia, and socially mandated "rational" suicide, are to be assessed in terms of whether rational self-interest maximizers behind the veil of ignorance would agree to accept such policies or not. However, despite the analogy between the lack of specific knowledge characteristic of parties to the original position and the lack of specific knowledge characteristic of ordinary persons who have not yet reached old age or death, what rational self-interest maximizers in the original position would agree to cannot be determined simply by inspecting the age and death-related choices of ordinary persons now. This is because the kinds of choices we ordinary persons make are very heavily determined by social expectation and custom, legal and religious restriction, paternalistic practices in medicine, financial limitations, and so on. Furthermore, as ordinary persons, we may fail both to realize what our own self-interests actually are and to choose the most efficient means of satisfying them. Consequently, it is necessary to consider—as far as possible independently of cultural constraints—what policies for putting age rationing into practice the hypothetical rational, self-interest-maximizing persons in the original position would accept, given that they have antecedently consented to policies assigning enhanced care to the early and middle years but reducing care to the aged. Parties to the original position have disenfranchised themselves, so to speak; but it remains to be seen what form they would agree this disenfranchisement should take.

Age Rationing by Denial of Treatment

Although parties to the original position will have already agreed to ration health care to the elderly (in order to enhance health care available to younger and middle-aged people and, thus, maximize the possibility of each person's reaching a normal life span at all), they must be assumed to have enough general information to see what the consequences of this antecedent agreement will be. First, under an appropriately thin veil of ignorance of this sort, they will know that a given measure of health care is not equally effective at all age ranges: it will be much more effective in younger years, much less effective in old age. Because old persons typically have more complex medical problems, compounded by a decline in the function of many organs and by reduced capacities for healing and homeostasis, trade-offs between earlier and later years cannot be made on a one-to-one basis: by and large, a unit of medical care consumed late in life will have much less effect in preserving life and maintaining normal species-typical function than a unit of medical care consumed at a younger age. It is this that in part will have induced the rational self-interest maximizers of the original position to consent to an age rationing policy in the first place; but it will also influence how they choose to put an age rationing policy into effect. Once the multiple infirmities of old age begin to erode an individual's functioning, comparatively larger amounts of health care are likely to be required to raise it again. Therapy that can successfully maintain comfort, or restore functioning, or preserve life may be very much more expensive in older patients, if indeed success is possible at all.

Parties to the original position will also know that under a rationing scheme it will be necessary, given their antecedent distributive decision, to restrict or eliminate most of the comparatively elaborate kinds of care. Presumably, if care is to be denied, it will be the highest-cost, least-gain varieties of care, including care that does not directly serve to maintain life. Of course, "cheap treatment" such as common antibiotics, could be retained for elderly patients, since these are low cost and, given their potential for saving life, high gain; but expensive diagnostic procedures and therapies like CAT scans or MRIs, renal dialysis, organ transplants, hip replacements, hydrotherapy, respiratory support, total parenteral nutrition, individualized physical therapy, vascular grafting, major surgery, and high-tech procedures generally would be ruled out.[24] Hospitalization, and the nearly equally expensive inpatient hospice care, might not be permitted, except perhaps briefly; sustained nursing home care (at $20,000 a year) would no doubt also be excluded. When the elderly person over an appropriate age ceiling or exceeding a predetermined level of deterioration begins to show symptoms of a condition more serious than a transitory, easily cured illness, he would simply be counted ineligible for treatment. "I'm sorry, Mr. Smith," we can expect the physician to say, "there is nothing more we can do."

Knowing these things, parties to the original position can then assess the impact of age rationing by denial of treatment. Although they will know that age rationing of some of the more expensive, elaborate treatment modalities, like renal dialysis and organ transplantation, is now prevalent in Britain[25] and is to an uneven extent also evident in the United States,[26] they will also understand that under the general age rationing policy to which they have agreed, the frequency and finality of such denials of treatment would be much more severe. Although allocations to the elderly would, of course, be a fluctuating function of scarcity in health-care resources as a whole, it is probably fair to estimate that were the degree of scarcity approximately equivalent to what it is now, a just distribution of health care would demand that a very large proportion of all health-care expenses now devoted to the elderly be reassigned to younger age groups. The elderly now use nearly a third of all health care.[27] Were these resources reassigned to the younger and middle-aged groups, the probability would be dramatically increased that all or virtually all these persons (except the worst-off newborns and those catastrophically injured or killed outright in accidents, homicide, or suicide) would not only reach a normal life span, but reach it in reasonably good health. Although the temporary life expectancy (or average number of years a group of persons at the beginning of an age interval will live during that age interval) is already very high, especially for the intervals zero to twenty and twenty to forty-five,[28] it is still the case that a sizable number of people do not reach a normal life span or reach it only in poor health.[29] Reallocation of substantial health-care resources would do a great deal to change this, particularly if the transfers were used for preventive medicine and support programs, such as prenatal nutrition and life-style change, as well as direct assaults on specific diseases. But, to achieve this effect, if the degree of overall scarcity of medical resources could not be altered, a substantial portion of the care now given the elderly would have to be withdrawn. At most, perhaps, minimal home hospice care and inexpensive pain relief could be routinely granted, together with some superficial care in transient acute illness not related to chronic conditions or interdependent diseases. But treatment for the elderly could not be escalated very much beyond this point if, within a fixed degree of scarcity, a just distribution of resources were still to be achieved: if only an insignificantly lesser portion of the care now devoted to the elderly were reassigned to younger age groups, there would be no substantial redistributive achievement and no significant increase in the propects for persons generally for reaching a normal life span. Minimal and erratic age rationing of the sort now practiced in the United States would accomplish virtually no redistributive goal at all.

In some cases, to deny the elderly treatment beyond minimal home hospice care and inexpensive pain relief would simply result in earlier deaths. This would, presumably, be the case in many sorts of acute conditions—heart attacks or sudden-onset renal failure, for instance—where emergency medical intervention is clearly lifesaving. But, especially in old age, such starkly life-versus-death episodes are less likely to occur in isolation; it is much more likely that an elderly person will already suffer from a number of related or unrelated chronic conditions, each of which could be relieved at least to some degree by treatment but which together make a fairly substantial and expensive list of complaints. Almost half of persons age sixty-five or older suffer from chronic conditions,[30] of which the most frequently reported for the noninstitutionalized elderly are arthritis, vision and hearing impairments, heart conditions, and hypertension.[31] The elderly over eighty-five in the community average 3.5 important disabilities per person, and those who are hospitalized 6.0.[32] Some of these chronic conditions, like visual impairment, arthritis, and loss of hearing, are extremely common, but they are not always inexpensive to treat. Many of the conditions associated with increasing age, such as Alzheimer's disease, certain types of arthritis and cancers, osteoporosis, or stroke, may require extended medical, nursing, or rehabilitative care. But extended, substantial medical, nursing, and rehabilitative care is expensive; consequently, these are precisely the conditions in which, in a just health-care system under conditions of scarcity, the elderly would be denied care.

Clearly, even hypothetical parties to the original position, under an appropriately thin veil of ignorance, will be dismayed by the consequences of the initial distributive decision they have made. Total hip replacements, for instance, could no longer be offered the elderly; however, it will be evident that there is a substantial difference in the character of life for an elderly person who remains ambulatory and one no longer able to walk. It will be evident, too, that the person who needs, but does not get, a pacemaker or a coronary bypass may lead a quite restricted life, seriously limited in activities, and that life with renal failure or cardiac arrhythmias or pulmonary insufficiency can be restrictive, painful, and/or frightening. Indeed, what may be most dismaying to those peering through this thin veil of ignorance is that elderly persons who are not allocated treatment do not simply die; rather, they suffer their illness and disabilities without adequate aid. Even symptom control in conditions like cancer, if not simply obliterative of consciousness, can be quite expensive, since effective relief may require constant titration and monitoring; if so, it, too, would presumably be ruled out. Worse still, common antibiotics and the few other kinds of cheap treatment that would still be available may simply serve to prolong this period of decline, not to reduce its discomforts, whereas labor-intensive care that might make it tolerable—like physical therapy or psychiatric support and counseling—would also be ruled out. To deny treatment does not always simply bring about earlier deaths that maximal care would postpone; denial of treatment also means denial of expensive palliative measures, both physical and psychological, which maximal care would permit at whatever age death occurs.

Nor can it be supposed that to deny care to the elderly is to simply allow them to die as their fathers and forefathers did; to deny care now is to subject persons to a medically new situation. Not only has it been comparatively unlikely until quite recently that a person would reach old age at all (in the United States, life expectancy at birth in 1900 was only 47.3 years, compared to 74.5 in 1982),[33] but in the past, most deaths were caused by parasitic and infectious diseases, many of which were rather rapidly fatal. Modern sanitation, inoculation, and antibiotic therapy have changed that, and for the first time the specter of old age as a constellation of various sublethal but severely limiting and discomforting conditions has become the norm. Hence, any notion that denial of treatment to the elderly will simply allow a return to the more "natural" modes of death enjoyed by earlier, simpler generations is a dangerously romanticized misconception. To ration health care by denial of treatment is not simply to abandon the patient to death but, often, to abandon him to a prolonged period of morbidity, only later followed by death.

But, of course, this is a prospect that the rational self-interest maximizer, behind the veil of ignorance about whether he or she will succumb quickly in an acute crisis or be consigned without substantial medical assistance to a long-term decline, will be concerned to protect against. Parties to the original position will thus find many reasons to reject policies that ration health care by denying treatment to the aged; the question for them will be whether they can devise better alternative methods.

Squaring the Curve

Since the publication in 1980 of James Fries's provocative article on the compression of morbidity,[34] there has been a good deal of discussion of the prospects for the reduction of senescence, or the end-of-life morbidity characteristic of old age. Although the average life span in the United States has increased by more than twenty-seven years between 1900 and the present, as Fries points out, the maximum life span has not increased; there is no greater percentage of centenarians, for instance, and there are no documented cases of survival, he claims, beyond 114 years. The result is an increasingly "rectangularized" mortality curve, as more and more people reach old age, but the maximum old age is not extended. Furthermore, since this rectangularization results from postponement of the onset of chronic illness, it means an increasingly rectangularized morbidity curve as well. On this basis, Fries optimistically predicts that the number of extremely old persons will not increase, that the average period of diminished physical vigor or senescence will decrease, that chronic disease will occupy a smaller proportion of the typical life span, and that the need for medical care in late life will decrease. Good health, in short, will extend closer and closer to the ideal average life span of about eighty-five, but life will not be extended much beyond this point (see Figure 3.1).

Fries's conclusions about "squaring the curve," as it is often called, have been vigorously disputed by Edward Schneider and Jacob Brody,[35] among others. They see no evidence of declining morbidity and disability in any age group, particularly those just prior to old age, but they do observe that increasing numbers of people are reaching advanced ages and point out that this fast-growing segment of the population is the one most vulnerable to chronic disease. While some writers set the biologic limit to the human life span at about one hundred, much higher than Fries's original estimate of eighty-five, others believe that there is no such limit. In either case, most of these comparatively pessimistic writers fear that a large increase in the number of individuals who reach old age will mean a large increase in the number of persons who spend long proportions of their lives afflicted with chronic disease. Advances in medicine will, they believe, prolong old age rather than delay its onset.

Clearly this issue is one with enormous consequences for health-care planning. But it has been debated as an empirical issue only; nowhere has it been recognized that the empirical question cloaks a central moral issue as well. What is crucial to

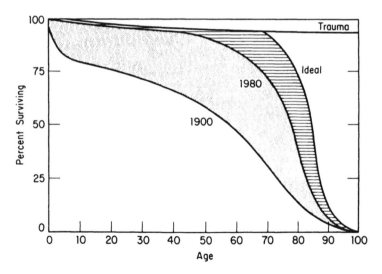

Figure 3.1. Fries's increasingly rectangular survival curve. About 80 percent (stippled area) of the difference between the 1900 curve and the ideal curve had been eliminated by 1980. Trauma, followed by homicide and suicide, are now the dominant causes of death in early life [AIDS had not yet appeared when this curve was drawn]. From James F. Fries, "Aging, Natural Death, and the Compression of Morbidity," *New England Journal of Medicine* 303 (July 17, 1980): 131, Fig. 2.

note is that both the optimistic and pessimistic parties to this dispute agree, or tacitly agree, on one thing: that a squared morbidity curve is a desirable thing. This is by no means surprising: the squared curve represents a situation in which life is, as Fries puts it, "physically, emotionally, and intellectually vigorous until just before its close."[36] Death without illness, or without sustained, long-term illness, rational self-interest maximizers would surely agree, is a desirable thing. But if this is so, the empirical disagreement between the optimists and the pessimists grows irrelevant. For regardless of whether or not changes in life-style or improvements in medical care would naturally flatten or square the mortality and morbidity curves, these curves can also be deliberately altered by other distributive and policy-based interventions as well—including those which implement age-rationing schemes.

As seen in the previous section, rationing that proceeds by denial of treatment may have the effect of not only hastening both the onset and termination of the drop-off or downhill slope of the morbidity curve—patients become impaired earlier and die sooner—but also in many cases flattening this downslope: the period of senescence, or chronic old-age disability, occupies a longer proportion of life, since it is endured without treatment. The morally significant feature of rationing policies that deny treatment is not simply their effect on mortality rates but their effect on the ways in which people die (see Figure 3.2).

But the curve can also be artificially squared—by deliberately bringing about death before the onset of serious morbidity, while the quality of life remains comparatively high. This, too, means that the onset and termination of the drop-off slope are both earlier—the termination a good deal earlier—but the slope itself is now perpendicular, not gradual, and life is terminated with only incipient decline. This is

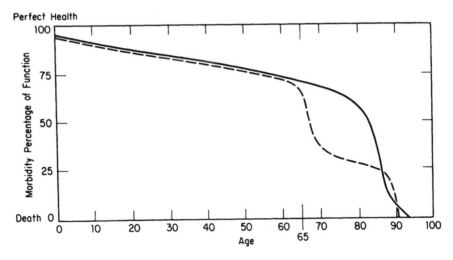

Figure 3.2. The effect of denying treatment in old age. Solid line shows morbidity curve characteristic for a representative individual where treatment is supplied; dotted line shows conjectural morbidity curve where treatment is denied after age sixty-five in sublethal chronic conditions.

precisely the effect of the primitive and historical practices mentioned earlier: senicide, euthanasia, and socially mandated "rational" suicide, at least where they are practiced early in the downhill course of a long-term degenerative disease. The squared curve will be produced, of course, by denial of treatment in sudden-onset life-threatening conditions, but these are much less characteristic of old age, and the more frequent effect of denying treatment is a flattened, prolonged decline. Practices that guarantee a squared curve, on the other hand, involve direct killing and, in particular, killing of persons whose quality of life is still comparatively high; nevertheless, these practices do achieve what is agreed by all to be desirable, namely, death without prior sustained, long-term disease (see Figure 3.3).

Under the assumptions employed here, parties to the original position have antecedently contracted for age rationing policies, even though these will have the effect of reducing the remaining length of life for those who reach old age. In virtue of this initial agreement, these parties are now also in a position to agree upon the sorts of policies by means of which this age rationing will be put into effect. Hence, they must choose between treatment-denying policies and those that impose death; constrained by their earlier decision in favor of age rationing, they no longer have the option of choosing policies that allocate extensive resources to the elderly and thus make possible the extension of life. To put it in the familiar terms of bioethics, they must choose between policies that involve "killing" and those that involve "allowing to die," and their agreement will serve to identify which policy is more just.

For the most part, the age rationing practices now followed in Britain and the United States, as well as elsewhere, involve denial of treatment, for instance, in the form of age ceilings for organ transplants, renal dialysis, or joint replacement. But I

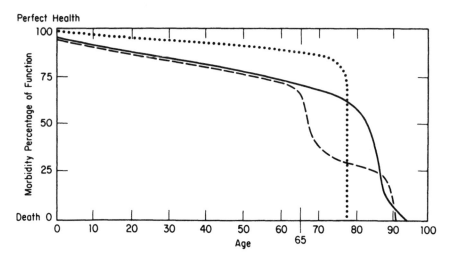

Figure 3.3. Morbidity curve in direct-termination practices. Solid line shows morbidity curve in old age with treatment, dashed line without treatment after age sixty-five, and dotted line shows conjectural morbidity curve in direct-termination practices such as senicide, early euthanasia, and culturally mandated "rational" suicide, displaying early redistributive gain.

wish to argue that rational self-interest maximizers in the original position would prefer the direct-killing practices that are the contemporary analogs of the historical and primitive practices of senicide, early euthanasia, and culturally encouraged suicide to those that involve allowing to die. Parties to the original position, after all, are fully informed about the possible societal consequences of their choices (except about the impact on themselves) and are not hesitant—as rational persons—to look the circumstances of death squarely in the face. There are, I think, two principal reasons why they would agree on direct-termination policies involving the causing of death, that is, on "squaring the curve."

Avoidance of Suffering

Except for persons who believe, on religious or other grounds, that suffering is of intrinsic merit or is of extrinsic value in attaining salvation or some other valued goal, rational persons eager to maximize their self-interests seek to avoid discomfort, disability, and pain. Of course, a good deal of suffering may willingly be endured by those who hope to survive a critical episode and return to a more normal condition of life; but terminal suffering known to be terminal is not prized. In medical situations where the prognosis is uncertain and sophisticated techniques are employed to support survival, the risk of suffering is one the rational person may well wish to take, since the odds of survival may be either unknown or large enough to make it worth the risk. But under an age rationing system that proceeds by denial of treatment, medical support will be minimal and, hence, comparatively ineffective in supporting survival; the chance of survival of an episode of illness is thereby drastically reduced. Thus, the possible gains to be achieved by enduring suffering disappear. Willingness to endure suffering may be a prudent, self-interest-favoring posture in a medical climate in which support is provided—even if that support is erratic or the chance of success is unknown—but it is not a prudent posture where age rationing precludes nearly all such support across the board.

Maximization of Life

Parties to the original position will also give preference to a policy that involves an overall distributive gain, benefiting all but giving the greatest benefit to the least advantaged. Since the allocation of resources may affect the overall total of resources available, they will prefer policies that maximize resources in a just distribution, and it is this that "squaring the curve" would accomplish. Of course, individuals surveying the possibility of policies that permit or require the direct termination of the existence of human beings may believe that their lives are to be sacrificed in the interests of other, younger people, and, were this the case, they would rightly resist this sort of utilitarian trade-off. But individuals who view these prospective policies in this way make a fundamental error: they view the effects of these policies from their own immediate perspective only and fail to see the larger impact these policies have. Quite the contrary, the overall effect of direct-termination policies is to *maximize* the preservation of life, not reduce it. This is a function of the fact, as pointed out earlier, that medical care is less efficient in old age and more efficient at younger ages, and that a unit of medical care consumed late in life will have much less effect in preserving life and maintaining normal species-typical function than a unit of medical care consumed at a younger age. The effect of rationing policies that allocate care away from elderly persons to younger ones is to increase the effectiveness of these resources, and thus greatly increase the chances for younger persons to reach a normal life span. Of course, since mortality in the zero to twenty and twenty to forty-five age ranges is already quite low (at least before the AIDS epidemic), the increase in temporary life expectancy will be greatest for those forty-five to sixty-five; but, it must be remembered, the veil of ignorance for those in the original position excludes all but the vaguest knowledge of likelihoods of their own positions,[37] and *any* possibly preventable mortality or morbidity in these younger age ranges will constitute a situation rational self-interest maximizers will work to avoid.

Furthermore, and for the same reasons of efficiency, the reallocation decreases by a much smaller amount the chances for older persons to live beyond a normal life span, since, after all, those chances were never very great. For example, ten units of medical care given to a ninety-two-year-old man with multiple chronic conditions might make it possible for him to live an additional two years, but ten units of care given to an eight-year-old girl in an acute episode might make it possible for her to live a normal life span, or about sixty-four additional years. The mistake the disgruntled elderly individual facing a rationing-mandated death makes is in failing to calculate not only the immediate loss he faces but also the benefit he has already gained from policies that have enhanced his chances of reaching his current age: his temporary life expectancy in the ranges zero to twenty, twenty to forty-five, and forty-five to sixty-five will have been much elevated, even though his total life expectancy may decline. The less care provided at the end of life and, hence, the greater the amount of transfer to earlier ages, the greater his gain in life prospects will have been. (Of course, this effect could not be achieved in the first generation of the implementation of such policies.) Furthermore, direct-termination policies are more effective in maximizing overall gains in life saved than denial-of-treatment policies. Since denial of treatment still always involves some costs as persons with multiple conditions in interrelated degenerative diseases are granted even minimal hospice and palliative care during their downhill courses, the proportion of savings is smaller, and less is transferred to earlier age groups.

Consequently, the disgruntled individual also makes a second mistake: he fails to see that because direct termination, rather than denial of treatment, maximizes the amount of transfer to younger age groups, such a policy will have maximized his own chances (except in the first generation) not just of reaching old age but also of entering it with fewer chronic, preexisting conditions. Furthermore, this policy will have done the same for all other persons as well. But as the number of persons entering old age with chronic conditions decreases, the normal life span will tend to increase (at least to any natural limit there may be) and, with it, the chances of any individual's reaching this mark. The long-term effect of such policies—despite the fact that they involve deliberately causing death in people who might continue to live—is to gradually increase the normal life span by delaying the onset of seriously debilitating and eventually fatal disease.

The rational person in the original position, then, who counts among his self-interests both the avoidance of suffering and the preservation of his life, will correctly see that social policies providing for the direct termination of his life at the onset of substantial morbidity in old age will more greatly enhance his prospects in satisfying these self-interests than any alternative available in a scarcity situation. After all, as a party to the original position, he has no knowledge of his own medical condition or age at any given time. Of course, if there were no benefits to older as well as to younger persons from this reallocation but, rather, merely the sacrifice of the interests of some people for those of others, parties to the original position could not agree to such policies; but this is not the case. Because such policies do provide benefits for all, and, indeed, the greatest benefits for the least advantaged (i.e., those who would otherwise die young), they will receive the agreement of all rational persons in the original position. This agreement, then, provides the basis for counting such policies just.

Attitudes toward Direct-Termination
Age Rationing

But of course, the rational self-interest maximizer in the original position can consent only to policies that are psychologically benign and that do not impose lifelong anguish or fear; this is because parties to the original position are rational in the sense that they will not enter into agreements they know they cannot keep or can do so only with great difficulty.[38] Age rationing policies that involve direct killing of the elderly may seem to invite just such anguish, as one cowers a lifetime in fear of being brutally extinguished by the unscrupulous physician or the naked power of the state. Certainly some of the primitive and historical policies mentioned earlier have engendered just this sort of fear: the early Nazi "euthanasia" program, although reserved for Aryans and initially performed with relatives' consent, comes to mind.

Nevertheless, whether death in old age is feared or welcomed is very much a product of social beliefs and expectations, and these not only undergo spontaneous transformations but can be quite readily altered and engineered.[39] Transformations in social practices in earlier historical periods make it evident that beliefs about whether there is such a thing as a time to die can change; transformation can be equally well imagined in the present. Aristotle's dictum notwithstanding, whether death is believed to be the worst of evils, or whether some circumstances—say, extreme incapacitation, inability to communicate, or continuous pain—are believed to be worse than death is much influenced by the surrounding society. Mary Rose Barrington speculates about an attitudinal change that, in the contemporary cost-conscious climate, seems an increasingly real possibility: "What if a time came when, no longer able to look after oneself, the decision to live on for the maximum number of years were considered a mark of heedless egoism? What if it were to be thought that *dulce et decorum est pro familia mori?*"[40]

Many sorts of prevailing social expectations serving the interests of society at large, and hence the long-term interests of individuals, are readily cooperated with, even at some immediate and direct cost to the individuals involved: for example, expectations about getting married, pursuing careers, supporting children, and so on. All of these involve a good deal of societal and institutional support. Marriage is encouraged in part by elaborate ceremonies and religious services; universities and technical schools not only provide employment skills but also socialize students to want to pursue careers; the support of children is enforced not only by legal penalties for failure to do so but also by extremely strong social sanctions. It is not at all difficult to imagine the development of social expectations around the notion that there is a time to die, or, indeed, that it is a matter of virtue or obligation to choose to die.[41] To be effective, these expectations would presumably be coupled with supportive social practices—for instance, pre-death counseling, physician assistance in providing the actual means of inducing death, or ceremonial recognition from such institutions as churches. Clearly, societal expectations concerning the time to die need not be dysphoric or condemn the members of an age rationing society to lifetimes of anguish or fear. Indeed, Daniels suggests that a view very like this characterized Aleut society: "The elderly, or the enfeebled elderly, are sent off to die, sparing the rest of the community from the burden of sustaining them. From descriptions of the practice, the elderly quite willingly accept this fate, and it is fair that they should."[42]

Nor need direct-termination rationing policies be viewed as a violation of rights. In an age rationing society there is no *right* to live maximally on, nor to receive the necessary medical care. Of course, an individual may have rights to many sorts of things, even in a society that rations by age—for instance, a right to termination procedures that are dignified and humane. A person will also have rights to freedom from abuse (to be discussed in the next section). And it will also be the case that younger persons have rights to medical care and the prolongation of life. Consequently, direct-termination age rationing policies, fairly applied, would not violate that Rawlsian principle of justice which stipulates that each person has an equal right to basic rights and liberties compatible with equal rights and liberties for all, since each person will have had an equal right to medical prolongation of life and equal liberty to live in his or her younger and middle years, and each person will be equally subject to the expectation that his or her life shall come to an end before sustained terminal morbidity sets in. This policy does not entail that elderly people no longer have rights; they continue to enjoy the rights of persons in society, but the right to extensive medical continuation of their lives is not among them.

The Issue of Abuse

Not only would rational self-interest maximizers in the original position require that any direct-termination rationing policies adopted neither be dysphoric in their application nor violate rights, but they will also require that these policies not invite abuse. To abuse a policy includes using it not only to cause harms to individuals but also to alter the practices it permits in such a way as to render the policy itself inherently unstable. Needless to say, virtually any policy can be abused, but some policies invite abuse in a much stronger way, and policies permitting or requiring direct killing may seem to make the strongest possible invitation of all. The issue, then, is whether parties to the original position could devise direct-termination policies that resist abuse or provide adequate protection against it.

Direct-termination age rationing policies would need to incorporate at least three features as protections against abuse. Without these features, rational self-interest maximizers in the original position could not consent to them.

Preservation of Choice

First, compliance with direct-termination policies would need to be experienced as essentially voluntary at the level of individual choice. This does not mean that individual choice would not be shaped by more general social expectations, but the individual could not be coerced, either legally or socially, into ending his life. Any individual who chose to resist the social expectation that it is time to die, and hence to endure the disenfranchisement from treatment that would be his lot, would have to be guaranteed the freedom to do so. Hence, in such a world, it could not be said that the ill, elderly individual has a "duty to die"; what he has is a duty to refrain from further use of medical resources. He may then think it prudent to avail himself of the support in direct, painless termination of his life that such a society would offer, instead of being abandoned to die without substantial medical help; but, of course, conceptions of prudence may vary from one individual to another. Indeed, if social acceptance of direct-termination policies were widespread enough to yield sufficient redistributive savings, this would perhaps permit giving those few persons who chose to tough it out additional medical care; this would further underscore the voluntary nature of response to a direct-termination social expectation. Preservation of choice is crucial because state or social coercion not only causes harms but also invites rebellion; it is inherently unstable. But the justice of age rationing in the first place depends on stable enough functioning of the scheme so that the distributive gains in overall life prospects are actually realized, and a scheme that is clearly unstable enough to make such redistributive effects impossible cannot be said to be just.

Rejection of a Fixed Age of Death

Second, the timing of direct-termination rationing policies must be based on expected time left until death, not on a fixed cutoff age such as sixty-five (as on the Greek island of Ceos), seventy-two (the approximate average life expectancy), eighty-five (Fries's conjecture)—or, for that matter, any other fixed age. This is because the underlying purpose of rationing is to enhance the length of life span for *all* members of society; though it will most greatly benefit those who now die earliest, it must also benefit the elderly as well. The central mechanism of redistributive age rationing is reallocation of treatment from older years to younger ones, where treatment is more efficacious and where the prospects of a longer life span are enhanced for all, especially for those whose life spans would otherwise be quite short. But if a fixed age cutoff point for the elderly were selected, whereby persons below that cutoff receive full treatment and persons above it were expected to end their lives, the fundamental purpose of rationing would be undermined. The use of a fixed-age cutoff point would be extraordinarily inefficient, since it would allocate some resources to persons on a clearly terminal course, where the possibility of extension of life is small, and it would also exterminate life where there was no medical treatment required to sustain it. It is not old age itself which is medically expensive; it is the last month, six months, or year or two of life. Variations in costs and efficacy of treatment are not so much a function of time since birth as time to death.[43] Many octogenarians are vigorously healthy; so are some people in their nineties and beyond. On the other hand, dying can be expensive and medical efforts futile even for those whose ages are not advanced. Still more important, avoidance of a fixed-age cutoff point protects the health-care system from political encroachments, particularly those that seek cost containment or other political objectives by adjusting the cutoff age downward.

Consequently, parties to the original position would not favor a fixed-age rationing policy but, rather, one that, depending on the degree of scarcity, encouraged direct termination via senicide, early euthanasia, or rational suicide only during the last month, half-year, or year of life. Of course, the precise antemortem period can be identified with certainty only retrospectively. However, even this does not constitute a fully effective counterargument, since it is usually possible for the experienced physician to recognize with at least a fair degree of accuracy the onset of what is likely to be a downhill course ending in death—especially in an elderly patient. Nevertheless, even if such predictions are sometimes inaccurate, the rational self-interest maximizer will still prefer reliance on them in order to maximize his opportunities for continuing life and normal functioning, something that would be jeopardized much more severely by a rigid age cutoff.

Furthermore, since some declines are comparatively rapid, even if not instantaneous, and some prolonged, parties to the original position will seek to maximize their overall opportunities not by agreeing to a policy in which a fixed amount of time at the end of life is held ineligible for care and in which direct termination may be practiced, but by supporting a policy in which disenfranchisement begins only at the onset of profound illness or irremediable chronic disease. After all, the precise duration of a downhill course can rarely be predicted with accuracy, although it can typically be accurately predicted that the course will indeed be downhill. Consequently, parties to the original position will consent to policies that impose disenfranchisement not long after the diagnosis and onset of symptoms of an eventually terminal disease, or at least long enough after the onset to confirm the diagnosis and for the need for medical care to have become pronounced. Hence, the curve in fact would never be perfectly squared, and individuals would not have their lives discontinued while they remained in full health, but the timing of disenfranchisement from care and the expectation that it is "time to die" would fall just after the onset of a characteristic downhill course. Just how far down this slope the cutoff point might come would be a function, of course, of the scarcity situation itself and also of individual, voluntary choices mentioned previously.

Public Awareness

Third, it is crucial that not only parties to the original position but also actual persons affected by such policies both know the policies and understand the rationale for them; secretive or propagandistic policies cannot be rationally chosen, nor can ill-founded ones. It is crucial for the stability and, hence, justice of "time to die" policies that persons affected by them understand their own distributive gain; without this understanding, they will remain in the posture of the disgruntled individual mentioned previously, who sees only his own loss. But individuals who see only their own losses under a policy constitute a force for change. This in turn renders the policy itself unstable in practice, and an unstable policy cannot operate in a way to produce a just distribution. It is crucial that the ordinary person who reaches old age understands that the very fact that he or she has been able to do so is in part the product of cooperation with policies that have him or her accept the claim that it is time to die when serious morbidity sets in. As mentioned earlier, the rational person will choose policies that promise both freedom from pain and as long a life as possible; it is only if the man in the street understands the theory and the operations of the policy that he will be able to see that it accomplishes both.

Conclusion: A Warning

This argument, that in an age rationing system direct termination of the lives of the elderly more nearly achieves justice than denying them treatment, may seem to be a reductio, but it is not. In a society characterized by substantial scarcity of resources, this contemporary analogue of ancient practices is the only fair response. However, this view does not—*repeat, NOT*—entail that contemporary society should impose age rationing or exterminate those among its elderly who are in poor health. For one thing, it is by no means clear that rationing either by denial of treatment or direct termination is better than providing full medical care for all the elderly who wish it, even at the expense of other social goods. Age rationing is a rationally defensible policy only if the alleged scarcity is real and cannot be relieved without introducing still greater injustices. But it may well be that the very scarcity assumption that gives rise to the issue of justice in health care in the first place is not accurate. Certainly some of the pressure on resources could be reduced by pruning waste and by greater attention to patients' actual desires, reducing the rather substantial amount of health-care expense attributable to the paternalistic imposition of treatment and to "defensive medicine" practices by physicians seeking to protect themselves from legal liability. More important, the degree of scarcity in health-care resources is itself a function of larger distributive choices among various kinds of social goods, including education, art, defense, welfare, and so on; the position of contemporary society does not resemble the economically precarious position of most of the primitive societies in which direct-termination practices have developed. Consequently, the appropriate response to the apparent cost-containment crisis in health care is not necessarily to devise just policies for enacting rationing, by age or in any other way, but to reconsider the societal priorities assigned various social goods. Given a world very much like the present one, it may be asked, what ceiling would parties in the original position assign to health care? This might obviate the necessity for rationing at all.

Second, a redistributive policy cannot be just without adequate guarantees that resources will, in fact, be redistributed as required. To deprive the elderly of health care without reassigning the savings in the form of health care for younger age groups is not just and ought not to be advertised in this way. Inasmuch as the erratic age rationing practiced in the United States (perhaps unlike that in a closed system, such as within the British National Health Service)[44] is not tied directly to redistribution of this care to others, it can hardly be described as just but, rather, as the product of ordinary, socially entrenched age bias. Furthermore, a just rationing system requires a background of just institutions to ensure its operation, and neither the United States nor Great Britain can boast a full set of these—nor, for that matter, can any of the primitive or historical societies mentioned at the outset. Consequently, although I believe there is a cogent argument for the moral preferability of a quite startling form of age rationing in a scarcity situation—voluntary but socially encouraged killing or self-killing of the elderly as their infirmities overcome them, in preference to the medical abandonment they would otherwise face—this is in no way a recommendation for the introduction of such practices in our present world. As Daniels remarks, if the basic institutions of a given society do not comply with acceptable principles of distributive justice, then rationing by age may make things worse[45]—and surely age rationing by direct-termination practices could make things very much worse indeed. Thus, while this essay argues that direct-termination practices would be just in a scarcity-characterized ideal world, it casts a quite skeptical eye on the sorts of arbitrary, unthinking age rationing we are toying with now.

Notes

I would like to thank Bruce Landesman, Leslie Francis, Tim Smeeding, Dan Wikler, Tom Reed, Virgil Aldrich, and the participants at the Health, Technology, and Environment Working Group Conference on Age Rationing in Health Care, Alta, Utah, September 1985. Some material for this chapter is drawn from an earlier paper, "Choosing the Time to Die: The Ethics and Economics of Suicide in Old Age," in *Geriatrics and Ethics: Value Conflicts for the 21st Century,* ed. I. Lawson, S. Spicker, and S. Ingman (Dordrecht: D. Reidel Publishing Co., 1987).

1. Euripides, *Suppliants* 1109, as quoted by [pseudo-] Plutarch in "A Letter of Condolence to Apollonius," 110C, in *Plutarch's Moralia,* vol. 2, trans. Frank Cole Babbitt (London: William Heinemann; Cambridge, Mass.: Harvard University Press, 1928), 153.

2. Colorado's Governor Richard D. Lamm was widely (mis)quoted in March 1984 as claiming that the terminally ill elderly "have a duty to die," engendering extremely vigorous controversy. Lamm's own account of what he actually did say appears in *New Republic* (August 27, 1984), as well as in a variety of speech and press corrections around this time.

3. Plato, *Republic* III.406C.

4. Thomas More, *Utopia,* bk. 2, "Their Care of the Sick and Euthanasia," trans. H. V. S. Ogden (Northbrook, Ill.: AHM, 1949), 57.

5. Friedrich Nietzsche, *The Twilight of the Idols*, sec. 36, in *The Complete Works of Friedrich Nietzsche*, vol. 16, trans. Anthony M. Ludovici (London: George Allen & Unwin, 1927), 88.

6. See Alexander H. Leighton and Charles C. Hughes, "Notes on Eskimo Patterns of Suicide," *Southwestern Journal of Anthropology* 11 (1955): 327–338, for a description of suicide practices from Yuit Eskimo informants on St. Lawrence Island, Alaska, and a survey of the literature on Eskimo suicide generally.

7. This practice is movingly depicted in Shohei Imamura's film *The Ballad of Narayama*, but there remains considerable controversy concerning whether the practice in fact has historical roots or is the product of legend imported at a later period.

8. The Hippocratic Oath reflects opposition to this practice on the part of a minority school. See Ludwig Edelstein, "The Hippocratic Oath: Text, Translation, and Interpretation," in *Supplements to the Bulletin of the History of Medicine*, no. 1 (Baltimore: Johns Hopkins University Press, 1943), and in *Ancient Medicine: Selected Papers of Ludwig Edelstein*, ed. Owsei and C. Lillian Temkin (Baltimore: Johns Hopkins University Press, 1967). Also see Danielle Gourevitch, "Suicide Among the Sick in Classical Antiquity," *Bulletin of the History of Medicine* 43 (1969): 501–518.

9. See Gitta Sereny, *Into that Darkness: From Mercy Killing to Mass Murder* (New York: McGraw-Hill Book Co., 1974), and Robert J. Lifton, *The Nazi Doctors: Medical Killing and the Psychology of Genocide* (New York: Basic Books, 1986) for accounts of the development of "euthanasia" policies under Hitler and their relationship to the mass extermination programs.

10. S. Jay Olshansky and A. Brian Ault, "The Fourth Stage of the Epidemiological Transition: The Age of Delayed Degenerative Diseases," *Milbank Memorial Fund Quarterly/Health and Society* 64 (1986): 355–391.

11. Norman Daniels, "Justice Between Age Groups: Am I My Parents' Keeper?" *Milbank Memorial Fund Quarterly/Health and Society* 61 (1983): 515.

12. U.S. Senate Special Committee on Aging, *Aging America, Trends and Projections* (1984), 70.

13. B. B. Torrey, "The Visible Costs of the Invisible Aged: The Fiscal Implications of the Growth in the Very Old" (Paper presented to the American Association for the Advancement of Science, New York, 1984), 1.

14. Ibid., 6.

15. J. H. Schultz, *The Economics of Aging* (Belmont, Calif.: Wadsworth Publishing Co., 1985), 140.

16. Ibid., 73.

17. J. W. Rowe, "Health Care of the Elderly," *New England Journal of Medicine* 312 (March 27, 1985): 831.

18. Schultz, *Economics of Aging*, 141.

19. Rowe, 828, quoting Sidney Katz et al., "Active Life Expectancy," *New England Journal of Medicine* 309 (November 17, 1983): 1218–1224.

20. James Lubitz and Ronald Prihoda, "The Use and Costs of Medicare Services in the Last 2 Years of Life," *Health Care Financing Review* 5 (1984): 119.

21. W. Hines, *Chicago Sun-Times*, 9 February 1983.

22. Daniels, "Justice between Age Groups," *passim*.

23. John Rawls, *A Theory of Justice* (Cambridge, Mass.: Harvard University Press, 1971), sec. 24, p. 138.

24. Parties to the original position are not only hypothetical but ahistorical, having no knowledge of what historical period they live in. The parties described here, however, seem to have an extraordinary amount of information about health-care costs in the 1980s. But this

is simply part of the general information such parties are assumed to have (ibid., sec. 24, p. 142); it can be assumed that they also have similarly detailed information about health-care costs in other historical periods, both before and after the 1980s. Regardless of the degree of technological development of medicine in these historical periods, however, in all of them, providing extensive care in end-of-life illness is more costly than denying care or directly terminating life; hence, in all of them, the age rationing problem will look very much like it does now.

25. See H. J. Aaron and W. B. Schwartz, *The Painful Prescription: Rationing Hospital Care* (Washington, D.C.: Brookings Institution, 1984) for an account of age rationing in Britain.

26. I have in mind nonmedically indicated age ceilings for heart transplants at Stanford, waiting lists in the Veterans Administration system for hip replacements, Medicaid's reduction of physical therapy for nursing home patients from twice daily to once daily, and the like.

27. Health-care expenditures for the elderly were estimated to reach 3.3 percent of the GNP in 1984, or nearly a third of the 10.5 percent of the GNP that represents all health care. See Daniel R. Waldo and Helen C. Lazenby, "Demographic Characteristics and Health Care Use and Expenditures by the Aged in the United States: 1977–1984," *Health Care Financing Review* 6 (1984): 8.

28. Olshansky and Ault, "The Fourth Stage," 4–5.

29. The "normal life span" is not to be confused with the "average life span," the latter of which 50 percent of the people do not reach and 50 percent exceed. The conception of "normal life span" employed by Daniels and others is not defined as a statistical notion but appears to have to do with the rough boundary between middle and old age or between early old age and late old age.

30. See Charles R. Fisher, "Differences by Age Groups in Health Care Spending," *Health Care Financing Review* 2 (Spring 1980): 69, Fig. 1.

31. John K. Iglehart, "The Cost of Keeping the Elderly Well," *National Journal* 12 (October 23, 1978): 1729.

32. Rowe, "Health Care of the Elderly," 830.

33. See Waldo and Lazenby, "Demographic Characteristics," 2.

34. James F. Fries, "Aging, Natural Death, and the Compression of Morbidity," *New England Journal of Medicine* 303 (July 17, 1980): 130–135.

35. Edward L. Schneider and Jacob A. Brody, "Aging, Natural Death, and the Compression of Morbidity: Another View," *New England Journal of Medicine* 309 (October 6, 1983): 854–855.

36. Fries, "Aging," 135.

37. Rawls, *Theory of Justice,* sec. 26, p. 155.

38. Ibid., 145.

39. See M. Pabst Battin, "Manipulated Suicide," in *Suicide: The Philosophical Issues,* ed. M. Pabst Battin and David J. Mayo (New York: St. Martin's Press, 1980, 172–173. [Chapter 10 in this volume.]

40. M. R. Barrington, "Apologia for Suicide," in *Suicide,* ed. Battin and Mayo, 97.

41. Battin, 172–173 ff.

42. Daniels, "Justice between Age Groups," 513.

43. Victor Fuchs, " 'Though Much Is Taken': Reflections on Aging, Health, and Medical Care," *Milbank Memorial Fund Quarterly/Health and Society* 62 (1984): 151–152.

44. See Norman Daniels, "Why Saying No to Patients in the United States Is So Hard: Cost Containment, Justice, and Provider Autonomy," *New England Journal of Medicine* 314 (May 22, 1986): 1380–1383.

45. Daniels, "Justice between Age Groups," 519.

4

Dying in 559 Beds:
Efficiency, "Best Buys," and the Ethics
of Standardization in National Health Care

In *The Notebooks of Malte Laurids Brigge,* the "heavy, difficult book" that he began in Rome during the winter of 1903–1904 and did not finish until 1910 in Paris, Rainer Maria Rilke employs a series of rapid, jolting impressions to express his pervasive concern with death and his distress about the institutional character of death among the poor. To convey an image of poverty, he describes the worn furniture of a cheap rented room:

> if I were not poor I would rent another room with furniture not so worn out, not so full of former occupants, as the furniture here. At first it really cost me an effort to lean my head on this arm-chair; for there is a certain greasy-grey hollow in its green covering, into which all heads seem to fit.[1]

To portray the nature of dying in medical institutions for the poor, he describes the Hôtel-Dieu, the poor-hospital, across the plaza from the Cathedral of Paris:

> This excellent hôtel is very ancient. Even in King Clovis' time people died in it in a number of beds. Now they are dying there in 559 beds. Factory-like, of course. Where the production is so enormous an individual death is not so nicely carried out; but then that doesn't matter. It is quantity that counts.[2]

And to describe the actual medical course of dying among the poor and sometimes even the rich, he creates the notion of what might be called the "official" death for a given disease, that is, its standard or most likely outcome:

> the wish to have a death of one's own is growing ever rarer . . . One dies just as it comes; one dies the death that belongs to the disease one has, for since one has come to know all diseases, one knows, too, that the different lethal terminations belong to the diseases and not to the people; and the sick person has so to speak nothing to do.[3]

In this short chapter, I'd like to take Rilke's rather enigmatic, impressionist descriptions seriously, not just to discover what it is that disturbs him about the medical

From *The Journal of Medicine and Philosophy* 17:1 (1992): 59–77. Copyright © 1992 by *The Journal of Medicine and Philosophy.* Reprinted by permission of the publisher.

character of dying among the turn-of-the-century European poor, but to see what this extraordinary poet's intuitions might tell us about turn-of-the-next-century national health care.

What troubles Rilke most, I think, is what we might call the prospect of *standardization:* the tendency of a system to treat people under its control in a uniform, regulated, unindividualistic way—robbing them, Rilke hints, of the capacity to function fully as persons. The poor are the immediate victims, since they are economically powerless to resist; but even the rich can be coopted by expectations in medicine that have the same standardizing and hence dehumanizing effect.

The prospect of standardization is, in Rilke's view, associated with large numbers and severe cost pressures: the poor are "dying in 559 beds" in a dismally equipped hospital funded only by charity. But it is this association of numbers and costs that invites us to consider the relevance of Rilke's concerns for contemporary national health-care systems: after all, national health systems involve both very large numbers and very severe cost pressures. Nor is there any way to relieve either of these pressures: by definition, a national health system involves the largest possible numbers, since everyone is to be eligible for care; and, as in any health system, a national health system is continuously subject to increasing cost pressures for which there is no natural solution. Since there is always need for more rapid and effective cure of disease, for better ways of controlling chronic conditions, for more reliable relief of pain with fewer side effects, and for more effective preventive efforts, and since there are always more patients who would benefit from these developments, there will always be cost pressures associated with providing better health care. Furthermore, since all patients eventually die, there is no natural bound to the resources in labor or technology that could be used to try to ease or postpone this event.

Efficiency in National Health Care

In the face of very large numbers and continuing cost pressures, a national health system will have, at least in principle, a predictable goal: the development of greater efficiency (also often called cost-effectiveness[4]) in the treatment and cure of disease and in the control of chronic conditions. It will continuously work to restructure its practices, including its medical practices, so as to achieve cure or control for less money. The early symptoms of this tendency are already apparent, in the current transitional medical climate, in the so-called "outcomes revolution"[5] evident in some sectors of U.S. medicine and followed with interest by many European observers. This reorientation of treatment evaluation practices seeks to change medicine's conservative reliance on conventional patterns of practice to direct inspection of the results obtained from specific procedures; that is, it looks not so much at whether the procedures physicians employ conform to a standard of practice, but at what results these procedures actually get. As outcomes are correlated with procedures, it is then possible to formulate efficient, cost-effective practice guidelines for the profession. For example, the federal Agency for Health Care Policy and Research has already begun the development of practice guidelines for six common conditions—angina pectoris, benign prostatic hypertrophy, gallstones, arthritis of the hip, conditions of the uterus, and low back pain—which now occasion treatment amounting to more than half of inpatient surgery.[6] The effort here, at least in principle, is to identify those procedures that are effective in treatment, discarding those that are not; to identify criteria under which they should be performed; and to stipulate ways of measuring morbidity and mortality that will realistically reflect the effectiveness of the procedure, given a specific severity of illness—or, in short, to identify the most effective way to achieve cure or control of these disease conditions, which can then be correlated with cost considerations.

A similar though unnamed emphasis on outcomes has long been at work in the development of associated practices such as preventive guidelines and early diagnosis programs, including screening programs, prophylactic care, instruction in self-help, genetic counseling, and so on. Here, it is assumed that by making possible prevention or early identification of disease, such measures offer a more efficient way of controlling or curing it than medical intervention could provide at a later point in the expected course of the disease. The impulse behind these programs might be described as akin to the concerns to be expected in a national health program, inasmuch as the effort is to save money, as well as human costs, for the population as a whole. To be sure, some authors have pointed out that screening and early risk identification programs can prove more expensive because they identify disease that then requires treatment but that would otherwise go untreated;[7] partisan bickering then begins when it is observed that money to be expended in prevention programs comes out of different pockets in a non-national system than those that would realize the savings.[8] Nevertheless, in a well-designed national system this need not be so, and it remains the case that such programs are in general both more humane and more efficient—if not initially cheaper—ways of responding to disease.

Thus, it appears that both the development of practice guidelines and the development of prevention and early-risk identification programs have in common that feature which Rilke suggests is the root of the problem of dehumanization in medicine: they invite "standardization." After all, practice guidelines have the effect of stipulating to the physician how a given disease condition is to be managed; prevention and early-risk programs initially treat all subjects uniformly, subjecting them to the same screening procedures, and then feed those identified as positive risk into the health-care system for treatment under its practice guidelines. Both thus increase the likelihood that all patients with a given condition will be treated in a uniform, "standardized" way. To be sure, similar developments may also occur in market-based, non-national health-care organizations; nevertheless, the distinctive problem of standardization will be most acute in a national health system for which efficiency in care is the principal objective.

Of course, to suggest that a national health system will predictably make efficiency in cure or control of disease its central objective is in certain ways an ideal view: it assumes that the system's administrators and professionals, including physicians, are not functioning primarily from greed or other ulterior motives, that the system is well run and efficiently administered, that the development of bureaucracy within the system is not so complete as to take on self-perpetuating characteristics, and that other distortions have not corrupted the system. It overlooks the bells and whistles a national health system might have to add, perhaps at the cost of other efficient care, in order to maintain political support. It also assumes that available funds are limited and that, as we have seen, health needs are never fully satisfied. But these conditions aside, a well-run national health system nevertheless should be more likely than a commercial health system to promote efficiency in providing health care. Were it not the case that the various factors involved are much too complex to admit such simplistic comparisons, it would be tempting to suggest that the substantially better health status of the populations of the major industrialized national-health nations than that of the United States suggests just such results: these populations, it would seem, get more efficient health care that is as good or better than that of the United States at substantially less cost.

Well-run competitive commercial health-care systems also seek to be efficient, of course, but they seek to be efficient in ways that enhance their own profitability. For example, providers are likely to try to increase their market share in providing a particular service—whether or not it is a service that is actually effective in curing or controlling disease. Providers, at least those who are not also payors, have less incentive to seek effective care than to expand the quantity of care provided, especially where the patient has little way of determining whether the care is necessary, because providing care is the source of their profit. This is the familiar phenomenon of overtreatment, a phenomenon directly addressed by federal controls such as the DRG reimbursement system, which pays hospitals for the costs of care for Medicaid and Medicare patients on the basis of their "diagnosis-related group," not their actual length of stay or treatment. Originally intended as an average of patients with a given condition, DRGs have quickly come to function as a ceiling. Other strategies, such as offering amenities and advertising directly to patients, represent additional techniques for stimulating demand for services in a profit-motivated system. In contrast, payors in a profit-motivated system, unlike providers, seek to limit their obligations as a way of enhancing their profits; this strategy is currently most evident in the insurance industry's attempt to move away from community rating to refusing to cover specific individuals and members of high-risk groups. But a national health system, though both provider and payor, will pursue neither of these strategies; it cannot seek to increase market share by overtreatment because there are no competitors from whom to take away business; and it cannot seek to exclude high-risk individuals because it is mandated to cover everyone. Thus, it is forced to seek efficiency in providing the services it is required to give to all, because under limited funding there is no other way for it to function.

Thus, the essential features of a national health system, and those features that encourage it to strive for "health-targeted" efficiency in providing care, are that the system attempt to provide care under a limited resource pool for very large numbers—everybody—and that it be without competitors in doing so. These features will be especially pronounced in a well-run national provider system under which physicians and other providers are employees of the state; they will also characterize a national insurance system in which reimbursement schedules are tight and explicit enough to control physician and other provider autonomy by limiting options for practice. In either form of national system, if it is the case that physician and other provider activity is controlled by practice guidelines that have been developed on the basis of demonstrated effectiveness in achieving specific outcomes, and if, furthermore, the system is mandated to provide care for all, there will be no internal incentive to provide more care in general or more care for some people than is needed. While there will still be pressures to exclude some types of treatment, there can be no pressures to exclude individuals or high-risk groups. In general, neither overtreatment nor risk-exclusion will be favored. To be sure, we already notice some of these altered trends in our current transitional system: quelling overtreatment is already a goal in some components of U.S. health care, including federal and state programs like Medicaid and Medicare, the VA, and large health-maintenance organizations that, operating almost like mini-national health systems, are their own payors as well as providers. Resisting exclusion is also becoming a goal in some states, for instance in those that have been attempting to expand Medicaid coverage or to develop insurance pools for those individuals deemed uninsurable by commercial firms.

Efficiency and "Best Buys"

If health-targeted efficiency is predictably to be the central goal in a national health system, as distinct from the profit-targeted efficiency to be expected in competitive commercial systems, it is essential to explore what forms health-targeted efficiency might take and to consider whether these forms of efficiency will give rise to the kind of standardization and consequent dehumanization against which Rilke warns. In the absence of corrupting features, we can expect a national health system to be a system in which cost pressures operate to influence the formulation of practice guidelines, and in which the least expensive way of achieving the best outcomes will be designated as the standard regulating all medical care. Leaving aside for the moment the scientific and research difficulties of measuring outcomes and developing practice guidelines, as well as the administrative difficulties of promoting universal use of them, one way a national health system's tendency to favor health-targeted efficiency might take shape is in selecting not the *best* way to achieve cure or control of disease, but the most efficient, cost-effective way to do so. A national health system operating under substantial cost pressures might thus employ—to use the term *Consumer Reports* made famous—not the best procedures for curing illness, but the "best buy" in procedures for doing so. Examples of "best buys" in procedures, as distinguished from the best procedures for treating the same conditions, include a number of modalities that are markedly cheaper than their "best" counterparts but give nearly as good results. These might include the use of hydroclorothyazide versus ACE inhibitors for hypertension; the use of medical rather than surgical methods of treating appendicitis; the use of traditional rather than low-osmolality contrast mediums in radiologic imaging; the use of cheaper, nonprescription niacin versus the prescription drug cholestyramine in controlling serum cholesterol; the use of medical rather than surgical methods of treating coronary heart disease; reliance on nonrepair rather than reconstruction in ACL-MCL knee injuries; medical rather than surgical methods of treating ulcer disease; the use of aspirin versus NSAIDs; and many others. Perhaps the most visible controversy over best versus "best-buy" options has been that involving the thrombolytic agents TPA and streptokinase. The enormous 1993 GUSTO study showed that accelerated TPA with heparin (at $2,300 a dose) is best, but streptokinase may be a best buy: at $320 a dose, it saves just one life less among a hundred heart attack victims.[9] Traditionally, considerations of the effectiveness of a procedure have in principle been given greater weight in the United States than considerations of cost: this is why the United States has developed a medical system providing care that, while very, very good, is also very, very expensive: its medical system has been providing first-class care, at least for some people, and has not, until recently, worried much about the price: it has insisted on the best, not on best buys. The prospect of a national health system seeking full efficiency in providing care for all but operating under budget limitations, however, forces us to consider whether it ought to turn to "best buys" in medicine rather than the traditional best in order to make ends meet.

To be sure, what counts as a "best buy" is a function of the amount of resources available, following the intuitive notion that a best buy is the best item of its kind one can get for the money one has available. If resources are not very limited the best buy will be nearly as good as the best; under greater scarcity, however, the difference between them will be pronounced. In either case, a national health system relying on fully demonstrated cost-effective "best-buy" practice guidelines or standards of practice for all medical and associated services would provide, in theory at least, the most benefits at the least cost for all persons. This would provide an alternative way of putting into practice the notion of "decent minimum": access to all services for all persons, but services of lesser efficacy.

Developing practice guidelines or standards of practice based either on "best" or on "best buy" treatments is itself a form of standardization: such guidelines attempt to describe and put into practice a uniform way of providing care for each disease condition, thus producing results for each patient that are uniformly effective to the same degree. In general, by codifying and regularizing uniform ways of treating specific conditions, well-developed practice guidelines benefit all patients with such conditions except the few statistical outliers—that is, patients who would have responded better to some less orthodox form of treatment. But a carefully developed practice guideline will have few, if any, such patients and, more importantly, it will be impossible to predict which individuals they are; for if it were possible to predict which patients would respond better to some other form of treatment, this fact would call for the development of a new practice guideline for this specific subgroup. Thus practice guidelines, in principle, are maximally effective. Of course in real life, under any system, practice guidelines in some contentious areas of medicine are likely to be adopted not just on the basis of unequivocal, exhaustive reporting of clinical experience and impeccable scientific research, but on the basis of political pressure from various groups partial on less-than-scientific grounds to one form of treatment or another. Then, too, the development of practice guidelines presents other problems—most notably, the problems of how such guidelines can be challenged, if accepted practice is uniform and there is no way, short of formal controlled trials, of gathering contrary findings; whether the disincentives for challenging guidelines would stifle clinical progress in medicine; whether they would provide too easy a target for litigation; and the problem mentioned earlier of ensuring universal compliance.[10] Furthermore, there are continuing problems about measuring the efficacy of treatment, about weighing the value of various objectives (e.g., pain control vs. rehabilitation), and about weighing nonmedical factors such as the value of privacy or confidentiality. Yet these problems do not outweigh the overwhelming utility of efficient practice guidelines in a cost-pressured system. In contrast to a market system in which some patients get precisely the treatment they need but other patients are undertreated, overtreated, treated inappropriately, or not treated at all, depending on what incentives affect the physicians who provide their care, a system based on practice guidelines—uniform throughout the medical system, and universally observed—would provide the most efficient care for all patients.

But of course, the development of ''best buy'' practice guidelines under cost constraints involves standardization at a lower level of effectiveness than when ''best'' guidelines are used. Discussion of disparate levels of care in medicine is already familiar talk in proposals for two-tiered health-care systems, but the conjecture here about what a national health program would favor is different. It considers an alternative form of two-tiered national health system, one that relies for cost savings neither on excluding individuals from treatment (as would be prohibited in a national health system in any case) nor on excluding certain conditions or procedures, such as transplants (a form of tiering that invites political pressure from patient disease-related advocacy groups), but that instead establishes two (or perhaps more) sets of practice guidelines to be employed, depending on whether the patient is receiving publicly funded or privately paid care. Of course, two-tiered systems provide little protection against erosion of the lower tier; if overall funding for a publicly supported system is meagre, the gap between highest-quality-possible care and most-efficient-given-the-budget-limitations care (i.e., between ''best'' and ''best buy'' care) could be quite large indeed, even though all persons would be eligible for care. Nevertheless, this form of two-tier system, under which ''best-buy'' care would be provided for the publicly funded and ''best care'' for those who could cover the additional cost, is demonstrably more just than other forms of public/private tiering (if any tiered system can be said to be just), since it imposes the liabilities of less adequate, lower-tier care equally on all publicly funded persons rather than, as in an exclusion system, on some few individuals from that group.

Rilke's Paradox? "Best" and "Best-Buy" Systems

Is it possible that a gap of this sort is the real problem that Rilke's concerns with standardization would have us address, though of course there were no practice guidelines in turn-of-the-century France? The Hôtel-Dieu, committed to providing for all the poor with limited charitable resources, would no doubt have had to practice a crude kind of cost-efficiency, of which standardization of practice would have been an earmark. Perhaps it is this standardization that Rilke observes: ''They are dying in 559 beds,'' he writes, ''factory-like, of course.'' He continues this ironic industrial metaphor: ''Where production is so enormous an individual death is not so nicely carried out; but then that doesn't matter. It is quantity that counts.''

Of course, Rilke might be objecting simply to the medicalization of death generally or to a kind of crude regimentation in medicine that pays little real attention to outcomes or the results of health care—that is, socially or medically callous warehousing of the dying—but his argument is still more interesting if we assume that the Hôtel-Dieu is doing the best it can to treat its patients' illnesses and that the standardization Rilke is objecting to involves practices as efficient as possible, given the medical science of the time. Whether or not this is what Rilke saw, it is what Rilke lets us see.

Yet what we see is paradox. If we look closely at Rilke's concerns, we see that the issue of standardization in medical care is much more complex than we might at first expect, and that even his images of illness and poverty do not support any general rejection of standardization or the apparent claim that it dehumanizes people. Consider, for instance, his image for the depersonalized condition of the poor: If he were not poor he would rent another room, he says, and describes the effort it has cost him to lean his head on the armchair in the room he currently occupies. The armchair had a greasy gray hollow into which all heads seem to fit—the heads of the previous, equally poor and transitory occupants of this shabby room. Not all of these occupants have been of the same physical size, but they have all been obliged to accommodate themselves to the same green armchair; and it is the fact that persons are forced by circumstances to accommodate themselves to a standardized item neither chosen by them nor suited to them that is the basis of Rilke's complaint. But is it a complaint that would also apply to an efficient national health system based on ''best-buy'' standards of practice, even one stretched by an inadequately funded attempt to provide health care for all to the point where its ''decent minimum,'' as stipulated by its lower-tier standards, is set quite low? To be sure, complaints about standardization, uniformity, and regimentation are a staple of naive objection to social welfare systems generally; but Rilke's objection is much more subtle in its comment on the special nature of health care.

After all, Rilke's argument against standardization initially appears altogether inadequate in the health-care context. Indeed, it doesn't even work for the furniture of rooming-houses. However dispiriting a thing it may be, an item of furniture like the green armchair in his room is remarkably efficient. Given cost pressures so severe that an armchair appropriately adapted to each new occupant cannot be provided, this unappealing green chair manages to accommodate everyone: ''all heads seem to fit.'' It would of course be preferable for each individual to live in a better equipped room with furniture of his or her own; but for the poor, it is this shabby room or nowhere at all. And it is this chair, used by all the previous down-and-out tenants, or no chair at all. Given no possibility of expanding the pool of resources available in this situation, the green armchair actually serves its purpose remarkably well: ''all heads seem to fit.''

Analogously, in health care, it is preferable to receive standardized lower-tier health care, including treatment stipulated in standards of practice and in mass prevention and identification programs, than to receive no care at all. Better to fit one's head into the greasy-grey hollow in the green armchair than to sit on the floor. Of course, one might idealistically spurn the armchair, preferring to camp on the floor, but the analogy does not work in medicine: unless one rejects health care altogether or some components of it for extraneous reasons (for example, on religious grounds, on the basis of fears about specific procedures, or on the basis of differing values about risk) or because the risk of iatrogenic complication is quite high, some health care is better than none at all. After all, the consequences of no treatment may be dysfunction, pain, or death, and it is never rational to prefer these to probable cure or restoration of function, except perhaps on outside grounds.

Thus, in a cost-pressured national health system, one may imagine a two-tiered system with dual practice guidelines. In such a system, for example, appendicitis patients in the lower tier, who would be treated medically rather than surgically, might have a slightly greater chance of dying than those in the upper tier, but nobody would risk the substantially greater chance of dying that exclusion from treatment altogether would entail. Patients in the lower tier would use niacin rather than cholestyramine, but would still be getting medical supervision of their cholesterol levels. Knee patients in the lower tier could expect conservative treatment of their ACL-MCL injuries, and although this would leave them unable to play certain sports and risk some instability, they could still function fairly well in most activities. Patients getting medical rather than surgical treatment of their ulcers would do nearly as well; and in all these circumstances, no patient would risk being entirely excluded from treatment. Although patients undergoing radiologic contrast studies would get traditional rather than low-osmolality contrast mediums and would therefore be at greater risk of anaphylactic reactions, no patient would be denied necessary diagnostic procedures. And whether or not TPA might eventually prove to have some therapeutic advantage over streptokinase, lower-tier patients would get streptokinase while upper-tier patients (or their physicians) might be permitted a choice; yet all heart attack patients would receive effective thrombolytic therapy.[11] Of course, a two-tier system risks allowing a substantial gap to develop between the upper and the lower tiers; on the other hand, if, as in Canada, the system prohibited a second tier (as I believe justice ultimately requires), political pressures would operate to keep the level of the single tier as high as possible. In either case, however, incentives characterizing a system under cost pressures, without competition, mandating care for all, would—if it were a system attentive enough to the requirements of justice to reject exclusion practices that impose unequal liabilities on persons— encourage the development of practice standards for maximally efficient health-targeted care. Thus, whether a national health system is a single-tiered or two-tiered one (or perhaps has multiple tiers), standardization is not the disadvantage a cursory reading of Rilke or inspection of our own stereotypes might seem to suggest, but is, on the contrary, the mechanism of its principal advantage. Of course, standardization does not mean utter uniformity in every detail of medical practice, and it does not require routinized interactions, inflexible schedules, physicians with indistinguishable smiles and identical bedside manners, or examining rooms all painted the same color. It refers only to adoption of the most effective practice where differences in practice make demonstrable differences in outcome, and it requires only the discarding of demonstrably ineffective, less effective, or damaging ways of doing things. Variety can flourish, but not uselessness or harmfulness, and because uselessness and harmfulness do not flourish, such a system provides the most effective care for all. Tied to considerations of cost, such a system will provide the most efficient care under cost-limiting constraints. This, I have argued, would most likely be the case, barring other corruptions, in a national health system that is noncompetitive but cost-pressured and mandated to provide care for all.

But it would be hasty to conclude that Rilke's intuitions are simply wrong, and that there is no moral problem raised by the prospect of standardization—even by the prospect of the sort of thoroughgoing standardization one might expect from a genuinely efficient national health system. Rilke describes dying at the Hôtel-Dieu as "factory like," a situation where "production is enormous" and it is "quantity that counts." But if it is "factory-like" that all items of a kind are treated in the same way, and if "production is enormous" means that everyone gets what he or she needs, then there is no moral problem here. Quantity *does* count: that is the whole point of national health systems, to ensure that everyone gets the health care he or she needs. Yet there is something else to notice about Rilke's observations: they are focused on a specific kind of health care, and the point he has to make has special application in this setting. What the patients in the 559 beds of the Hôtel-Dieu are doing is *dying:* this is a hospital for incurables, for terminal cases, as distinct from the Maison d'Accouchement, the obstetric hospital, and the Val-de-Grâce, the military hospital, down the street. The division of these hospitals in Rilke's turn-of-the-century Paris reflects a distinction central in his observations: there is something different about dying, and it is in dying as distinct from other medical events that the moral problems raised by standardization arise. It is not just that Rilke is obsessed with the notion of death—as not only Rilke but the Existentialists influenced by him would also be—but that he sees that there is something different from other medical situations about this process.

Efficiency in Dying

What, then, is disturbing about the factory-like production of deaths in the 559 beds of the Hôtel-Dieu? No one cares anymore for a "finely-finished death," Rilke laments: "No one. Even the rich, who could after all afford this luxury of dying in full detail, are beginning to be careless and indifferent; the wish to have a death of one's own is growing ever rarer."[12]

But if my account of efficiency in medical care is correct, surely the "factory-like production" of deaths would not raise any moral problem, unless, of course, it were accompanied by callousness, abuse, or cruelty, all peripheral institutional problems that are not part of the focus here.

But this presents the central problem: the very notions of "standard of practice" and "practice guideline" cannot function in the same way in dying as they do for the treatment of other medical conditions, because these are concepts that make central reference to the medical outcome to be attained. The procedure or medical treatment to be designated as standard in a practice guideline for a given condition is the one that is most effective in producing cure or control of the condition within the limits of resources available: it is the most efficient, cost-effective manner of producing a given outcome. But the sense in which death is the "outcome" of medical treatment is a very different one from the one associated with measurements of efficacy in standards of practice, as, for instance, cure of appendicitis is the outcome of an appendectomy or control of kidney failure is the outcome of dialysis. Unlike cure or the control of a chronic condition, death is not the *objective* of medical treatment and not the outcome in terms of which efficacy can be measured. Medical treatment does not *aim* at death; medical treatment aims at cure or the control of a condition, and death occurs only if it fails rather than succeeds. Thus, there can be no such thing as an "efficient" or "cost-effective" way of dying, since, except in the specific final procedure of euthanasia, death cannot be the objective of treatment. Even in hospice care provided terminally ill patients, death is not the objective, although it is the expected, unresisted outcome; on the contrary, the objective, to use the rhetoric associated with this important movement, is the fullest, best possible living of the last moments of life. If death were the objective, either in ordinary medical care or in hospice care, efficient dying would be that which gets the process completed in the shortest, and hence cheapest, possible time—but this is what few patients or physicians would regard as ideal and what no national health or similar system ought to encourage. This is not to encourage the prolongation of life, but not to encourage arbitrarily abrupt termination either. Cheap, rapid dying may be a personal goal for some patients, but ought not be imposed as an institutional or societal one.

But if there can be no such thing as "efficient dying," there can be no standard of practice for dying either, even when the dying is expected to follow the usual pattern of a predictable downhill course in a familiar fatal disease—advanced colon cancer, for instance, or kidney failure, or lung disease. At best, one could string together a series of procedures, each governed by its own practice guidelines, for the events or medical episodes along the way of this downhill course—for example, a procedure to relieve tumor pressure on a nerve, therapy for congestive heart failure, a procedure to relieve respiratory distress—but this is to view dying as a series of isolated, discrete events and to miss, as it were, the forest for the trees. If dying is seen as an integral process, not just as a series of interconnected medical failures, understanding it in the terms appropriate to other areas of medicine cannot fully succeed. There is no "best buy" in dying, although there may be "best buys" in specific sorts of symptom relief; there is no standard, efficient pattern that dying ought to follow. This is not to romanticize dying, but only to remark that viewing it in the way appropriate to other medical conditions is to cut off from view what we most ought to see: it is a circumstance in which efficiency is beside the point.

It might be suggested that Rilke's overwhelming concern with death raises only a tangential issue in medicine. But this is hardly so, especially given the cost-related issues that fuel pressures for national health care. After all, according to all the various figures so frequently cited in discussions of health care's high cost, an immense proportion of health-care dollars are spent in the last month, two months, or half-year of life. Of course, the last month, two months, or half-year of life can be identified only retroactively and not all patients were "dying" during those periods. Nevertheless, in a society in which approximately three of every four deaths occur as a result of degenerative disease (cancer, heart disease, stroke, liver, kidney and other organ failure, AIDS, neurological diseases, etc.)[13] and deaths from acute, rapidly fatal parasitic and infectious diseases and trauma are comparatively few, the issue of how dying is to take place in a cost-pressured, efficiency-oriented system, as a just national health system must be, is no trivial matter and cannot remain of peripheral interest only.

In Rilke's view, most systems—not only that of charity care for the poor of Paris at the Hôtel-Dieu but also Europe's private sanatoria for the wealthy—do function in effect by imposing standardized practices, even in terminal cases. "One dies the death that belongs to the disease one has," Rilke remarks, "for since one has come to know all diseases, one knows too, that the diferent lethal terminations belong to the diseases and not to the people; and the sick person has so to speak nothing to do." This is what I've called the notion of the "official" death, and it is what one might expect were standards of practice formulated to govern the whole scope of that series of medical events characteristic of specific downhill, terminal courses. It is this standardization in dying that Rilke sees as particularly dehumanizing; he writes, sarcastically, "In sanatoria, where people die so willingly and with so much gratitude to doctors and nurses, they die from one of the deaths attached to the institution; that is favorably regarded."[14]

Of course, one might argue that the objective of medical care in dying is the achievement of the longest life possible consistent with the least suffering; thus, there is a "standard of practice" in the broader sense even for dying. Indeed, this seems to be the assumption of contemporary terminal care: there is an easiest course the patient can be expected and encouraged to follow, one that will maximize "good" life but avoid terminal pain. But Rilke—and here it is difficult and important to be sensitive to his intuition—would regard this as an imposition of values where, because there is no objective goal for medical care, there is no legitimate basis for doing so: while some dying patients might regard a terminal period weighing maximized life against minimized pain as preferable, others might prefer it some other way. As an illustration, Rilke creates the extraordinary character Chamberlain Christoph Detlev Brigge, whose death was "two months long and so loud that it could be heard as far off as the manor farm."[15] To be sure, Rilke romanticizes a vigorous, rebellious, almost athletic dying—a value judgment there is no need for us to accept—but what he thus succeeds in pointing out is that there is *no reason at all why everyone should die in the same way.* Such contemporary devices as living wills may seem to protect individual choice, but they are not very robust: in general, advance directives mean only that one's course through the standard progression of dying can be interrupted after one is no longer competent, typically quite late in the game. The wish to have "a death of one's own" ought to be recognized, indeed admired, Rilke insists, and in this he is clearly right, since because it is not like other medical processes, there is no compelling reason for it to be any one, uniform way. Indeed, diversity may be the best protection against manipulation and abuse. However, it is precisely the having of "a death of one's own" that the standardization of practice—clearly so efficient and beneficial in other areas of medicine—would preclude. Being treated for appendicitis or hypertension or ulcer disease or ACL-MCL knee injuries or myocardial infarction "factory-like in 559 beds" (assuming the personal character of the care provided is humane, not literally factory-like, and the institutional environment reasonably pleasant) would present no moral problem, because treating these conditions in the most efficient way would increase all 559 patients' chances of cure, especially since no patients risk nontreatment. But dying is different, and it is not morally appropriate for a system governed by principles of efficiency to impose a standard expectation of how this final period of an individual's life should play itself out. Perhaps it is appropriate for a society to reassess its communal expectations about the nature of old age and medical responses to dying, as Daniel Callahan would recommend,[16] but it is not the role of a single, sole-provider system in effect to decide or enforce this.

What Rilke sees is not entirely easy to grasp. It is tempting to raise two further objections: first, that even if death is not the outcome sought, there can still be such a thing as efficiency in dying; and second, that a universal health-care system with pressures for efficiency can still tolerate diversity and individual choice.[17]

The first objection insists that although it is not death that is the objective sought, there is still an objective: a "good" dying process, one that minimizes indignity, pain, social isolation, etc., and maximizes the individual's personal values; and the second objection, that because an efficient health-care system can let patients refuse high-tech, intrusive means of prolonging life and thus allow them to choose death on their own terms, it can offer more control, more individuality, and greater "user satisfaction." These objections are closely related, and they both demand that we see in greater detail the point that Rilke invites us to recognize. To be sure, the "objective" of medical care for the terminally ill can be described as a "good" dying process, but this is a social goal, not a medical one. It depends on what the individual takes to be good (or "least worst") in dying, but this is a matter of individual judgment, not medical dictate. No doubt, many—perhaps most—patients will prefer a dying process that minimizes indignity, pain, and social isolation, and maximizes individual choice in promoting the values he or she espouses. But there is more to dying than this.

The problem arises as a function of the "institutional" character of death (whether one actually dies in a hospital or at home); it is the result of the fact that dying—in the view Rilke would have us see—typically involves following the usual trajectory of one's specific illness in a way shaped or dictated by the institutions in which or from which one receives care. One "dies from one of the deaths attached to the institution," Rilke observes; "that is favorably regarded." The deaths we have all come to expect, and will no doubt seek to achieve when our own time comes, are indeed deaths that preserve dignity, minimize pain, counteract social isolation, and allow us expression of our values, because these are the sorts of deaths that our institutions—hospitals, hospices, family environments, and cultural institutions more generally—regard favorably, even if they are not always achieved.

But there is a large range of possibilities *not* open to us in the deaths that are favorably regarded by the institutions in which we are situated. For instance, we may not take unproven therapies, such as Laetrile, whether or not we are persuaded they will work: Food and Drug Administration regulations preclude this choice by prohibiting the sale of such drugs. We may not volunteer for very high-risk medical experimentation, and certainly not for experimentation that would result in death (though we perhaps can imagine someone choosing to do so in order to benefit medical science or to have some sense that his or her life had been worth living); IRB regulations prevent self-sacrifice of this sort, even if death is around the corner in any case. We may not take cannabis or heroin for symptomatic relief in late-stage terminal illness, even though the British have been using the latter with great effectiveness in Hospice's famous Brompton's Mixture for many years. We may not ask our physicians for assistance in suicide, nor for euthanasia to end our lives in a controlled, painless way; at least, these requests have no legal protection.

Nor, at the other extreme of choices our institutions do not regard favorably, may we easily ask for all-out, maximal treatment in the face of an evidently hopeless condition, where treatment is viewed as futile and of no benefit to the patient. Although the *Wanglie* case may seem to have established a right to maximal treatment (in this case, respirator support for an eighty-six-year-old woman in a persistent vegetative state with permanent respiratory dependency—a patient permanently unconscious, and with, all physicians agreed, no chance of recovery), it is well worth noting that *Wanglie* was a hard-fought case.[18] Playing a major role in the case was the fact that Mrs. Wanglie's private supplementary insurance plan announced itself as prepared to assume the costs for maximal care; Medicare would not have covered her hospitalization. If our institutions tolerate choices like that made on behalf of Mrs. Wanglie at all, it is partly because it was made on religious grounds and partly because the financial arrangements were already contractually covered; and whether they would permit such a choice or not, such a choice would hardly be "favorably regarded." In short, individual choices at both extremes of the spectrum of possible responses to death are strongly discouraged or ruled out—both actively abbreviated and actively prolonged care.

What, then, is the death that is "favorably regarded" by our medical and social institutions? The details differ, of course, depending on whether one's illness is cancer, heart disease, stroke, various sorts of organ failure, one of the neurological diseases, or AIDS, but the "official" deaths all have many things in common: they typically involve initial aggressive therapy in an attempt to reverse the condition; then, when aggressive measures fail, a series of palliative procedures designed to control symptoms; and then, toward the end of the downhill course, a decision—sometimes made by the patient, but more often made by family members or by physicians with family consent, after the patient is no longer competent—to withhold further treatment or to withdraw treatment already in progress. Any symptomatic distress this may cause is relieved by the heavy administration of morphine. At the very end, the patient is managed in accord with DNR or "do not resuscitate" orders, and no attempt is made to stave off death when it occurs.

It is thus the norm that the patient endures nearly, but not entirely, the full downhill course of the disease, until, when treatment is withheld or withdrawn, the disease kills the patient. Of course, we are encouraged to go through the stages of denial, anger, bargaining, depression, and what is called "acceptance," since these are the stages—originally described by Elizabeth Kübler-Ross[19]—of what we now view as "normal" coming to terms with death. We are also encouraged to make our wills, draft living wills or durable-powers-of-attorney, contact Hospice, and voluntarily request that we be put on DNR status. The only exception to this pattern occurs when heavy doses of morphine, administered under a kind of secular version of the principle of double effect in order to control pain (not, we insist, to shorten life!), brings about death a little sooner than might otherwise be the case, but this is by no means a major deviation in the standard picture; it simply cuts the very final phases a little bit shorter. This scenario is rapidly becoming the ubiquitous American death: some 70 percent of deaths in U.S. health-care institutions involve elective decisions to withhold or withdraw some form of life-sustaining treatment, it is estimated, and 85 percent of deaths in the United States occur in these institutions.[20] Indeed, this pattern is part of the developing specialty of "terminal care." Of course, different diseases necessitate slightly different variations, but radically different options are not favorably regarded. Except, perhaps, for allowing earlier refusals and withdrawals of treatment, they are likely to be even less favorably regarded in a system in which dying may be regarded as a medical scenario with expectations of efficiency that are appropriate and just.

In seeing what is at stake in a system in which expectations of efficiency may function to reinforce patterns of the "official" deaths attached to various diseases, we may also need to explore the roots of our conventional postures towards death in general. Our attitudes about death, reflected in our medical and legal institutions, are based on what I think we may call the "passivity," "acquiescence," or "submission" model of approach to death; this is the traditional model of approach to death with which, as members of a common culture, we—as well as Rilke and the patients he portrays—are all familiar. Indeed, our language richly suggests the posture we adopt. We "succumb," "submit," or "accede" to death; we "wait" until death "comes," and when we can hold out no longer, we "give in" to death. We praise each other for our courage, and urge each other to accept the fact that "our time has come."

In its roots, the acquiescence or submission model is a religious, characteristically Christian one, though because it has been so pervasive in Western culture we do not usually identify it in this way. It derives, originally, from the theological conception of death as God's punishment for sin; death is understood as the curse that the fall of Adam and Eve brought upon the human race, though it is also seen as the gateway to a redemptive afterlife. It is central in this theological conception of death as in part punishment that it is imposed by God; it therefore is understood as a punishment from which one ought not flinch, since the believing Christian should (joyfully) accept what God metes out to him or her. Of course, as David Hume pointed out, a full-fledged acquiescence view of death would require that I not "turn aside a stone which is falling upon my head,"[21] and it is clear that the submission model we do accept is not an absolutely passivist one; on the contrary, it directs that where death is clearly preventable and there is no other reason for allowing it to occur, we should attempt to prevent it. Yet where death is clearly unavoidable, as in the terminal illness cases at issue here, this model holds that we should submit as gracefully as we can.

This acquiescence or submission model of death is what lies in the background of the turn-of-the-century hospitals Rilke describes; it lies in the background of our own contemporary hospitals as well. This is our cultural legacy—our model of how to approach death. It informs many of our practices; for instance, it is what is involved in rationing strategies where patients are denied potentially lifesaving care and are expected to "accept" this denial of treatment. To be sure, we sometimes violate this legacy; Dan Callahan in particular has pointed to the ways in which our "modernizing" attitudes of seeking indefinite life extension, characteristic of "heroic" life-prolonging care, have corrupted any defensible conception we may have had of the meaning of old age,[22] but much of the current protest against the excesses of life-prolongation reveals, I think, our underlying commitment to a much more passivist understanding of our role in death. Although this is rarely phrased in religious terms and often argued for cost reasons instead, it strongly resembles the traditional Christian notion that when death is approaching and not preventable, one's proper role is to accept death as God's plan when it comes. Dylan Thomas's "rage, rage against the dying of the light" notwithstanding, the traditional religious model of the proper stance toward oncoming death, one of ultimate, accepting submission, still informs contemporary secular culture's attitudes about dying.

If we contrast this view with what we might call an autonomist view of death, we find striking differences: the autonomist view assigns the individual whose death it is to be an active rather than passive role, but a role that emphasizes personal responsibility in choosing a course of action. This view too has historical roots: it is an essentially Stoic view—a view prevalent among both the late Greek Stoics and in Rome, especially evident in such figures as Seneca and Marcus Aurelius. However, because this autonomist view of death (together, of course, with Stoic philosophy generally) was eclipsed by the rise of Christianity and supplanted by Christianity's passivist view, it has left no continuous historical legacy for contemporary culture in the way that Christianity has. As we rediscover this view, late in the twentieth century, it seems alien to us, since we do not recognize that in fact it is part of our historical roots.

On the autonomist view, one is to assume responsibility for the character of one's own death, rather than allow its character to be dictated by external circumstances. Assuming an active role in one's own death may include controlling its timing, circumstances, manner, and the amount of suffering one is willing to endure; it also permits one to attempt to anticipate and shape its effect on others. It need not stipulate that one cause one's own death or commit suicide, as the Stoics favored but did not require, but simply that one assume an active, responsible role in the design of one's own death, whatever causal form it might actually take. One becomes the *agent* of one's own death, on this view, not the *patient*. For the Stoics, assuming this responsibility was one of the primary obligations of the wise man.

It is this contrast that allows us to see what form the efficiency pressures of a national health system can be expected to take, and in what way they can be expected to exacerbate the problem of the "official" death Rilke identifies for us. Autonomist, Stoic postures will be discouraged, except when the choices made under them happen to coincide with the "normal" progression of dying encouraged under the passivist model—first aggressive treatment, then palliative care, then withholding and withdrawal of treatment, and finally DNR—since autonomist choices may seek to encompass a much wider range of possibilities. They would need to encompass those who choose suicide or voluntary active euthanasia; they would also need to encompass those who choose, Wanglie-style, maximal care even when it yields no evident benefit. But, of course, the cost differential between these two choices would be enormous, and it is consequently hard to imagine that in a cost-pressured system, choices like the Wanglies' could be allowed—certainly not "favorably regarded"—or that the much, much cheaper choice of others for suicide or euthanasia far earlier in the trajectory of dying would not come to be regarded in a much better light. Yet this is just what a national health system, as I said earlier, ought not do: understand as most efficient, and hence favor, that form of care, including those practice guidelines, which get dying finished in the shortest, cheapest possible time. An autonomist model under a cost-pressured system will always be unstable, since the system will necessarily favor the cheaper choice yet do so in conflict with what we may take to be its most basic purposes. Retreat to a passivist model in which standardized choices are essentially dictated by the system—in which one does follow the standard pattern of care, in which one travels along the expected trajectory, in which one dies from "one of the deaths attached to the institution"—may well be "favorably regarded" for a reason, since it may be inevitable as a bulwark against the continuous erosion threatened by continuous cost pressures. Yet this easy retreat to a uniform passivist model is not an entirely defensible move; it is, rather, a central dilemma raised by the appropriate demands of justice for efficiency in health care.

This, I think, is what Rilke lets us see. "Now they are dying there in 559 beds," he had said of the Hôtel-Dieu, ". . . Where the production is so enormous an individual death is not so nicely carried out . . ." But he does not worry that the Hôtel-Dieu is inhumane in any conventional sense, and that is not our worry about efficient health-care systems either; what Rilke has in mind instead is a much more subtle erosion of human dignity, the way in which such circumstances preclude having "a death of one's own."

A national health-care system may certainly be greeted with enthusiasm on many grounds (and I strongly support its adoption in the United States), but, especially where very large proportions of its resources are at stake, it may also pose substantial moral problems. I think these risks are greatest in matters of dying. Of course, competitive, for-profit health-care systems also pose moral risks concerning dying, though these risks will differ as a function of the various incentives under which these systems operate. A particular risk in competitive free-market systems is a function of incentives to increase the quantity and technical quality of care performed: this may take the form of lengthening the process of dying so as to be able to provide more care, and is a practice that has been the focus of much public sentiment against the prolongation of dying. (To be sure, such prolongation, too, may jeopardize having what Rilke called "a death of one's own.") I think the risks in dying we can expect to see posed under a national health-care system will be less damaging to individual welfare than those we are now subject to in our current health-care environment, even in the more complex real world than the idealized versions considered here, but that does not mean we can pretend there are none. Nor is it the case that the ethical issues a national health-care system will generate, for all its advantages, will be limited to the matter of dying, but they will be particularly conspicuous in this difficult area.

Notes

I would like to thank Robert P. Huefner, Larry Brown, Paul Menzel, Dan Brock, Allen Buchanan, and participants in the Seventh Utah Conference on Ethics and Health, January 17–19, 1991, where an earlier version of this chapter was originally presented, for their comments.

1. Rainer Maria Rilke, *The Notebooks of Malte Laurids Brigge* (New York: Norton, 1964), 49.

2. Ibid., 17.

3. Ibid., 17–18, punctuation slightly altered.

4. Although it is equivalent to the sense in which I will be using the term "efficient," I will generally avoid the term "cost-effective" because it is so frequently misapplied and misunderstood. For instance, "cost-effective" is variously used to mean "cost saving," "effective," "cost saving, with an equal (or better) outcome," and "having an additional benefit worth the additional cost." See Peter Doubilet, Milton C. Weinstein, and Barbara J. McNeil, "Use and Misuse of the Term 'Cost Effective' in Medicine," *New England Journal of Medicine* 314 (January 23, 1986): 253–255.

5. Arnold S. Relman, M.D., "Assessment and Accountability: The Third Revolution in Medical Care," *New England Journal of Medicine* 319 (November 3, 1988): 1220–1222.

6. John E. Wennberg, "Outcomes Research, Cost Containment, and the Fear of Health Care Rationing," *New England Journal of Medicine* 323 (October 25, 1990): 1202.

7. See, for example, Louise B. Russell, *Is Prevention Better than Cure?* Studies in Social Economics (Washington, D.C.: Brookings Institution, 1986).

8. On why national and non-national systems are different, see Norman Daniels, "Why Saying No to Patients in the United States Is So Hard," *New England Journal of Medicine* 314 (May 22, 1986): 138–183.

9. The GUSTO Investigators, "An International Randomized Trial Comparing Four Thrombolytic Strategies for Acute Myocardial Infarction," *New England Journal of Medicine* 329 (September 2, 1993): 673–682.

10. On the problem of litigation, see Paul M. Ellwood, M.D., "Outcomes Management: A Technology of Patient Experience" (Shattuck Lecture), *New England Journal of Medicine* 318 (June 9, 1988): 1555. On universal compliance, see Jonathan Lomas et al., "Do Practice Guidelines Guide Practice?" *New England Journal of Medicine* 321 (November 9, 1989): 1306–1311.

11. On the discussion of these last two examples in one Canadian province, see Adam L. Linton and C. David Naylor, "Organized Medicine and the Assessment of Technology: Lessons from Ontario," *New England Journal of Medicine* 323 (November 22, 1990): 1463–1467.

12. Rilke, *Notebooks*, 17.

13. S. Jay Olshansky and A. Brian Ault, "The Fourth Stage of the Epidemiologic Transition: The Age of Delayed Degenerative Diseases," in *Should Medical Care Be Rationed by Age?* ed. Timothy M. Smeeding et al. (Totowa, N.J.: Rowman & Littlefield, 1987), 17.

14. Rilke, *Notebooks*, 18.

15. Ibid.

16. Daniel Callahan, *Setting Limits: Medical Goals in an Aging Society* (New York: Simon and Schuster, 1987), and his subsequent *What Kind of Life? The Limits of Medical Progress* (New York: Simon and Schuster, 1990).

17. I'd like to thank an anonymous reviewer for Oxford University Press for doing so.

18. See the group of articles on the Wanglie case in the July–August 1991 issue of *The*

Hastings Center Report, including pieces by Ronald Cranford, Michael Rie, and Daniel Callahan, as well as the articles by Marcia Angell and Steven Miles in the *New England Journal of Medicine* 325, no. 7 (August 15, 1991).

19. Elizabeth Kübler-Ross, *On Death and Dying* (New York: Macmillan, 1969).

20. Steven Miles and Carlos Gomez, *Protocols for Elective Use of Life-Sustaining Treatment* (New York: Springer Verlag, 1988).

21. David Hume, "On Suicide," (posthumously published in 1777) in *The Philosophical Works of David Hume,* vol. 4 (Edinburgh: Printed for Adam Black and William Tait, 1826).

22. See Callahan, *Setting Limits,* and *What Kind of Life?*

II

Euthanasia

5

Euthanasia: The Fundamental Issues

Because it arouses questions about the morality of killing, the effectiveness of consent, the duties of physicians, and equity in the distribution of resources, euthanasia is one of the most acute and uncomfortable contemporary problems in medical ethics. It is not a new problem; euthanasia has been discussed—and practiced—in both Eastern and Western cultures from the earliest historical times to the present. But because of medicine's new technological capacities to extend life, the problem is much more pressing than it has been in the past, and both the discussion and practice of euthanasia are more widespread. Despite this, much of contemporary Western culture remains strongly opposed to euthanasia: doctors ought not kill people, its public voices maintain, and ought not let them die if it is possible to save life.

I believe that this opposition to euthanasia is in serious moral error—on grounds of mercy, autonomy, and justice. I shall argue for the rightness of granting a person a humane, merciful death, if he or she wants it, even when this can be achieved only by a direct and deliberate killing. But I think there are dangers here. Consequently, I shall also suggest that there is a safer way to discharge our moral duties than relying on physician-initiated euthanasia, one that nevertheless will satisfy those moral demands upon which the case for euthanasia rests.

The Case for Euthanasia, Part I: Mercy

The case for euthanasia rests on three fundamental moral principles: mercy, autonomy, and justice.

The principle of mercy asserts that *where possible, one ought to relieve the pain or suffering of another person, when it does not contravene that person's wishes, where one can do so without undue costs to oneself, where one will not violate other moral obligations, where the pain or suffering itself is not necessary for the sufferer's attainment of some overriding good, and where the pain or suffering can be relieved without precluding the sufferer's attainment of some overriding good.*[1] (This principle might best be called the principle of medical mercy, to distinguish it

From D. VanDeVeer and T. Regan, eds., *Health Care Ethics* (Philadelphia: Temple University Press, 1987). Copyright © 1987 by Temple University Press. Reprinted by permission of the publisher.

from principles concerning mercy in judicial contexts.[2]) Stated in this relatively weak form, and limited by these provisos, the principle of (medical) mercy is not controversial, though the point I wish to argue here certainly is: contexts that require mercy sometimes require euthanasia as a way of granting mercy—both by direct killing and by letting die.

Although philosophers do not agree on whether moral agents have positive duties of beneficence, including duties to those in pain, members of the medical world are not reticent about asserting them. "Relief of pain is the least disputed and most universal of the moral obligations of the physician," writes one doctor. "Few things a doctor does are more important than relieving pain," says another.[3] These are not simply assertions that the physician ought "do no harm," as the Hippocratic Oath is traditionally interpreted, but assertions of positive obligation. It might be argued that the physician's duty of mercy derives from a special contractual or fiduciary relationship with the patient, but I think that this is in error: rather, the duty of (medical) mercy is generally binding on all moral agents,[4] and it is only by virtue of their more frequent exposure to pain and their specialized training in its treatment that this duty falls more heavily on physicians and nurses than on others. Hence, though we may call it the principle of *medical* mercy, it asserts an obligation that we all have.

This principle of mercy establishes two component duties:

1. the duty not to cause further pain or suffering; and
2. the duty to act to end pain or suffering already occurring.

Under the first of these, for a physician or other caregiver to extend mercy to a suffering patient may mean to refrain from procedures that cause further suffering— provided, of course, that the treatment offers the patient no overriding benefits. So, for instance, the physician must refrain from ordering painful tests, therapies, or surgical procedures when they cannot alleviate suffering or contribute to a patient's improvement or cure. Perhaps the most familiar contemporary medical example is the treatment of burn victims when survival is unprecedented;[5] if with the treatments or without them the patient's chance of survival is nil, mercy requires the physician not to impose the debridement treatments, which are excruciatingly painful, when they can provide the patient no benefit at all.

Although it is increasingly difficult to determine when survival is unprecedented in burn victims, other practices that the principles of mercy would rule out remain common. For instance, repeated cardiac resuscitation is sometimes performed even though a patient's survival is highly unlikely; although patients in arrest are unconscious at the time of resuscitation, it can be a brutal procedure, and if the patient regains consciousness, its aftermath can involve considerable pain. (On the contrary, of course, attempts at resuscitation would indeed be permitted under the principle of mercy if there were some chance of survival with good recovery, as in hypothermia or electrocution.) Patients are sometimes subjected to continued unproductive, painful treatment to complete a research protocol, to train student physicians, to protect the physician or hospital from legal action, or to appease the emotional needs of family members; although in some specific cases such practices may be justified on other grounds, in general they are prohibited by the principle of mercy. Of course, whether a painful test or therapy will actually contribute to some overriding good for the patient is not always clear. Nevertheless, the principle of mercy directs that where such procedures can reasonably be expected to impose suffering on the patient without overriding benefits for him or her, they ought not be done.

In many such cases, the patient will die whether or not the treatments are performed. In some cases, however, the principle of mercy may also demand withholding treatment that could extend the patient's life if the treatment is itself painful or discomforting and there is very little or no possibility that it will provide life that is pain-free or offers the possibility of other important goods. For instance, to provide respiratory support for a patient in the final, irreversible stages of a deteriorative disease may extend his or her life but will mean permanent dependence and incapacitation; though some patients may take continuing existence to make possible other important goods, for some patients continued treatment means the pointless imposition of continuing pain. "Death," whispered Abe Perlmutter, the Florida patient with amyotrophic lateral sclerosis—"Lou Gehrig's Disease"—who pursued through the courts his wish to have the tracheotomy tube connecting him to a respirator removed, "can't be any worse than what I'm going through now."[6] In such cases, the principle of mercy demands that the "treatments" no longer be imposed, and that the patient be allowed to die.

But the principle of mercy may also demand "letting die" in a still stronger sense. Under its second component, the principle asserts a duty to act to end suffering that is already occurring. Medicine already honors this duty through its various techniques of pain management, including physiological means such as narcotics, nerve blocks, acupuncture, and neurosurgery, and psychotherapeutic means such as self-hypnosis, conditioning, and good old-fashioned comforting care. But there are some difficult cases in which pain or suffering is severe but cannot be effectively controlled, at least as long as the patient remains sentient at all. Classical examples include tumors of the throat (where agonizing discomfort is not just a matter of pain but of inability to swallow); "air hunger," or acute shortness of breath; tumors of the brain or bone; and so on. Severe nausea, vomiting, and exhaustion may increase the patient's misery. In these cases, continuing life—or, at least, continuing consciousness—may mean continuing pain. Consequently, mercy's demand for euthanasia takes hold here: mercy demands that the pain, even if with it the life, be brought to an end.

Ending the pain, though with it the life, may be accomplished through what is usually called "passive euthanasia": withholding or withdrawing treatment that could prolong life. In the most indirect of these cases, the patient is simply not given treatment that might extend his or her life—say, radiation therapy in advanced cancer. In the more direct cases, lifesaving treatment is deliberately withheld in the face of an immediate, lethal threat—for instance, antibiotics are withheld from a cancer patient when an overwhelming infection develops; either the cancer or the infection will kill the patient, but the infection does so sooner and in a much gentler way. In all of the passive euthanasia cases, properly so called, the patient's life could be extended; it is mercy that demands that he or she be "allowed to die."

But the second component of the principle of mercy may also demand the easing of pain by means more direct than mere allowing to die; it may require *killing*. This is usually called "active euthanasia," and despite borderline cases (for instance, removing a respirator or a lifesaving IV), it can in general be conceptually distinguished from passive euthanasia. In passive euthanasia, treatment is withheld that could support failing bodily functions, either in warding off external threats or in performing its own processes; active euthanasia, in contrast, involves the direct interruption of ongoing bodily processes that otherwise would have been adequate to sustain life. However, although it may be possible to draw a conceptual distinction between passive and active euthanasia, this provides no warrant for the ubiquitous view that killing is morally worse than letting die.[7] Nor does it support the view that withdrawing treatment is worse than withholding it. If the patient's condition is so tragic that continuing life brings only pain, and there is no other way to relieve the pain than by death, then the more merciful act is not one that merely removes support for bodily processes and waits for eventual death to ensue; rather, it is one that brings the pain—and the patient's life—to an end *now*. If there are grounds on which it is merciful not to prolong life, then there are also grounds on which it is merciful to terminate it at once. The easy overdose, the lethal injection (successors to the hemlock used for this purpose by non-Hippocratic physicians in ancient Greece[8]), are what mercy demands when no other means will bring relief.

But, it may be objected, the cases I have mentioned to illustrate intolerable pain are classical ones; such cases are controllable now. Pain is a thing of the medical past, and euthanasia is no longer necessary, though it once may have been, to relieve pain. Given modern medical technology and recent remarkable advances in pain management, the sufferings of the mortally wounded and dying can be relieved by less dramatic means. For instance, many once-feared or painful diseases—tetanus, rabies, leprosy, tuberculosis—are now preventable or treatable. Improvements in battlefield first aid and transport of the wounded have been so great that the military coup de grace is now officially obsolete. We no longer speak of "mortal agony" and "death throes" as the probable last scenes of life. Particularly impressive are the huge advances under the hospice program in the amelioration of both the physical and emotional pain of terminal illness,[9] and our culture-wide fears of pain in terminal cancer are no longer justified: cancer pain, when it occurs, can now be controlled in virtually all cases. We can now end the pain without also ending the life.

This is a powerful objection, and one very frequently heard in medical circles. Nevertheless, it does not succeed. It is flatly incorrect to say that all pain, including pain in terminal illness, is or can be controlled. Some people still die in unspeakable agony. With superlative care, many kinds of pain can indeed be reduced in many patients, and adequate control of pain in terminal illness is often quite easy to achieve. Nevertheless, complete, universal, fully reliable pain control is a myth. Pain is not yet a "thing of the past," nor are many associated kinds of physical distress. Some kinds of conditions, such as difficulty in swallowing, are still difficult to relieve without introducing other discomforting limitations. Some kinds of pain are resistant to medication, as in elevated intracranial pressure or bone metastases and fractures. For some patients, narcotic drugs are dysphoric. Pain and distress may be increased by nausea, vomiting, itching, constipation, dry mouth, abscesses and decubitus ulcers that do not heal, weakness, breathing difficulties, and offensive

smells. Severe respiratory insufficiency may mean—as Joanne Lynn describes it—
"a singularly terrifying and agonizing final few hours."[10] Even a patient receiving
the most advanced and sympathetic medical attention may still experience episodes
of pain, perhaps alternating with unconsciousness, as his or her condition deterio-
rates and the physician attempts to adjust schedules and dosages of pain medication.
Many dying patients, including half of all terminal cancer patients, have little or no
pain,[11] but there are still cases in which pain management is difficult and erratic.
Finally, there are cases in which pain control is theoretically possible but for various
extraneous reasons does not occur. Some deaths take place in remote locations
where there are no pain-relieving resources. Some patients are unable to communicate the nature or extent of their pain. And some institutions and institutional
personnel who have the capacity to control pain do not do so, whether from inatten-
tion, malevolence, fears of addiction, or divergent priorities in resources.

In all these cases, of course, the patient can be sedated into unconsciousness; this
does indeed end the pain. But in respect of the patient's experience, this is tantamount to causing death: the patient has no further conscious experience and thus can
achieve no goods, experience no significant communication, satisfy no goals. Furthermore, adequate sedation, by depressing respiratory function, may hasten death.
Thus, although it is always technically possible to achieve relief from pain, at least
when the appropriate resources are available, the price may be functionally and
practically equivalent, at least from the patient's point of view, to death. And this, of
course, is just what the issue of euthanasia is about.

Of course, to see what the issue is about is not yet to reach its resolution, or to
explain why attitudes about this issue are so starkly divergent. Rather, we must
examine the logic of the argument for euthanasia and observe in particular how the
principle of mercy functions in the overall case. The canon "One ought to act to end
suffering," the second of the abstract duties generated by the principle of mercy, can
be traced to the more general principle of beneficence. But its application in a given
case also involves a minor premise that is ostensive in character: it points to an
alleged case of suffering. This person is suffering, the applied argument from mercy
holds, in a way that lays claim on us for help in relieving that pain.

It may be difficult to appreciate the force of this argument if its character is not
adequately recognized. By asserting the abstract duty of mercy and pointing to
specific occasions of pain, the argument generates the conclusion that we ought not
let these cases of pain occur: not only ought we to prevent them from occurring if we
can, but also we ought to bring them to an end if they do. In practice, most
arguments for euthanasia on grounds of mercy are pursued by the graphic evocation
of cases: the tortures suffered by victims of awful diseases.

But this argument strategy is problematic. The evocation of cases may be very
powerful, but it is also subject to a certain unreliability. After all, pain is, in general,
not well remembered by those not currently suffering it, and though bystanders may
be capable of very great sympathy, no person can actually feel another's pain.
Suffering that does not involve pain may be even harder for the bystander to assess.
Conversely, however, bystanders sometimes seem to suffer more than the patient:
pain, particularly in those for whom one has strong emotional attachments, is noto-
riously difficult to watch. Furthermore, sensitivity on the part of others to pain and

suffering is very much subject to individual differences in experience with pain, beliefs concerning the purpose of suffering and pain, fears about pain, and physical sensitivity to painful stimuli. Yet there is no objective way to establish how seriously the ostensive premise of the argument from mercy should be taken in any specific case, or how one should respond. Clearly, such a premise can be taken too seriously—so that concern for another's pain or suffering outweighs all other considerations—or one can be far too cavalier about the facts. To break a promise to a patient—say, not to intubate him—because you perceive that he is in pain may be to overreact to his suffering. However, it is morally repugnant to stand by and watch another person suffer when one could prevent it; it is a moral failing, too, to be insensitive, when there is no overriding reason for doing so, to the fact that another person is in pain.

The principle of mercy holds that suffering ought to be relieved—unless, among other provisos, the suffering itself will give rise to some overriding benefit or unless the attainment of some benefit would be precluded by relieving the pain. But it might be argued that life itself is a benefit, always an overriding one. Certainly life is usually a benefit, one that we prize. But unless we accept certain metaphysical assumptions, such as "life is a gift from God," we must recognize that life is a benefit because of the experiences and interests associated with it. For the most part, we prize these, but when they are unrelievedly negative, life is not a benefit after all. Philippa Foot treats this as a conceptual point: "Ordinary human lives, even very hard lives, contain a minimum of basic goods, but when these are absent the idea of life is no longer linked to that of good."[12] Such basic goods, she explains, include not being forced to work far beyond one's capacity; having the support of a family or community; being able to more or less satisfy one's hunger; having hopes for the future; and being able to lie down to rest at night. When these goods are missing, she asserts, the connection between *life* and *good* is broken, and we cannot count it as a benefit to the person whose life it is that his or her life is preserved.

These basic goods may all be severely compromised or entirely absent in the severely ill or dying patient. He or she may be isolated from family or community, perhaps by virtue of institutionalization or for various other reasons; he or she may be unable to eat, to have hopes for the future, or even to sleep undisturbed at night. Yet even for someone lacking all of what Foot considers to be basic goods, the experiences associated with life may not be unrelievedly negative. We must be very cautious in asserting of someone, even someone in the most abysmal-seeming conditions of the severely ill or dying, that life is no longer a benefit, since the way in which particular experiences, interests, and "basic goods" are valued may vary widely from one person to the next. Whether a given set of experiences constitutes a life that is a benefit to the person whose life it is, is not a matter for *objective* determination, though there may be very good external clues to the way in which that person is in fact valuing them; it is, in the end, very much a function of subjective preference and choice. For some persons, life may be of value even in the grimmest conditions, for others, not. The crucial point is this: when a suffering person is conscious enough to have any experience at all, whether that experience counts as a benefit overriding the suffering or not is relative to that person and can be decided ultimately only by him or her.[13]

If this is so, then we can no longer assume that the cases in which euthanasia is indicated on grounds of mercy are infrequent or rare. It is true that contemporary pain-management techniques do make possible the control of pain to a considerable degree. But unless pain and discomforting symptoms are eliminated altogether without loss of function, the underlying problem for the principle of mercy remains: how does *this* patient value life, how does he or she weigh death against pain? We are accustomed to assume that only patients suffering extreme, irremediable pain could be candidates for euthanasia at all and do not consider whether some patients might choose death in preference to comparatively moderate chronic pain, even when the condition is not a terminal one. Of course, a patient's perceptions of pain are extremely subject to stress, anxiety, fear, exhaustion, and other factors, but even though these perceptions may vary, the underlying weighing still demands respect. This is not just a matter of differing sensitivities to pain, but of differing values as well: for some patients, severe pain may be accepted with resignation or even pious joy, whereas for others mild or moderate discomfort is simply not worth enduring. Yet, without appeal to religious beliefs about the spiritual value of suffering, we have no objective way to determine how much pain a person *ought* to stand. Consequently, we cannot assume that euthanasia is justified, if at all, in only the most severe cases. Thus, the issue of euthanasia looms larger, rather than smaller, in the contemporary medical world.

That we cannot objectively determine whether life is a benefit to a person or whether pain outweighs its value might seem to undermine all possibility of appeal to the principle of mercy. But I think it does not. Rather, it shows simply that the issue is more complex, and that we must recognize that the principle of mercy itself demands recognition of a second fundamental principle relevant in euthanasia cases: the principle of autonomy. If the sufferer is the best judge of the relative values of that suffering and other benefits to him- or herself, then his or her own choices in the matter of mercy ought to be respected. To impose ''mercy'' on someone who insists that despite his or her suffering life is still valuable to him or her would hardly be mercy; to withhold mercy from someone who pleads for it, on the basis that his or her life could still be worthwhile for him or her, is insensitive and cruel. Thus, the principle of mercy is conceptually tied to that of autonomy, at least insofar as what guarantees the best application of the principle—and hence, what guarantees the proper response to the ostensive premise in the argument from mercy—is respect for the patient's own wishes concerning the relief of his or her suffering or pain.

To this issue we now turn.

The Case for Euthanasia, Part II: Autonomy

The second principle supporting euthanasia is that of (patient) autonomy: *one ought to respect a competent person's choices, where one can do so without undue costs to oneself, where doing so will not violate other moral obligations, and where these choices do not threaten harm to other persons or parties.* This principle of autonomy, though limited by these provisos, grounds a person's right to have his or her own choices respected in determining the course of medical treatment, including those relevant to euthanasia: whether the patient wishes treatment that will extend life, though perhaps also suffering, or whether he or she wants the suffering relieved, either by being killed or by being allowed to die. It would of course also require respect for the choices of the person whose condition is chronic but not terminal, the person who is disabled though not dying, and the person not yet suffering at all, but facing senility or old age. Indeed, the principle of autonomy would require respect for self-determination in the matter of life and death in any condition at all, provided that the choice is freely and rationally made and does not harm others or violate other moral rules. Thus, the principle of autonomy would protect a much wider range of life-and-death acts than those we call euthanasia, as well as those performed for reasons of mercy.

Support for patient autonomy in matters of life and death is partially reflected in U.S. law, in which a patient's right to passive voluntary euthanasia (though it is not called by this name) is established in a long series of cases. In 1914, in the case *Schloendorff v. New York Hospital*, [14] Justice Cardozo asserted that "every human being of adult years and sound mind has a right to determine what shall be done with his own body" and held that the plaintiff, who had been treated against his will, had the right to refuse treatment; more recent cases, including *Yetter*, [15] *Perlmutter*, [16] and *Bartling*, [17] establish that the competent adult has the right to refuse medical treatment, on religious or personal grounds, even if it means he or she will die. (Exceptions include some persons with dependents and persons who suffer from communicable diseases that pose a risk to the public at large.) Furthermore, the patient has the right to refuse a component of a course of treatment, even though he or she consents to others; this is established in the Jehovah's Witnesses cases in which patients refused blood transfusions but accepted surgery and other care. In many states, the law also recognizes passive voluntary euthanasia of the no longer competent adult who has signed a refusal-of-treatment document while still competent; such documents, called "natural death directives" or living wills, protect the physician from legal action for failure to treat if he or she follows the patient's antecedent request to be allowed to die. Additionally, the durable power of attorney permits a person to designate a relative, friend, or other person to make treatment decisions on his or her behalf after he or she is no longer competent; these may include decisions to refuse life-sustaining treatment. Many hospitals have adopted policies permitting the writing of orders not to resuscitate, or "no-code" orders, which stipulate that no attempt is to be made to revive a patient following a cardiorespiratory arrest. These policies typically are stated to require that such orders be issued only with the concurrence of the patient, if competent, or the patient's family or legal guardian. In theory, at least, living wills, no-code orders, durable powers of attorney, and similar devices are designed to protect the patient's voluntary choice to refuse life-prolonging treatment.

These legal mechanisms for refusal of treatment all protect individual autonomy in matters of euthanasia: the right to choose to live or to die. But it is crucial to see that they all protect only passive euthanasia, not any more active form. The Natural Death Act of California, like similar legislation in other states, expressly states that "nothing in this [Act] shall be construed to condone, authorize, or approve mercy killing."[18] Likewise, the living will directs only the withholding or cessation of treatment, in the absence of which the patient will die.[19] A durable power of attorney permits the same choices on behalf of the patient by a designated second party. These legal mechanisms are sometimes said to protect the "right to die," but it is important to see that this is only the right to be *allowed* to die, not to be helped to die or to have death actively brought about. However, we have already seen that allowing to die is sometimes less merciful than direct, humane killing: the principle of mercy demands the right to be killed, as well as to be allowed to die. Thus, the protections offered by the legal mechanisms now available may be seen as truncated conclusions from the principle of patient autonomy that supports them; this principle should protect not only the patient's choice of refusal of treatment but also a choice of a more active means of death.

It is often objected that autonomy in euthanasia choices should not be recognized in practice, whether or not it is accepted in principle, because such choices are often erroneously made. One version of this argument points to physician error. Physicians make mistakes, it holds, and since medicine in any case is not a rigorous science, predictions of oncoming, painful death with no possibility of cure are never wholly reliable. People diagnosed as dying rapidly of inexorable cancers have survived, cancer-free, for dozens of years; people in cardiac failure or long-term irreversible coma have revived and regained full health. Although some of this can be attributed simply to physician error, we must also guard against the more pernicious phenomenon of the "hanging of crepe," in which the physician (usually not intentionally) delivers a prognosis dimmer than is actually warranted by the facts. If the patient succumbs, the physician cannot be blamed, since that is what was predicted; but if the patient survives, the physician is credited with the cure.[20] Other factors interfering with the accuracy of a diagnosis or prognosis include impatience on the part of a physician with a patient who is not doing well, difficulties in accurately estimating future complications, ignorance of a treatment or cure that is about to be discovered or is on the way, and a host of additional factors arising when the physician is emotionally involved, inexperienced, uninformed, or incompetent.[21]

A second argument pointing to the possibility of erroneous choice on the part of the patient asserts the very great likelihood of impairment of the patient's mental processes when seriously ill. Impairing factors include depression, anxiety, pain, fear, intimidation by authoritarian physicians or institutions, and drugs used in medical treatment that affect mental status. Perhaps a person in good health would be capable of calm, objective judgments even in such serious matters as euthanasia, so this view holds, but the person as patient is not. Depression, extremely common in terminal illness, is a particular culprit: it tends to narrow one's view of the possibilities still open; it may make recovery look impossible, it may screen off the possibilities, even without recovery, of significant human relationships and important human experience in the time that is left.[22] A choice of euthanasia in terminal illness, this view holds, probably reflects largely the gloominess of the depression, not the gravity of the underlying disease or any genuine intention to die.

If this is so, ought not the euthanasia request of a patient be ignored for his or her own sake? According to a limited paternalist view (sometimes called "soft" or "weak" paternalism), intervention in a person's choices for his or her own sake is justified if the person's thinking is impaired. Under this principle, not every euthanasia request should be honored; such requests should be construed, rather, as pleas for more sensitive physical and emotional care.

It is no doubt true that many requests to die are pleas for better care or improved conditions of life. But this still does not establish that all euthanasia requests should be ignored, because the principle of paternalism licenses intervention in a person's choices just *for his or her own good*. Sometimes the choice of euthanasia, though made in an impaired, irrational way, may seem to serve the person's own good better than remaining alive. Thus, since the paternalist, in intervening, must act for the sake of the person in whose liberty he or she interferes, the paternalist must take into account not only the costs for the person of failing to interfere with a euthanasia decision when euthanasia was not warranted (the cost is death, when death was not in this person's interests) but also the costs for that person of interfering in a decision that was warranted (the cost is continuing life—and continuing suffering—when death would have been the better choice).[23] The likelihood of these two undesirable outcomes must then be weighed. To claim that "there's always hope" or to insist that "the diagnosis could be wrong" in a morally responsible way, one must weigh not only the cost of unnecessary death to the patient but also the costs to the patient of dying in agony if the diagnosis is right and the cure does not materialize. But cases in which the diagnosis is right and the cure does not materialize are, unfortunately, much more frequent than cases in which the cure arrives or the diagnosis is wrong. The "there's always hope" argument, used to dissuade a person from choosing euthanasia, is morally irresponsible unless there is some quite good reason to think there actually *is* hope. Of course, the "diagnosis could be wrong" argument against euthanasia is a good one in areas or specialties in which diagnoses are frequently inaccurate (the chief of one neurology service admitted that on initial diagnoses "we get it right about 50 percent of the time"), or where there is a systematic bias in favor of unduly grim prognoses—but it is not a good argument against euthanasia in general. Similarly, "a miracle cure may be developed tomorrow" is also almost always irresponsible. The paternalist who attempts to interfere with a patient's choice of euthanasia must weigh the enormous suffering of those to whom unrealistic hopes are held out against the benefits to those very few whose lives are saved in this way.

As with limited paternalism, extended "strong" or "hard" paternalism—permitting intervention not merely to counteract impairment but also to avoid great harm—provides a special case when applied to euthanasia situations. The hard paternalist may be tempted to argue that because death is the greatest of harms, euthanasia choices must always be thwarted. But the initial premise of this argument is precisely what is at issue in the euthanasia dispute itself, as we've seen: is death the worst of harms that can befall a person, or is unrelieved, hopeless suffering a still worse harm? The principle of mercy obliges us to relieve suffering when it does not serve some overriding good; but the principle itself cannot tell us whether sheer existence—life—is an overriding good. In the absence of an objectively valid answer, we must appeal to the individual's own preferences and values. Which is the greater evil—death or pain? Some persons may adopt religious answers to this question, others may devise their own; but the answer always is tied to the person whose life it is, and cannot be supplied in any objective way. Hence, unless he or she can discover what the suffering person's preferences and values are, the hard paternalist cannot determine whether intervening to prolong life or to terminate it will count as acting for that person's sake.

Of course, there are limits to such a claim. When there is no evidence of suffering or pain, mental or physical, and no evidence of factors like depression, psychoactive drugs, or affect-altering disease that might impair cognitive functioning, an external observer usually can accurately determine whether life is a benefit: unless the person has an overriding commitment to a principle or cause that requires sacrifice of that life, life *is* a benefit to him or her. (But such a person, of course, is probably not a patient.) Conversely, when there is every evidence of pain and little or no evidence of factors that might outweigh the pain, such as cognitive capacities that might give rise to other valuable experience, then an external observer generally can also accurately determine the value of this person's life: it is a disbenefit, a burden, to him or her. (Given pain and complete cognitive incapacity, such a person is almost always a patient.) It is when both pain and cognitive capacities are found that the person-relative character of the value of life becomes most apparent, and most demanding of respect.

Thus, if we view the spectrum of persons from fully healthy through severely ill to decerebrate or brain dead, we may assert that the principle of autonomy operates most strongly at the middle of this range. The more severe a person's pain and suffering, when his or her condition is not so diminished as to preclude cognitive capacities altogether, the stronger the respect we must accord his or her own view of whether life is a benefit or not. At both ends of the scale, however, paternalistic considerations come into play: if the person is healthy and without pain, we will interfere to keep him or her alive (preventing, for instance, suicide attempts); if his or her life means *only* pain, we act for the person's sake by causing him or her to die (as we should for certain severely defective neonates who cannot survive, but are in continuous pain). But when the patient retains cognitive capacities, the greater is his or her suffering, and the more his or her choices concerning it deserve our respect. When the choice that is faced is death or pain, it is the patient who must choose which is worse.

We saw earlier that in euthanasia issues the principle of mercy is conceptually tied to the principle of autonomy, at least for its exercise; we now see that the principle of autonomy is dependent on the principle of mercy in certain sorts of cases. It is *not* dependent in this way, however, in those cases most likely to generate euthanasia requests. That someone voluntarily and knowingly requests release from what he or she experiences as misery is sufficient, other things being equal, for the request to be honored; although this request is rooted in the patient's desire for mercy, we cannot insist on independent, objective evidence that mercy would in fact be served, or that death is better than pain. We can demand such evidence to protect a perfectly healthy person, and we can summon it to end the sufferings of someone who can no longer choose; but we cannot demand it or use it for the seriously ill person in pain. To claim that an incessantly pain-racked but conscious person cannot make a rational choice in matters of life and death is to misconstrue the point: he or she, better than anyone else, can make such a choice, based on intimate acquaintance with pain and his or her own beliefs and fears about death. If the patient wishes to live, despite such suffering, he or she must be allowed to do so; or the patient must be granted help if he or she wishes to die.

But this introduces a further problem. The principle of autonomy, when there are no countervailing considerations on paternalistic grounds or on grounds of harm to others, supports the practice of voluntary euthanasia and, in fact, any form of rational, voluntary suicide. We already recognize a patient's right to refuse any or all medical treatment and hence correlative duties of noninterference on the part of the physician to refrain from treating the patient against his or her will. But does the patient's right of self-determination also give rise to any positive obligation on the part of the physician or other bystander to actively produce death? Pope John Paul II asserts that "no one may ask to be killed";[24] Peter Williams argues that a person does not have a right to be killed even though to kill him might be humane.[25] But I think that both the Pope and Williams are wrong. Although we usually recognize only that the principle of autonomy generates rights to noninterference, in some circumstances a right of self-determination does generate claims to assistance or to the provision of goods.

We typically acknowledge this in cases of handicap or disability. For instance, the right of a person to seek an education ordinarily generates on the part of others only an obligation not to interfere with his or her attendance at the university, provided the person meets its standards; but the same right on the part of a person with a severe physical handicap may generate an obligation on the part of others to provide transportation, assist in acquiring textbooks, or provide interpretive services. The infant, incapable of earning or acquiring its own nourishment, has a right to be fed. There is a good deal of philosophic dispute about such claims, and public policies vary from one administration and court to the next. But if, in a situation of handicap or disability, a right to self-determination can generate claim rights (rights to be aided) as well as noninterference rights, the consequences for euthanasia practices are far-reaching indeed. Some singularly sympathetic cases—like that of Elizabeth Bouvier, who is almost completely paralyzed by cerebral palsy—have brought this issue to public attention. But notice that in euthanasia situations, *most* persons are handicapped with respect to producing for themselves an easy, "good," merciful death. The handicaps are occasionally physical, but most often involve lack of knowledge of how to bring this about and lack of access to means for so doing. If a patient chooses to refuse treatment and so die, he or she still may not know what components of the treatment to refuse in order to produce an easy rather than painful death; if the person chooses death by active means, he or she may not know what drugs or other methods would be appropriate, in what dosages, and in any case he or she may be unable to obtain them. Yet full autonomy is not achieved until one can both choose and act upon one's choices. It is here, in these cases of "handicap" that afflict many or most patients, that rights to self-determination may generate obligations on the part of physicians (provided, perhaps, that they do not have principled objections to participation in such activities themselves[26]). The physician's obligation is not only to respect the patient's choices but also to make it possible for the patient to act upon those choices. This means supplying the knowledge and equipment to enable the person to stay alive, if he or she so chooses; this is an obligation physicians now recognize. But it may also mean providing the knowledge, equipment, and help to enable the patient to die, if that is his or her choice; this is the other part of the physician's obligation, not yet recognized by the medical profession or the law in the United States.[27]

This is not to say that any doctor should be forced to kill any person who asks that: other contravening considerations—particularly that of ascertaining that the request is autonomous and not the product of coerced or irrational choice, and that of controlling abuses by unscrupulous physicians, relatives, or patients—would quickly override. Nor would the physician have an obligation to assist in "euthanasia" for someone not severely ill. But when the physician is sufficiently familiar with the patient to know the seriousness of the condition and the earnestness of the patient's request, when the patient is sufficiently helpless, and when there are no adequate objections on grounds of personal scruples or social welfare, then the principle of autonomy—like the principle of mercy—imposes on the physician the obligation to help the patient in achieving an easy, painless death.

The Case for Euthanasia, Part III: Justice

Although the term euthanasia originates from Greek roots meaning "good death," especially the avoidance of suffering, in recent years use of the term has been extended to cover cases in which the patient is neither suffering nor capable of choosing to die. Ruth Russell, for instance, includes among cases of euthanasia the ending of "a meaningless existence."[28] For Tom Beauchamp and Arnold Davidson, euthanasia can be the termination of an irreversibly comatose state.[29] Termination of the lives of the brain dead, the permanently comatose, and those who are, as Paul Ramsey puts it, "irretrievably inaccessible to human care"[30] is justified, it is argued, under the principle of justice: euthanasia permits fairer distribution of medical resources in a society that lacks sufficient resources to provide maximum care for all. Once this principle is invoked, however, it may seem that it also applies in cases in which the patient is still competent: to permit earlier, easier dying will be favored not only on grounds of mercy and autonomy but on grounds of justice as well.

Drawing on the principle of mercy advanced earlier, we may assert that each person, by virtue of his or her medical illness, injury, disability, or other medical abnormality that causes pain or suffering, has a claim on whatever medical resources might be effective in the full treatment of his or her condition: because we have an obligation (subject to the provisos mentioned previously) to relieve the person's suffering, he or she has a correlative claim (subject to corresponding provisos) to whatever medical treatment can be used. But since there are not enough resources to supply full treatment for every condition for every person, and since the resources typically cannot be subdivided in a way that makes equal apportionment of them possible (half an operation will do you no good), full treatment can be devoted only to some conditions, or only to some persons. In a scarcity situation, not all competing claims can be satisfied, and a principle of distributive justice must be invoked to adjudicate among them.

Various principles can be proposed for allocating medical resources: to those in greatest medical need, to those for whom restoration of function would be most complete; to those who can pay; to those whose societal contributions are or have been greatest; to those who have been most deprived of medical care in the past; to those whose conditions are not self-induced (this might rule out people suffering from smokers' diseases, conditions exacerbated by obesity, suicide attempts, and perhaps venereal diseases and high-risk sports injuries); or to those who are the winners in a coin toss, lottery, or other system of random selection. Alternatively, treatment could be allocated on the basis of the medical condition involved: to end-stage kidney patients, for instance, but not to those with deteriorative heart disease. But, unless we expand the size of the resources pool, treatment will still be denied to some, *whatever* distributive principle is adopted. Hence, whatever the principle (except perhaps one that allocates all available resources simply to staving off death for the last few minutes in every medical condition), some of those denied treatment will die sooner than otherwise would be the case. But this, it can be argued, would be unjust, since it would impose earlier death on some persons on the basis of characteristics that are not legitimate grounds for death—ability to pay, and so on. Rather, it is often argued, if treatment is to be denied to some people with the result that they will die, it is better to deny it just to those people who are (loosely speaking) medically unsalvageable and will die soon anyway: the terminally ill, the extremely aged, and the seriously defective neonate. The practices of euthanasia in accord with this principle—which can be called the salvageability principle—is justified, this argument then concludes, by the demands of justice in a scarcity situation.

Of course, to deny treatment to a dying patient on grounds of justice cannot properly be called euthanasia in the traditional sense, since it is not done for the sake of the patient or to provide a "good death." A congressional decision not to fund artificial heart research or not to provide Medicaid/Medicare payments for heart transplants can hardly be called euthanasia for those heart patients who will die. However, as we saw at the outset of this section, policies involving withholding treatment are frequently called euthanasia when practiced on the permanently comatose, the brain dead, the profoundly retarded, or others in nonsapient states. Despite the abuse of the term under the Nazi regime, our linguistic usage is again undergoing rapid change, and it is apparent that we are coming to use the term euthanasia not just for pain-sparing deaths but for resource-conserving deaths as well. It is in this newer sense that we can consider whether justice requires the practice of euthanasia in certain kinds of scarcity situations.

The argument from justice, though not always put forward in a coherent, comprehensive way, is often initiated with a recitation of facts. The hospital bill [in 1985] for a 500-gram newborn with serious deficits, it is said, may run somewhere between $60,000 and $80,000, or even more than $100,000; this does not by any means guarantee that the infant will survive or live a normal life. Ths cost of a coronary bypass, a procedure frequently employed even when it does not extend life expectancy (though it greatly increases the quality of life), is somewhere around $30,000. The bill for a series of bone marrow transplants may run to $80,000, even though the transplants may not succeed in staving off death. According to a study published late in 1981, the average intensive care unit bill (total hospital charges, plus ancillary charges) was $7,112—for patients who survived.[31] But for patients who died, the bill was more than double, a staggering $15,874. A vast proportion of medical costs are incurred during the final year of life (this includes unsalvageable neonates as well as adults), most of it in the last few weeks or days. Justice, under the distributive principle articulated previously, demands that the dying be allowed to die, and these resources be given instead to other, salvageable competitors for full health care.

This is not to suggest that the dying should be denied palliative and comfort care: indeed, if their claims to therapeutic treatment diminish, the principle of mercy demands that their claims to palliative care increase. Nor is it to suggest that the dying "do not deserve" medical care that could prolong their lives. *All* parties in the distribution have prima facie claims to care, under the principle of justice, but the claims of the dying are weakest.

This argument from justice is usually employed only to justify the denial of treatment, that is, to justify passive euthanasia, but similar considerations also favor active euthanasia. Passive euthanasia is often practiced upon unsalvageable patients by withholding treatment if a medical crisis occurs: for instance, no-code orders are issued, or pneumonias are not treated, or electrolyte imbalances not corrected if they occur. If justice demands that, despite the prima facie claims of these patients, the resources allocated to their care are better assigned somewhere else, then we must notice that *passive* euthanasia does not provide the most just redistribution of these resources. To "allow" the patient to die may still involve enormous expenditures of money, scarce supplies, or caregiver time. This is most evident in cases of "irretrievably inaccessible" patients, for whom no considerations of mercy or autonomy override the demands of justice in weighing claims. The cost [in 1985] of maintaining a coma patient in a nursing home without heroic treatment is somewhere around $15,000 a year; the cost for a profoundly retarded resident of a state institution is more than $20,000. Whole-brain dead patients may survive on life supports in hospital settings from several hours to a few days or more; upper-brain dead patients may live for years. The total cost of maintaining a permanently comatose woman, who was injured in a riding accident in 1956 at age twenty-seven and died eighteen years later, has been estimated at just over $6,000,000; this care provided her with not a single moment of conscious life.[32] The record survival for a coma patient is 37 years and 111 days.[33] The argument from justice demands that these patients, since their claims for care are so weak as to have virtually no force at all, be killed, not simply allowed to die.

Objection to the Argument from Justice: The Slippery Slope

But if justice, under the salvageability principle considered here, licenses the killing of permanently comatose patients, will it not also license the killing of still-conscious, still-competent dying patients, perhaps still salvageable, close or not so close to death? What extensions of the scope of this principle might be made, should resources become still more scarce? These concerns introduce the "wedge" or "slippery slope" argument, which holds that although some acts of euthanasia may be morally permissible (say, on grounds of mercy or autonomy), to allow them to occur will set a logical precedent for, or will causally result in, consequences that are morally repugnant.[34] Just as Hitler's 1938 "euthanasia" program for mentally defective, senile, and terminally ill Aryans paved the way for the establishment of the extermination camps several years later, it is argued, so permissive euthanasia policies invite irreversible descent down that slippery slope that leads to mass murder. Indeed, to permit even the most humane euthanasia may do more than set a precedent: by accustoming doctors to ending life, by supplying death technology, by changing the expectations of family members or other guardians of those who become candidates for death, and by changing the expectations of patients themselves, the practice of euthanasia even in humane cases may lead to moral holocaust.

As it is usually posed, the form of the argument that points to the Nazi experience does not succeed: the forces that brought the mass extermination camps into being were not *caused* by the earlier euthanasia program, and, other things being equal, the extermination camps for Jews would no doubt have been established had there been no euthanasia program at all. To argue that permitting euthanasia now will lead to death camps like Hitler's is to overlook the many other political, social, and psychological factors of the Nazi period. Yet the wedge argument cannot be simply discarded; the factors operating to favor the slide from morally warranted euthanasia to murder are probably much stronger than we realize. They are best seen, I think, as misunderstandings or corruptions of the very principles that favor euthanasia: mercy, autonomy, and perhaps most prominently, justice.

A contemporary version of the wedge argument holds that to permit euthanasia at all—including cases justified on grounds of mercy, autonomy, or justice—will in the presence of strong financial incentives lead to circumstances in which people are killed who are not suffering or who do not wish to die. Furthermore, to permit some doctors to allow their patients to die or to kill them would invite cavalier attitudes concerning the lives of the patients and, in addition to financial incentives, ordinary greed, insensitivity, hastiness, and self-interest, would cause some doctors to let their patients die—or kill them—when there was no moral warrant for doing so.[35] Doctors treating difficult or unresponding patients would find an easy way out. Medical blunders could be more easily covered up, and doctors might use euthanasia as a way of avoiding criticism in cases that were medically difficult to treat. Particularly important, perhaps, are societal and political pressures, most evident in cost-containment policies, to which doctors might respond. After all, to permit earlier, less expensive death would ease the enormous pressure on third-party insurers, hospitals, and the Medicaid/Medicare system: euthanasia is less expensive than continuing medical care. The diagnosis-related group reimbursement system would particularly favor this since a hospital profits most from the patient who remains hospitalized for the shortest amount of time, but loses money on the one who remains longer than what is average for the DRG. Although passive euthanasia is cheaper than continuing life-prolonging treatment, active euthanasia is cheaper still: killing is the least expensive, most resource-conserving treatment of intractable disease.

Is there any reason to think such practices would actually occur? The reasons are closer to hand than one might imagine. Rather than predicting the future, we need simply look to our present practices for evidence that violations of the moral limits to euthanasia can occur. It is tempting to reply to a wedge argument against any social practice that we will always be able to draw a moral line when the time comes, but the clear evidence in the case of euthanasia is that we are not managing to do so now.

First, contemporary euthanasia practices sometimes involve violations of the principle of mercy. These violations are of two forms, neither conspicuous because neither involves evident physical cruelty. Nevertheless, both are cases of euthanasia that the principle of mercy does not endorse. First, there are cases in which the rhetoric of euthanasia, with its concept of painless, easy death, is used though considerations of mercy cannot possibly apply: these are the cases of the permanently comatose or brain dead. Since these persons do not suffer, euthanasia as the granting of mercy cannot be practiced upon them, and we mislead ourselves if we claim that they are "better off" dead. Second, there are cases in which the principle of mercy is violated when more than enough relief is given to those who do suffer. The principle of mercy demands euthanasia *only* when no other means of relieving pain will suffice. Yet we fail to acknowledge that the continuous, very heavy use of narcotizing drugs can be functionally equivalent to mercy killing itself: when used in a sustained way, without drug-free, conscious intervals or careful titration against alertness, such therapy effectively ends the patient's sentient life: his or her existence as a person ends when the drugging begins.[36] Of course, it may sometimes be difficult to obtain adequate and effective narcotics; nevertheless, because we do not recognize such drugging as equivalent in some respects to *active* euthanasia, we may be incautious and hasty in its use.

Contemporary euthanasia practices sometimes also involve violations of the principle of autonomy. It is true that much euthanasia, both passive and active, occurs at the request or with the consent of the individual who dies; passive euthanasia practices are provided for in natural death legislation and the use of durable powers of attorney and living wills. But we are also beginning to see the widespread development of hospital policies concerning nonresuscitation, and more frequent, routine physician exercise of this practice. It may even be fair to speak of a widespread consensus that in certain cases, nonresuscitation is the appropriate response. Official policies require that the patient—if competent—or his or her legal guardian be consulted before nonresuscitation orders are written. But such directives are by no means always followed. In Salt Lake City recently (though the story is universal), a physician reminded the granddaughter of an alert, competent eighty-nine-year-old nursing home patient, "You can always have 'do not resuscitate' orders written into her record." ("Why don't you ask her if that's what she wants?" was the granddaughter's reply.) A cardiologist at a major university says, in contrast, that he would not make such a suggestion to the family—because he "wouldn't want to put them through that"; this physician writes no-code orders on his own, without consulting either patient or family. In some places, no-code orders are written in pencil, so that they can be erased from records if desired; or circumlocutions not intelligible to laypersons ("consult primary physician before initiating treatment") are used.

Most significant among our current euthanasia practices may be the violations of justice. The argument from justice, as discussed so far, favors permitting euthanasia on the grounds that denial of treatment is morally permissible in certain specific cases: those in which the claims of a dying individual to medical resources are overridden by the claims of others in medical need. However, we often see the use of distributive policies that deny treatment to some but do not involve either the weighing of claims between the dying and others or the assurance that resources conserved would in fact be redistributed in accord with justice. The congressional decisions concerning artificial and transplant heart care may be one kind of example; arbitrary age minimums and ceilings for transplants, pacemakers, and dialysis, when they are not medically appropriate, may be another. Yet distributive justice concerns the point at which a dying person's right to medical treatment is outweighed by the claims of others; and the salvageability principle considered here does not hold that dying deprives one altogether of rights to medical care. In a situation of dire scarcity, such as urgent organ transplants, denying a transplant to one person usually means granting a transplant to someone else; if without it each person would die, the distributive principle of salvageability considered here holds that the person more likely to survive and benefit from the procedure has the stronger claim. But many distributive policies do not involve this kind of direct weighing of claims or assurances of reallocation, and much denial of treatment is done simply for thrift. *Thrift,* however, is not the same as *justice in distribution.* To deny treatment to the dying to "conserve resources" or to "save money" is not to show that the claims of the dying are overridden by stronger claims on the part of someone else, or a group of persons, to whom such resources would in fact be redistributed; yet it is this point that is essential in preserving the principle of justice as applied to euthanasia.

In all these areas, then, there is evidence of "euthanasia" practices not justified by moral principle. Given these facts, the wedge argument and its objection to permitting euthanasia may loom larger. The wedge argument forecasts a slide down the slippery slope from morally permissible practices to impermissible ones; but even if we accept its model, there is no reason to assume that we are still at the top of this slope. Indeed, the evidence available suggests that we are already slipping. We already engage in "euthanasia" practices not justified on grounds of mercy, autonomy, or justice, and there is no reason to think that such abuses will not become still more widespread.

Nevertheless, I do not agree with the conclusion of the slippery slope argument: that because permissible euthanasia practices would lead (or are leading) to impermissible ones, we ought not allow them at all. We should not cease no-coding; mercy demands it. We should not restrict refusal of treatment or insist that all who can conceivably benefit be given as much treatment as possible; respect for autonomy requires that the patient be permitted to determine what is done to him or her. We should not resist legislative protections for passive euthanasia, like living wills and natural death laws, or oppose legislation permitting voluntary active euthanasia: justice, mercy, and autonomy all demand that euthanasia—both passive and active—be legally protected. Although the wedge argument is a serious one, prohibiting euthanasia is not the appropriate conclusion.

Most advocates of the wedge argument overlook a crucial feature of the structure of the argument itself. The wedge argument is teleological in character: it points to the bad consequence of permitting a morally acceptable type of action (call it A), namely, that a morally unacceptable type (B) occurs. But users of the wedge argument err in failing to recognize that B's occurrence is not the sole outcome of A; A and B are *distinct* actions, each with its own set of consequences. Thus, in deciding whether to permit A, one must reckon in the bad consequences of the occurrence of B, but must also reckon in the other, possibly good consequences of A. Or, if one is deciding to prohibit A, the reckoning will include the (good) effects of avoiding B, but must also include the other (bad) effects of not having A occur. The wedge argument against euthanasia usually takes the form of an appeal to the welfare or rights of those who would become victims of later, unjustified practices. Usually, however, when the conclusion is offered that euthanasia therefore ought not be permitted, no account is taken of the welfare or rights of those who are to be denied the benefits of this practice. Hence, even if the causal claims advanced in the wedge argument are true and we are not able to hold the line or avoid the slide, they still do not establish the conclusion. Rather, the argument sets up a conflict. Either we ignore the welfare and abridge the rights of persons for whom euthanasia would clearly be morally permissible in order to protect those who would be the victims of corrupt euthanasia practices, or we ignore the potential victims in order to extend mercy and respect for autonomy to those who are the current victims of euthanasia prohibitions.

Thus, this conflict itself reveals an issue of justice still more fundamental than the distributive problems with which I began. The wedge argument assumes, without adequate justification, that the rights of those who may become the victims of abuses of a practice outweigh the rights of those who become victims if a practice is prohibited to whose benefits they are morally entitled and urgently need.

To protect those who might wrongly be killed or allowed to die might seem a stronger obligation than to satisfy the wishes of those who desire release from pain, analogous perhaps to the principle in law that "better ten guilty men go free than one be unjustly convicted."[37] However, the situation is not in fact analogous and does not favor protecting those who might wrongly be killed. To let ten guilty men go free in the interests of protecting one innocent man is not to impose harm on the ten guilty men. But to require the person who chooses to die to stay alive in order to protect those who might unwillingly be killed sometime in the future is to impose an extreme harm—intolerable suffering—on that person, which he or she must bear for the sake of others. Furthermore, since, as I have argued, the question of which is worse, suffering or death, is person-relative, we have no independent, objective basis for protecting the class of persons who might be killed at the expense of those who would suffer intolerable pain; perhaps our protecting ought to be done the other way around. Thus, I return to the recurrent problem throughout this discussion: which is the worse of two evils, death or pain? Since there are no prior agreements or claims that are relevant here, justice requires that rights to avoid the worse of the two evils be honored first, before others come into play. This, however, may be an obligation that, because it is person-relative and hence resistant to policy construction, we do not know how to meet.

Justice and Realistic Desire

Is there a workable solution to the problem that euthanasia poses? Certainly we can make some progress by attending to the violations of principle we have discovered. First, we must improve the conditions of dying; mercy will not demand euthanasia, nor the autonomous person choose it, when the conditions of dying are humane. Cicely Saunders, the founder of St. Christopher's Hospice in England and an ardent opponent of euthanasia, is perfectly right when she says of euthanasia, "one should be working to see that it is not needed."[38] Second, we need to improve the quality of the mercy we extend by attending to the element of autonomy in it: we must learn to respond to suffering in a way that takes account of the patient's own wishes and tolerances for pain, so that we give neither too little relief nor too much. Third, we must broaden our respect of autonomy in matters of dying by recognizing that the patient may choose active as well as passive means of coming to die—or none at all. It is crucial that the dying person receive full information about the consequences of accepting treatment or refusing it, so that he or she can rationally choose the way of dying—or staying alive—most in accord with his or her own values.[39] After all, a "good death" must always be a death that counts as good *for the patient*. For some it is the least painful, for others it is the quickest, for others one that permits final communication with family, and for still others the one that can be delayed the longest possible time. In this most personal of matters, a person's choice deserves the greatest respect.

But attention to mercy and autonomy does not yet seem to solve the problem of justice: the problems of whose rights are to be honored, and who is to be denied care. I mentioned earlier that all the workable distributive principles we might adopt would have the effect of forcing death on some persons who do not want it—those who cannot pay, those who have made no societal contributions, etc. Even the most plausible of these principles—the salvageability principle—would force earlier death upon the already dying, some of whom may wish to die but some of whom, under their own conception of the relative disvalue of suffering and death, want to continue as long as they possibly can. Thus, I think that the salvageability principle too is in error. Rather, we should favor a distributive principle that would allocate medical resources to whose who *want* treatment, where "wanting" is interpreted as "realistic desire." This is to say, realistic desire ought to be considered both a necessary and a sufficient condition for providing treatment for those who are seriously ill.

To desire medical treatment in a realistic, reasonable, or rational way, the patient must not only actually have or be about to contract the condition for which treatment is proposed but also must understand the treatment's intended purposes, its possible side effects, the probability of success or failure, and the possible end condition to which the treatment would lead. For, say, an appendectomy, the patient must not only have appendicitis but also must understand at least roughly the nature of the procedure, what could go wrong, the approximate likelihood of success, and the end condition: relief of the acute pain in the abdomen, avoidance of death, and a small scar on the side. In most cases of acute appendicitis, an appendectomy will be the object of realistic desire. In a few cases, however, it is not, such as when the patient believes on religious grounds that the end condition of accepting medical treatment or a blood transfusion includes eventual damnation. Although religious cases are comparatively rare, there are many cases in which the principle of realistic desire would require substantial changes in our current distribution of medical care. Life-prolonging care given to the permanently comatose, decerebrate, profoundly brain damaged, and others who lack cognitive function is not, even in the case of antecedently executed directives, realistically desired, since such patients cannot want it, they are not entitled to life-prolonging care. Not even supportive care—such as feeding or routine hygiene—should be supplied, since this too cannot be realistically desired; patients in these extreme conditions should be allowed—or perhaps caused—to die.

Withholding care from permanently comatose patients may not seem morally problematic. But in a serious illness in which a cure cannot be guaranteed yet the patient remains competent, the problem becomes much more complex. Do patients with cancer of the larynx, for instance, *want* surgical treatment that, while providing a better-than-half chance of survival three years later, entails the permanent destruction of the normal voice? Most do, but, according to one study, at least 20 percent do not.[40] In such situations, the new distributive principle articulated here apportions treatment solely on the basis of a patient's desires, not on characteristics such as age or social worth. Most patients will receive appendectomies; four-fifths will have surgery on the larynx; permanently comatose patients will receive no care at all.

Would a distributive principle of realistic desire be effective in a scarcity situation? Although one's initial impression may be to the contrary, I believe that it would. It is crucial to remember that medical treatment is not like any ordinary consumer good; getting more of it does not entail that your advantages are increased. (Indeed, in an ideal lifetime, the amount of therapeutic medical treatment a person realistically wants is zero; this is the mark of the perfectly healthy life.) The treatments that are less likely to be realistically desired are, generally speaking, precisely those likely to occur at the end of life—the heroic, last-ditch, odds-against measures, undertaken because nothing else has worked. The chances are that the procedures will be painful, that they will introduce new limitations, and that they will not succeed. And the chance is also that these treatments will be extremely expensive. It is not possible to tell whether the savings in treatment costs under such a distributive policy would make it possible to provide full treatment for all who do want it, but there is no reason to *assume* that such savings would not: we need only recall the huge financial costs for nonsurvivors in an intensive care unit, for severely defective, unsalvageable neonates, or for permanently comatose patients in a nursing home or institution. A vast proportion of medical costs, as stated before, occurs in the last year of life. Most of this can be described as "needed" treatment. No doubt much of this is also "wanted" treatment, but much of it is not.

If use of the distributive principle of realistic desire should prove inadequate to solve the scarcity problem, then an additional distributive principle would need to be adopted to resolve conflicting claims among competitors who all realistically desire treatment: the salvageability principle, denying treatment to those who will die soon anyway, might then be brought into play. But those who will die soon may nevertheless want every moment of life they can possibly get, and it is unacceptable to adopt a distributive principle that has the effect of depriving some persons of wanted life before there is clear need to do so.

Of course, a distributive principle of realistic desire must have built into it paternalistic proxy procedures for providing medical care for incompetents of a variety of sorts, including infants and children, unconscious accident victims, the mentally ill, and the retarded. But I believe that these procedures should *not* include persons who are capable of realistic desire in the matter of terminal care but who have failed to consider and articulate their desires. Rather, it is becoming apparent that the individual has an obligation, increasingly evident as advances in medical technology both exacerbate the scarcity situation and offer heroic life-prolonging treatment that may not be desired, to stipulate in advance which modes of treatment he or she will accept and which he or she will decline, insofar as the patient's probable future can be foreseen. Only about one death in ten is wholly unexpected, and most result from prolonged, chronic illnesses.[41] Thus, most deaths can be predicted, within a fairly limited range of possibilities, before the event, and the course of the dying in certain general ways anticipated. What, most basically, the patient is obliged to do is indicate, as fully as possible, which he or she takes to be worse in situations that can be forseen: pain or death. From this basic choice the treatment alternatives appropriate to the patient's condition can be deduced. By failing to exercise this obligation, the individual may force others—his or her physician, family members, or the courts—to make what are often morally precarious euthanasia decisions for him or her, perhaps on the basis of self-interest, societal pressure, or distributive principles for which there is no moral warrant. Because the patient has rights to medical treatment that he or she realistically desires and because it is the corresponding obligation of others to distribute treatment in accord with these desires, it is in turn the obligation of the patient to make his or her desires known whenever it is possible to do so.

However, it is particularly important to notice that continuous sedation is *not* an option the patient may choose, nor is it a defensible general solution to the problem of euthanasia. The patient's autonomous requests must still conform to the demands of justice, particularly as specified for medical situations by the principle of realistic desire. It is true that continuous sedation may satisfy both the principles of mercy and autonomy, but because there is no ongoing experience or sentient end state to which the treatment leads, the patient cannot realistically desire the treatment that would maintain him or her. Of course, there may be many cases in which the patient's condition is potentially reversible or the sedation can be interrupted to permit further personal experience, and in these circumstances sedation may indeed be realistically preferred to either pain or death (given the difficulty of accurately predicting circumstances in which continuous sedation will be permanently required without any hope of intervening lucidity, such cases may be the rule rather than the exception); in these cases the patient retains his or her claim to care. There may also be certain special situations in which the needs of, say, family members or transplant recipients outweigh the claims of other patients competing for resources, so that justice will permit maintaining a patient in continuous sedation on the same basis as it might in rare cases permit maintaining a patient who is permanently comatose. But when such conditions do not obtain, even the patient who articulates his or her choices in advance is not entitled to request *permanent* sedation, since the principle of realistic desire prohibits him or her, like the proverbial dog in the manger, from laying claim to resources he or she cannot possibly enjoy. Nor may physicians turn to continuous sedation as a way of avoiding difficult moral dilemmas in terminal care (except, of course, in the frequent situations in which they think that their predictions may be wrong); they are bound to honor the choices of a patient made in accord with the principle of realistic desire, but this principle does not permit such a choice. At least in any scarcity situation, the patient must choose either death or periodically sentient life, though this may involve pain; he or she cannot morally choose to be maintained in a permanently sedated or unconscious state when that means depriving someone else of care.

Conclusion: Euthanasia and Suicide

It may be objected that requiring the patient to choose between death and life, insofar as the patient must antecedently consider treatment decisions that affect the circumstances and timing of his or her own demise, is equivalent to requiring the patient's consideration of suicide. In a sense, it is; but this is also the more general solution to the euthanasia problem. Although euthanasia is indeed warranted on grounds of mercy, autonomy, and justice, these principles can be more effectively and safely honored by permitting suicide, perhaps assisted by the physician who has care of the patient or a family member under the advice of the physicians,[42] and supplemented by nonvoluntary euthanasia *only* when the patient is permanently comatose or otherwise irretrievably inaccessible. Not only do practical reasons like avoiding greed and manipulation on the part of physicians or the institutions controlling them speak for preferring physician-assisted suicide to physician-initiated euthanasia, but there are conceptual reasons as well. The conditions that distinguish morally permissible euthanasia from impermissible murder all involve matters that the patient, not the physician, is in a privileged position to know. To extend mercy, the physician must know how the patient weighs suffering against death, and at what point *for the patient* death becomes the lesser of two evils. To respect the patient's autonomy, the physician must know what his or her preferences are, given the alternatives available, in the matter of dying. And to exercise justice, the physician must know what treatment the patient realistically desires. Perhaps the physician who is painstakingly careful in listening to an articulate and self-aware patient may discover these things, but he or she cannot have the patient's knowledge. Consequently, since the risk of misinterpretation is great and the possibility of manipulation or coercion high, the physician should not be the one to *initiate* the choice. Rather, he or she must be prepared to assist the patient who chooses death, just as he or she is prepared to assist the patient who chooses continuing life. In physician-assisted suicide, it is the person whose death is in question who is responsible for the death; he or she originates and chooses this course of action, rather than having death chosen for him or her. Of course, to permit suicide in these situations may seem to increase the risk of encouraging ill-considered suicide among emotionally disturbed or mentally ill persons, but here the physician serves as a check: in the role of assistant to the suicide, the physician will refuse to assist whenever in his or her professional perception the circumstances clearly do not warrant such an act (such as in cases in which there is neither pain nor approaching death, but not in those exhibiting one or both). This is by no means a foolproof policy; the physician will no doubt often influence the patient. But this intrusion is still a far cry from having the physician decide when or why euthanasia is appropriate and initiate the act.

Furthermore, physician-assisted suicide is less subject to the erection of policy requirements than are euthanasia practices. The choices of patients about whether and how to die will vary widely; but then, there is no reason why they should not. These choices are influenced by an enormous range of individual values, past experiences, and moral and religious beliefs. Euthanasia policies developed by physicians or medical institutions may overlook individual differences in patients' wishes by establishing routine, common procedures for dealing with terminal illness, and in this way invite the continuing slide down the slippery slope. We must be prepared to permit and perform mercy killing when the patient desires it and when there is no other way to avoid the sufferings of death. But we do not want doctors to assume the responsibility for such killings, or to appeal to standardized, court-approved procedures, made under economic constraints, for determining when such killings are appropriate. Rather, mercy killing must ideally always be mercy killing of the patient by him- or herself, in which the patient is entitled to the assistance of the physician he or she has chosen. When proxy procedures are required, we must be sure that they approximate as nearly as possible what the person's own decision would have been. It is crucial to exercise mercy; it is essential to respect autonomy, and though we must submit to the demands of justice, we can hope to do so at no one's expense. It is extremely important to avoid any further slide down the involuntary thrift-euthanasia slope. Recognition of physician-aided suicide, as distinguished from physician-directed euthanasia, comes closest to satisfying all of these moral demands.

After all, we must not forget that we already practice euthanasia on quite a wide scale, but we do not always practice it in a morally defensible way. We practice passive euthanasia by withholding and withdrawing treatment, and we practice active quasi-euthanasia by using sedation sufficient to terminate the personal existence of a human being. Some of this is in accord with the principles of mercy, autonomy, and justice, but much of it is not. What grows dimmer in contemporary practice is the sense that euthanasia, as "good death," must be good *for the person whose death it is;* we are losing any sense that mercy must play a major role or that the patient's choice is crucial in determining whether that death counts as good. Already we are beginning to count resource-conserving deaths under this term. Paul Ramsey remarks that "it is better if you do not know the Greek language or the root meaning of the word";[43]—but, of course, knowing these things permits us to see the shifts in our use of the term, shifts that are perhaps symptomatic of the slide already under way down the slippery slope. Our very language invites us to overlook distinctions that we ought to make. The concept of euthanasia has come to include letting patients die and killings that are not required by mercy, autonomy, or justice, but are simply the product of thrift in medical affairs. Yet at the same time our discomfort with this fact leads us to claim, at least officially, that we reject any practice of euthanasia at all, though of course this is not true. In this way, the increasing distortion of the term itself leads us to overlook a double moral fault: often, we practice "euthanasia" when we should not, and very often, we fail to practice euthanasia when we should.

Notes

I'd like to thank Arthur G. Lipman, Pharm. D., and Howard Wilcox, M.D., as well as my colleagues in philosophy, Bruce Landesman and Leslie Francis, for comments on earlier drafts of this chapter.

1. Perhaps the principle of (medical) mercy is stronger than this and asserts a duty to relieve the suffering of others even at some substantial cost to oneself, or in violation of others of these provisos. The quite weak form of the principle, as I have stated it here, requires, for instance, that one ought not stand idly by (all other things being equal) when one could easily help an injured person but does not require feats of physical or financial heroism or self-sacrifice. This is not to say that I think a stronger version of the duty to relieve suffering (as defended, for instance, by Susan James, "The Duty to Relieve Suffering," *Ethics* [October 1982] 93:4–21), could not be supported, but that the stronger version is not necessary for the case I am making here: a prima facie duty to participate in both passive and active euthanasia, at least in a more permissive legal climate, is entailed even by the very weak form of the principle of mercy.

Incidentally, although much of the medical literature distinguishes between pain and suffering, I have not chosen to do so here: it would raise difficult mind/body problems, and in any case the two are clearly intertwined. I grant, however, that the principle of (medical) mercy would meet still broader assent if phrased to require the relieving of physical pain alone.

2. It is important not to confuse the principle of (medical) mercy with a principle permitting or requiring judicial mercy. In judicial and political contexts, such as pardons or amnesties, the individual on whom penalties have been or are about to be imposed may have no claim to benevolent treatment, and the issue concerns whether mercy may or should be granted. Many authors treat judicial mercy as a work of individual supererogation, not a requirement or duty, and some suggest that it is morally forbidden: one ought not excuse a person guilty of a crime. However, we are concerned here not with judicial mercy, but rather with mercy as it arises primarily in medical contexts: injuries, illnesses, disabilities, degenerative processes, and genetic defect or disease. Unlike pain or suffering inflicted in judicial contexts, in the medical context these are not warranted by the past actions of the suffering individual, but are usually of natural or accidental origin and in most cases are beyond the individual's control: pain and suffering are something that happen to him or her, not something the patient has earned. The principle of medical mercy is usually taken to apply even in cases in which a medical condition is caused or exacerbated by the individual's voluntary behavior, as in smokers' diseases or injuries from attempted suicide. It is consistent to hold that mercy is supererogatory (or perhaps morally forbidden) in judicial or political contexts, but also that it is required in medical ones.

3. Edmund D. Pellegrino, M.D., "The Clinical Ethics of Pain Management in the Terminally Ill," *Hospital Formulary* 17 (November 1982): 1495–96; and Marcia Angell, "The Quality of Mercy," *New England Journal of Medicine* 306 (January 1982): 98–99.

4. For instance, I take it to be a moral duty, and not merely a nice thing to do, to help a child remove a painful splinter from a finger when the child cannot do so alone and when this

can be done without undue costs to oneself. (I assume that the splinter case satisfies the other provisos of the principle of medical mercy.) Similarly, I take it to be a moral duty to stop the bleeding of a person who has been wounded or to pull someone from a fire, though in very many of the cases in which such circumstances arise (wars, accidents) this duty is abrogated because we cannot do so without risks to ourselves. The duty of medical mercy is not simply equivalent to either nonmaleficence or beneficence, though perhaps derived from them, since the former is understood as a duty to refrain from causing harm and the latter to do good in a positive sense; the duty of medical mercy requires one to counteract harms one did not cause, though it may not require conferring additional positive benefits.

5. See Sharon H. Imbus and Bruce E. Zawacki, "Autonomy for Burned Patients When Survival Is Unprecedented," *New England Journal of Medicine* 297 (August 11, 1977): 309–311.

6. See Mary Voboril, *Miami Herald,* Saturday, July 1, 1978, see also note 17.

7. An extensive discussion of the conceptual and moral distinctions between killing and letting die begins with Jonathan Bennett, "Whatever the Consequences," *Analysis* 26 (1966): 83–97, and, after the American Medical Association's stand prohibiting mercy killing but permitting cessation of treatment, continues in James Rachels's "Active and Passive Euthanasia," *New England Journal of Medicine* 292 (January 9, 1975): 78–80, and many subsequent papers.

8. See Ludwig Edelstein, "The Hippocratic Oath," in *Ancient Medicine: Selected Papers of Ludwig Edelstein,* ed. Owsei Temkin and C. Lilian Temkin (Baltimore: The Johns Hopkins University Press, 1967), esp. 9–15, on the Greek physician's role in euthanasia.

9. Hospice, founded and directed by Cicely Saunders, is a movement devoted to the development of institutions for providing palliative but medically nonagressive care for terminal patients. In additon to its extraordinary contribution in developing methods of prophylactic pain control, according to which analgesics are administered on a scheduled basis in advance of experienced pain, Hospice has also emphasized attention to the emotional needs of the patient's family. An account of the theory and methodology of Hospice can be found in various publications by Saunders, including "Terminal Care in Medical Oncology," in *Medical Oncology,* ed. K. D. Bagshawe (Oxford: Blackwell, 1975), 563–576.

10. Joanne Lynn, M.D., "Supportive Care for Dying Patients: An Introduction for Health Care Professionals," Appendix B of the President's Commission for the Study of Ethical Problems in Medicine and Biomedical and Behavioral Research, *Deciding to Forgo Life-Sustaining Treatment* (Washington, D.C.: Government Printing Office, 1983), 295.

11. Robert G. Twycross, "Voluntary Euthanasia," in *Suicide and Euthanasia: The Rights of Personhood,* ed. Samuel E. Wallace and Albin Eser (Knoxville: The University of Tennessee Press, 1981), 89.

12. Philippa Foot, "Euthanasia," *Philosophy & Public Affairs* 6 (Winter 1977): 95.

13. To discover what one's own views are, try the following thought experiment. Imagine that you have been captured by a gang of ruthless and superlatively clever criminals, whom you know with certainty will never be caught or change their minds. They plan either to execute you now, or to torture you unremittingly for the next twenty years and then put you to death. Which would be worse? Does your view change if the length of the torture period is reduced to twenty days or twenty minutes, and if so, why? How severe does the torture need to be?

14. 211 N.Y. 127, 129; 105 N.E. 92, 93 (1914).

15. *In re Yetter,* 62 Pa. D.&C. 2d 619 (1973).

16. *Satz v. Perlmutter,* 362 S. 2d 160 (Fla. App. 1978), affirmed by Florida Supreme Court 379 So. 2d 359 (1980).

17. *Bartling v. Superior Court,* 2 Civ. No. B007907 (Calif. App. 1984).

18. California Health & Safety Code, Sections 7195–7196.

19. The living will and durable power of attorney forms valid in different states are distributed by Choice in Dying, 200 Varig Street, New York, NY 10014. Copies are also available from hospitals and attorneys.

20. M. Siegler, "Pascal's Wager and the Hanging of Crepe," *The New England Journal of Medicine* 293 (1975): 853–857.

21. See also a study of other factors associated with differences in prognosis and treatment decisions: R. Pearlman, T. Inui, and W. Carter, "Variability in Physician Bioethical Decision-Making," *Annals of Internal Medicine* 97 (September 1982): 420–425.

22. The effects of depression on the choice concerning whether to live or die are described by Richard B. Brandt, "The Morality and Rationality of Suicide," in *A Handbook for the Study of Suicide*, ed. Seymour Perlin (New York: Oxford University Press, 1975), 61–76, and reprinted in part in M. Pabst Battin and David J. Mayo, eds., *Suicide: The Philosophical Issues* (New York: St. Martin's Press, 1980), 117–132.

23. I've considered elsewhere the symmetrical argument that if death is in some circumstances actually better than life, the paternalist should be prepared to override a patient's choice of life. See M. Pabst Battin, *Ethical Issues in Suicide* (Englewood Cliffs, N.J.: Prentice-Hall, 1982), 160–175.

24. Vatican Congregation for the Doctrine of the Faith, "Declaration on Euthanasia," June 26, 1980; see Section II, "Euthanasia."

25. Peter C. Williams, "Rights and the Alleged Right of Innocents to Be Killed," *Ethics* 87 (1976–77): 383–394.

26. This proviso may appear to resemble similar provisos exempting physicians, nurses, and other caregivers who have principled objections to participating in abortions. But I am much less certain that weight should be given to the scruples of physicians in euthanasia cases, at least at the time of need. As I will suggest in the final section of this chapter, the patient has an obligation to make his or her wishes concerning euthanasia known in advance in a foreseeable decline; if the physician objects, it is his or her duty to excuse himself or herself from the case and from the care of the patient altogether *before* the patient's deteriorating condition prevents or makes it difficult to transfer to another physician; the doctor cannot simply voice his or her objections when the patient finally reaches the point of requesting help in dying. The physician should of course object if, for instance, he or she believes that the patient is acting on faulty information; but the physician ought not introduce a principled objection to participation in euthanasia in general at this late date.

27. To this end, the British and Scottish voluntary euthanasia societies have published booklets of explicit information concerning methods of suicide for distribution to their members; the Dutch voluntary euthanasia society has published a handbook intended specifically for physicians, and voluntary physician-assisted euthanasia is legally tolerated in Holland. In the United States, Hemlock, a society advocating legalization of voluntary euthanasia and assisted suicide, also makes available similar information.

28. O. Ruth Russell, *Freedom to Die: Moral and Legal Aspects of Euthanasia*, rev. ed. (New York: Human Sciences Press, 1977), 19.

29. Tom L. Beauchamp and Arnold I. Davidson, "The Definition of Euthanasia," *The Journal of Medicine and Philosophy* 4 (September 1979): 301.

30. Paul Ramsey, *The Patient as Person* (New Haven: Yale University Press, 1970), 161.

31. Allan S. Detsky et al., "Prognosis, Survival, and the Expenditure of Hospital Resources for Patients in an Intensive-Care Unit," *The New England Journal of Medicine* 305 (September 17, 1981): 667–672; figures from Table 1.

32. This case, originally presented in the *Illinois Medical Journal* and reprinted in *Connecticut Medicine* with commentary from medical, ethical, and legal experts, is summarized

in *Concern for Dying* 8 (Summer 1982): 3. This patient did receive treatment for intervening infections, pneumonia, dermatitis, and convulsions, and for the ten days before her death was maintained on oxygen, respiratory therapy, and antibiotics.

33. President's Commission for the Study of Ethical Problems in Medicine and Biomedical and Behavioral Research, *Defining Death: Medical, Legal, and Ethical Issues in the Determination of Death* (Washington, D.C.: Government Printing Office, 1981), 18, citing the *Guinness Book of World Records* regarding the case of Elaine Esposito.

34. See the useful discussion of the form of the wedge argument in Tom L. Beauchamp and James F. Childress, *Principles of Biomedical Ethics* (New York: Oxford University Press, 1979), 109–117. I am concerned primarily with the second, empirical form of the argument here, but disagree with the conclusions Beauchamp and Childress reach.

35. As one physician has pointed out, objecting to the wedge argument's contention that greed would bring doctors to kill their patients, there is "not much financial incentive with a dead patient." In fact, greed may work the other way around: doctors strive to keep their patients alive, whatever the physical or financial costs to the patients, because their income is derived from services provided. As another physician has pointed out, however, not all patients are profitable, and the physician who has enough profitable ones will find that killing off the unprofitable ones further improves the bottom line. Needless to say, greed in any of these varieties will violate the principles of mercy, autonomy, and justice.

36. See the position of Pope Pius XII on the use of painkillers in "The Prolongation of Life," an address to an international congress of anesthesiologists, reprinted in Dennis J. Horan and David Mall, eds., *Death, Dying, and Euthanasia* (Frederick, Md.: University Publications of America, 1980), 281–287. The view of Pius XII is reemphasized by Pope John Paul II (see note 24). Although both permit the use of painkillers that shorten life, provided they are intended to relieve pain, not intended to produce death, both also warn against the casual use of painkillers that cause unconsciousness, since, in the words of the latter, "a person not only has to be able to satisfy his or her moral duties and family obligations; he or she also has to prepare himself or herself with full consciousness for meeting Christ" (Section III). Advanced pain-managemment techniques may be able to reduce the problem, but in practice the excessive use of painkillers remains common.

37. See the discussion of this analogy in John D. Arras, "The Right to Die on the Slippery Slope," *Social Theory and Practice* 8 (Fall 1982): 301 ff.

38. Cicely Saunders, "The Moment of Truth: Care of the Dying Person," in *Confrontations of Death: A Book of Readings and a Suggested Method of Instruction*, ed. Francis G. Scott and Ruth M. Brewer (Corvallis, Ore.: A Continuing Education Book, 1971), 119, quoted in Paul Ramsey, *Ethics at the Edges of Life* (New Haven: Yale University Press, 1978), 152. Dame Saunders is the founder and medical director of St. Christopher's Hospice near London, which has provided the stimulus and model for the contemporary hospice movement.

39. See chapter 1 of this book.

40. Barbara J. McNeil, Ralph Weichselbaum, and Stephen G. Pauker, "Speech and Survival: Tradeoffs between Quality and Quantity of Life in Laryngeal Cancer," *New England Journal of Medicine* 305 (October 22, 1981): 982–987. The study, however, was performed with healthy volunteers, not actual patients. See Correspondence, *New England Journal of Medicine* 306 (February 25, 1982): 482–483, for other criticisms of this study, including evidence that rehabilitation of speech may be quite satisfactory.

41. See Courtney S. Campbell, "'Aid-in-Dying' and the Taking of Human Life," *Journal of Medical Ethics* 18(1992): 128–134, for an estimate that 76–84 percent of deaths are caused by chronic conditions.

42. It is sometimes argued that physician assistance in a patient's suicide would violate the Hippocratic Oath. It is true that the oath, in its original form, does contain an explicit

injunction that the physician shall not give a lethal potion to a patient who requests it, nor make a suggestion to that effect (to do so was apparently common Greek medical practice at the time). But the oath in its original form also contains explicit prohibitions of the physician's accepting fees for teaching medicine, and of performing surgery—even on gallstones. These latter prohibitions are not retained in modern reformulations of the oath, and I see no reason why the provision against giving lethal potions to patients who request it should be. What is central to the oath and cannot be deleted without altering its essential character is the requirement that the physician shall come "for the benefit of the sick." Under the argument advanced here, physician assistance in patient suicide may in some cases indeed be for the benefit of the patient. What the oath would continue to prohibit is physician assistance in a suicide for the physician's own gain or to serve other institutional or societal ends.

43. Ramsey, *The Patient as Person*, 145.

6

A Dozen Caveats Concerning the Discussion of Euthanasia in the Netherlands

As the discussion of voluntary active euthanasia heats up in the United States, increasing attention is being given to its practice in the Netherlands. There, euthanasia (and with it, physician-assisted suicide) is more and more openly discussed and practiced; it is performed with the knowledge of the legal authorities; physicians who follow the guidelines are protected from prosecution; and, as a result of broad public discussions of the issue in the media, euthanasia is familiar to virtually all Dutch residents as an option in end-of-life medical care.

In the United States, those who think euthanasia should be legalized often cite the Netherlands as a model of conscientious practice; those who think it should not be legalized, on the other hand, often claim that Dutch practice already involves abuse and will inevitably lead to more. For the most part, these generalizations invite misunderstanding, and they often reflect only the antecedent biases of those who make them. I would like to offer a few caveats for those about to become embroiled in the discussion of euthanasia, as the United States debates whether it, too, will permit this practice—caveats offered in the hope of contributing to better mutual understanding rather than greater polarization over this extremely volatile issue.

1. *Legal claims are misleading, either way.* Many American observers of the Dutch practice of euthanasia are tempted to claim that euthanasia is legal in Holland; others insist that it is not. Both are right—but only partly so. Killing at the request of the person killed as well as assistance in suicide remain crimes under the Dutch penal code, punishable by imprisonment;[1] however, several lower court decisions, supported by a Supreme Court decision and reflected in the policies of the regional attorneys-general, and further promulgated by the Royal Dutch Medical Association, have held that when euthanasia meets a certain set of guidelines it may be

This list of a dozen caveats is an amalgam of my two earlier papers, "Seven Caveats Concerning the Discussion of Euthanasia in Holland," *Perspectives in Biology and Medicine* 34, no. 1 (Autumn 1990): 73–77, copyright © 1990 by the University of Chicago, reprinted in *Newsletter of the American Philosophical Association Committee on Philosophy and Medicine* 89, no. 2 (Winter 1990): 78–80 and "Seven (More) Caveats Concerning the Discussion of Euthanasia in Holland," *Newsletter of the American Philosophical Association Committee on Philosophy and Medicine* 92, no. 1 (Spring 1993): 76–80.

defended under a plea of *force majeure*[2] and so is reasonably sure of not being subjected to prosecution. In February 1993, these provisions were accepted by the Second Chamber of the Dutch Parliament, and, if accepted in the fall of 1993 by the First Chamber as well, will be enacted into law. While euthanasia will still remain technically illegal by statute, the physician who conscientiously meets the guidelines in practicing it can be sure he or she will not be prosecuted. These guidelines, sometimes called "rules of due care," are not to be understood as rules in a legal sense and are not themselves incorporated into any statute or regulation (this may explain why they are so variously stated), but rather as a set of "points for consideration," the questions the physician must answer to the Ministry of Justice as it decides whether he or she has met the guidelines, and hence whether a given case of euthanasia is to be prosecuted.[3] Nevertheless, these guidelines have come to define the Dutch consensus on when euthanasia is permitted. They are as follows; I've roughly divided them into two groups:

Substantive Guidelines
  (a) Euthanasia must be voluntary; the patient's request must be seriously considered and enduring.
  (b) The patient must have adequate information about his or her medical condition, the prognosis, and alternative methods of treatment.
  (c) The patient's suffering must be intolerable, in the patient's view, and irreversible (though it is not required that the patient be terminally ill).
  (d) It must be the case that there are no reasonable alternatives for relieving the patient's suffering that are acceptable to the patient.

Procedural Guidelines
  (e) Euthanasia may be performed only by a physician (though a nurse may assist the physician).
  (f) The physician must consult with a second physician whose judgment can be expected to be independent.
  (g) The physician must exercise due care in reviewing and verifying the patient's condition as well as in performing the euthanasia procedure itself.
  (h) The relatives must be informed unless the patient does not wish this.
  (i) There should be a written record of the case.
  (j) The case may not be reported as a natural death.

Is euthanasia legal or illegal? It is a violation of the statue but is *gedoogd* or "tolerated" if it meets these guidelines, and will not be prosecuted. Yet it is not excused in advance, and the plea of *force majeure,* although often compelling in single cases, does not easily serve as a basis for policy. Until 1990, it was required that any case of euthanasia be reported to the police and investigated after the fact, further prosecution being set aside if the case met the guidelines; in fact, comparatively few cases were reported, and physicians complained that they—and patients' families—were being treated as criminal suspects even when they had met all the guidelines. Policy changes in 1990 avoided the step of initial reporting to and investigation by the police; instead, the physician provides a written account of the case to the medical examiner, who then forwards it to the public prosecutor. If the

criteria are satisfied, a certificate of "no objection to burial or cremation" is issued
and there is no further investigation. These policy changes, however, have not
altered the delicate legal status of euthanasia in the Netherlands—prohibited by law,
but tolerated under guidelines developed in the courts, and now recognized though
not stated in the law—a delicate balance often misunderstood by outside commentators. This delicate legal status has been seen by many observers as a deterrent to
abuse; it is also seen by some as accounting for a great deal of the underreporting. In
any case, it is clear why the legal status of euthanasia in the Netherlands is so
frequently misinterpreted by American commentators: its delicate balance between
legality and illegality—the Dutch posture of "tolerance"—would be difficult to
replicate in the American legal system.

   2. *Exaggerations are frequent.* It is also sometimes supposed that euthanasia is
a routine, frequent, everyday practice in the Netherlands, a commonplace that
happens all the time. On the contrary, euthanasia is comparatively rare. There are
about 2,300 cases of euthanasia per year; these represent just 1.8 percent of the total
annual mortality, which in 1990, was 128,786 deaths in a population of about 15
million. In addition, there are about 400 cases of physician-assisted suicide, just 0.3
percent of the total annual mortality. Although a substantial proportion of patients,
about 25,000 a year, seek their doctors' reassurance of assistance if their suffering
becomes unbearable, only 9,000 explicit requests for euthanasia are made annually,
and of these, fewer than one third are honored. Thus, the contention sometimes
heard that there is widespread euthanasia on demand is seriously exaggerated. The
actual frequency of euthanasia is about 1 in 25 deaths that occur at home, about 1 in
75 in hospital deaths, and about 1 in 800 for deaths in nursing homes.[4]

   3. *The institutional circumstances of euthanasia in the Netherlands are easily
misunderstood.* Although many American observers of Dutch euthanasia risk misin-
terpreting many features of this practice, a particularly frequent error arises from
failing to appreciate differences between health-care delivery systems and other
social institutions in the Netherlands and those in the United States. In the United
States virtually all physician care is provided in a professional or institutional setting: an office, clinic, care facility, or hospital. By contrast, most primary care in the
Netherlands is provided in the patient's home or in the physician's home office by
the *huisarts,* the general practitioner or family physician. The family physician, who
typically serves a practice of about 2,300 people and is salaried on a capitation basis rather than paid on a fee-for-service basis, typically lives in the neighborhood
and makes frequent house calls when a patient is ill. This provides not only closer,
more personal contact between physician and patient but also an unparalleled opportunity for the physician to observe features of the patient's domestic circumstances,
including any family support or pressures that might be relevant in a request for
euthanasia.

   Furthermore, all Dutch have a personal physician; this is a basic feature of how
primary care is provided within the Netherlands' national health system. While
euthanasia is sometimes performed in hospitals (about 700 of the 2,300 cases),
usually when the family physician has been unable to control the patient's pain and it
has been necessary to readmit the patient to the hospital, or when the patient has had
extensive hospital care and feels most "at home" there, and while most hospitals

now have protocols for doing so, the large majority of cases take place in the patient's home, typically after hospitalization and treatment have proved ineffective in arresting a terminal condition and the patient has come home to die. In these settings, euthanasia is most often performed by the physician who has been the long-term primary care provider for the family, and it is performed in the presence of the patient's family and others whom the patient may request, such as the visiting nurse or the pastor, but outside public view. Yet the (non)institutional circumstances of euthanasia in the Netherlands are not easy for Americans to understand: whereas dying at home is not unusual in the Netherlands (about 40 percent of Dutch deaths occur at home, and 48 percent of cancer deaths),[5] in the United States as many as 85 percent of deaths occur in a hospital or other health-care institution, where attendance by a long-term family physician is far less frequently the case.

4. *Euthanasia isn't routine or anonymous.* Especially in the United States, euthanasia is often understood on the "It's Over, Debbie" model, derived from the notorious account in a 1988 issue of the *Journal of the American Medical Association,* which described a sleepy resident giving a lethal dose in the middle of the night to a young woman dying of ovarian cancer—a patient he'd never seen before, whose chart he had not actually examined, with whose unidentified companion sitting by the bed he had no communication, for whom he made no attempt to provide other treatment or better pain control, and with whom he exchanged only the briefest of words.

"Let's get this over with," Debbie said, in the midst of her pain. The resident ordered a syringe of morphine sulfate drawn and—telling Debbie only that he would give her something to "let her rest" and that she should say goodbye—killed her. In fact, "It's Over, Debbie" is a virtual compendium of all that is *not* tolerated in Holland. Euthanasia is typically performed by the patient's personal physician, not a stranger; it is performed within the context of an extended period of consultation and care. Not only is it usually performed at home with the patient's family present, but the physician remains with the patient or in an adjoining room throughout the process. The physician takes no fee for performing euthanasia. Nor will Dutch physicians perform euthanasia for patients from other countries, with whom they have had no prior contact. Fears sometimes voiced in the United States concerning the commercialization of euthanasia or the development of a death trade, practiced for profit by greedy physicians, have no place in Holland. Euthanasia remains a rare event, generally presupposing a long-term relationship between physician and patient, and it involves an often substantial commitment of time with no financial reward.

5. *There isn't enough hard data about the practice of euthanasia in the Netherlands.* Until the appearance of two large empirical studies in 1991–1992, very little hard data had been available about the practice of euthanasia in the Netherlands, even though the practice had become open, vigorously discussed, and legally tolerated. Despite the policy that cases of euthanasia were to be reported to the Ministry of Justice by physicians who performed them, in 1986 only 84 cases were reported (now estimated to have been 3 percent of the total), and by 1990 only 454 (about 17 percent). This generated an extensive amount of conjecture about the unreported cases, variously estimated to range in frequency between 2,000 and 20,000, and

invited the accusation that these cases were unreported because Dutch physicians had something to hide.

Two major empirical studies of the actual practice of euthanasia in the Netherlands were published in 1991–1992: the government-sponsored study popularly known as the Remmelink Commission report (named after Professor J. Remmelink, attorney general of the Dutch Supreme Court, who chaired the committee to which it was presented)[6] and a dissertation presented at the Free University in Amsterdam by Gerrit van der Wal.[7] Although the Remmelink Commission study involved a much more complex design, covered a wider range of physicians (including specialists and nursing home physicians), and received a great deal more attention than the van der Wal study of family-practice physicians only, the two studies were similar in many respects. Although their range was different, both sought to discover what Dutch physicians actually do and do not do as their patients approach death; both attempted to assess the frequency of euthanasia in the Netherlands; both attempted to assemble information about the characteristics of patients, the nature of their requests for euthanasia, and the nature of the physician's response; and both were alert to the possibility of abuse. Both studies involved surveys of physicians under the strictest guarantees of confidentiality, and both achieved high response rates. The Remmelink study included extensive direct interviews with a large sample of physicians; the van der Wal study examined police reports. Both studies were well designed, and both quite informative.

Furthermore, the two studies agreed in many of their results. Although based on extrapolations from different survey populations, they came very close in their estimates of the overall frequency of euthanasia in the Netherlands. According to the Remmelink report, of the approximately 2,300 cases of euthanasia a year, about 1,550 are performed by general practitioners, 730 by specialist physicians, and about 20 by nursing home physicians. In addition, there are another 400 cases of physician-assisted suicide. Van der Wal found a combined total of about 2,000 euthanasia and assisted-suicide cases per year in general practice alone. These studies thus revised the previously accepted best estimate of 6,000 cases a year (not to mention the extreme estimate of 20,000 cases a year) dramatically downward. Both studies agreed that euthanasia was far more frequent than assisted suicide. Both found that only a minority of requests for euthanasia are honored. Both studies examined the reasons why patients request euthanasia, and both found that pain is very seldom (about 5 percent in both studies) the sole reason, though pain is often (46 percent) one reason among others. Both found that the diagnosis in the majority of cases is cancer and that the average age of euthanasia patients is in the sixties. The Remmelink study found that euthanasia is slightly less common among men than women (48 percent males, though there was no significant difference) while assisted suicide is more common for men than women (61 percent males), and van der Wal found that euthanasia is about equal for both sexes. Both studies found that the estimated life expectancy for patients receiving euthanasia is usually a week or two, though in a small fraction of cases it is longer than six months and in another small fraction it is less than a day. And both also revealed the existence of cases that do not strictly fit the guidelines.

As extensive as the contributions of these two studies to the discussion of euthanasia in Holland have been, however, there still is not enough hard data. To be sure, some further information has become available: for example, the researchers who prepared the report to the Remmelink Commission have recently published a more intensive study of the findings in about a thousand cases that involve active termination but without explicit, current request from the patient; this took the form of three representative case scenarios.[8] But there is not yet a broad collection of what one might call phenomenological data: interior narrations by patients themselves of their experiences as they decide to request euthanasia—perhaps available from personal journals, dictations to family members, direct interviews, diaries, and the like—that might shed further light on the nature of such choices, though there have been a few documentaries and real-life interviews (for instance, on television) between physicians and patients. A participant-observer study of euthanasia is now in progress,[9] as well as a small, anecdotal study involving interviews of family members concerning their grieving processes following the euthanasia of a loved one.[10] But there are neither hard nor soft comprehensive data on the perceptions of family members, nurses, clergy, or others who might have played an observer's role, nor on the perceptions of patients themselves. In short, there is still a great deal more to be learned about the practice of euthanasia in Holland. The two studies now available should be understood as crucial first contributions of empirical information rather than as the last word.

6. *Terminological differences operate to confuse the issue.* By and large, Dutch proponents of euthanasia use the term to refer only to what in the United States would be called voluntary active euthanasia. The term *active euthanasia* is considered essentially redundant and the term *passive euthanasia* meaningless. The Remmelink study examined not only euthanasia and assisted suicide, but also drew distinctions between withdrawal and withholding of treatment (approximately 17.5 percent of deaths) and the use of opiates while "taking into account the probability of hastening death" (another 17.5 percent of deaths). The latter phrase was chosen deliberately to cover such actions as the heavy use of morphine to control pain, even though this might depress respiration and thus bring about death, which are understood under the principle of double effect. However, the Dutch also employ the term *levensbeëindigend handelen* ("life-terminating acts") to refer to practices that result in the death of the patient but cannot be considered voluntary active euthanasia; this term is sometimes used broadly to encompass all withholding or withdrawing treatment, including, for instance, that in severely defective newborns, permanent coma patients, and psychogeriatric patients (all of these are situations in which withholding or withdrawing treatment is also frequent in the United States), and it is sometimes used (as in the Remmelink study) to refer to direct termination. The Remmelink researchers defined a category of practices they more narrowly called "life-terminating acts without explicit request" or LAWER; this category includes the 1,000 cases (0.8 percent of the total annual mortality) of actively caused deaths where there was no current, explicit request. Since these cases do not fit the criteria for euthanasia, they are not labeled by that term. Thus, the claim that there is no nonvoluntary active euthanasia in Holland may seem to be merely analytically true.

On the other hand, it is clear that claims by some of the more vocal opponents of euthanasia also rest on terminological confusion. For instance, Dutch cardiologist

Richard Fenigsen's assertion that involuntary euthanasia outside the guidelines is widespread rests on his conflating what in the United States would be called active and passive euthanasia: Fenigsen, like many others of the opposition, does not always distinguish between causing death and withholding or withdrawing treatment, that is, what we call "allowing to die."[11] In the United States, withholding or withdrawal of treatment, including respiratory support, antibiotics, chemotherapy, cardiopulmonary resuscitation, and artificial nutrition and hydration, tends to be regarded as morally acceptable in certain circumstances, even when these decisions are not actually made by the patient but by second parties, perhaps following the patient's antecedent wish (a view reflected in many of the cases from *Quinlan* to *Cruzan*), whereas, on the other hand, the direct causing of death, even at the current, explicit request of the patient, is regarded as problematic in the extreme. In the Netherlands, the view tends to be the other way around. One suspects that much of the opposition in Holland to active voluntary euthanasia has actually been opposition to passive nonvoluntary euthanasia, a practice much more accepted in the United States than in the Netherlands. It is often said in the United States that the Dutch are stepping out onto the slippery slope in permitting active euthanasia; the Dutch, in contrast, think it is *we* who are already on the slippery slope, given our readiness to "allow to die" in ways that are not voluntary on the part of the patient. As the Dutch now begin more open discussion of decision-making concerning incompetent patients, they are entering a territory already heavily discussed in the United States in the cases from *Quinlan* to *Cruzan;* as Americans begin to debate the issues in first-party choices of euthanasia or assisted suicide, we are entering territory already well familiar to the Dutch.

7. *The Dutch don't want to defend everything.* The Dutch are sometimes accused of being self-serving or, alternatively, of being self-deceived in their efforts to defend the practice of euthanasia. To be sure, not all Dutch accept the practice. There is a vocal group of about a thousand physicians adamantly opposed to it, and there is some opposition among the public and within specific political parties (in particular, the Christian Democratic Party, which has for years controlled the Netherlands' coalition government) and religious groups (especially the Catholic church). Yet the practice is supported by a majority of the Dutch populace (rising from 40 percent in 1966 to 78 percent in 1992)[12] as well as a majority of Dutch physicians. Of physicians interviewed for the Remmelink study, 54 percent said they had practiced euthanasia at the explicit and persistent request of the patient or had assisted in suicide at least once (62 percent of the general practitioners, 44 percent of specialists, and 12 percent of nursing home physicians), and only 4 percent said they would neither perform euthanasia nor refer a patient to a physician who would. In the words of the Remmelink Commission's comment on the report, "a large majority of physicians in the Netherlands see euthanasia as an accepted element of medical practice under certain circumstances."[13]

But this is not to say that the Dutch seek to whitewash the practice. They are disturbed by reports of cases that do not fit the guidelines and are not explained by other moral considerations, although these may be quite infrequent. Of the approximately 1,000 cases of active termination in which there was no explicit, current request—the LAWER cases—36 percent of patients were competent, the physician knew the patient for an extended period (on average, 2.4 years for a specialist physician, or 7.2 years for a *huisarts* or general practitioner), and in 84 percent life was shortened somewhere between a few hours and a week.[14] Because there was no current, explicit request, these cases are sometimes described in the United States as cold-blooded murder, yet most are explained by other moral considerations. Of these 1,000 cases, according to the Remmelink researchers in both the initial and supplementary reports, about 600 did involve some form of antecedent discussion of euthanasia with the patient. These ranged from a rather vague earlier expression of a wish for euthanasia, as in comments like "If I cannot be saved anymore, you must give me something," or "Doctor, please don't let me suffer for too long," to much more extensive discussions, yet still short of an explicit request. (Thus, these cases are best understood in a way that approximates them to advance-directive cases in other situations.) In all other cases, discussion with the patient was no longer possible. In almost all of the remaining 400 cases, there was neither an antecedent nor current request from the patient, but at the time of euthanasia—"possibly with a few exceptions"—the patient was very close to death, incapable of communication, and suffering grievously. For the most part, this occurred when the patient underwent unexpectedly rapid deterioration in the final stages of a terminal illness. (These cases are best understood as cases of mercy killing, with emphasis on the motivation of mercy.) In these cases, the report to the Remmelink Commission continued, "the decision to hasten death was then nearly always taken after consultation with the family, nurses, or one or more colleagues." Most Dutch also defend these cases, though as critics point out, the danger here is that the determination of what counts as intolerable suffering in these cases is essentially up to the doctor.[15]

Direct termination of life is also performed in a handful of pediatric cases, about ten a year, usually involving newborns with extremely severe deficits who are not in the ICU and from whom, therefore, life-prolonging treatment cannot be withdrawn.[16] These cases are regarded as difficult and controversial. Equally controversial—and as rare or rarer—are cases concerning patients in permanent coma or persistent vegetative state; patients whose suffering, though intolerable and incurable, is mental rather than physical; and patients who have made explicit requests for euthanasia by means of advance directives, but after becoming incompetent no longer appear to be suffering.

The Remmelink study also provided some suggestion, though no clear evidence, that there may be a small fraction of cases in which there is no apparent choice by the patient and in which a merciful end of suffering for a patient *in extremis* is not the issue. These cases do disturb the Dutch: they are regarded as highly problematic, and it is clearly intended that if they occur, they should be stopped. In the Remmelink study, interviews with physicians revealed only two instances, both from the early 1980s, in which a fully competent patient was euthanized without explicit consent; in both, the patient was suffering severely. In the Remmelink study interview, the physician in one of these cases indicated that under present-day circumstances, with increased openness about these issues, he probably would have initiated more extensive consultations. There is no evidence of any patient being put to death *against* his or her expressed or implied wish.

The Dutch also distinguish between procedural and substantive or material failures to meet the guidelines, regarding the latter as much more problematic than the former. They note that failure to meet the procedural requirements of the guidelines is not uncommon; for instance, according to van der Wal, only 75 percent of family doctors asked another doctor for a second opinion, slightly fewer than half (48 percent) had kept written records, and 74 percent has issued a false death certificate, stating that the death was due to natural causes. Only around a quarter had reported performing euthanasia to the Ministry of Justice, and as van der Wal pointed out, "cases that reveal shortcomings are hardly ever reported to the Public Prosecutor."[17] Procedural failures do not particularly trouble the Dutch, but they are alert to cases in which euthanasia was performed against the wishes of the patient or for ulterior reasons. Neither study yielded concrete information about any such cases, although neither study denied that such cases ("a few exceptions") might occur.

To understand how the Dutch defend their practice of euthanasia, given the possibility of such cases, a domestic analogy may be helpful. We, like the Dutch, recognize and defend the practice of marriage: it is enshrined in our law, our religions, and our cultural norms. Among other things, we understand this practice to be quintessentially voluntary: in order to marry, the parties involved must each choose freely to do so, and their signatures on the marriage license serve to attest to this fact. But we also recognize that some marriages are not voluntary: shotgun weddings, for example, in which the groom has been threatened by the father of the pregnant bride or in which the bride sees no alternative to marrying the man who has impregnated her. Yet although we recognize that physically or socially coerced marriages do occur from time to time, we continue to defend the institution of marriage, claiming that coerced marriages aren't really central to the practice we otherwise respect. The Dutch attitude toward euthanasia is a bit like this, though coerced marriages are no doubt a good deal more frequent than problematic cases of euthanasia: it is the *practice* that is defended, not each single case that occurs within or around it. On the contrary, the Dutch seek to control these few problematic cases on the fringes—that is part of the point of bringing the practice out into the open. The Dutch government has recently indicated its intention that physicians performing LAWER will as a rule be prosecuted (though this does not guarantee that all prosecutions will result in conviction), presumably as a way of asserting more thorough control over this practice and eliminating the risk of abuse.

8. *There are no "indications" for euthanasia.* In the Netherlands, euthanasia is understood by definintion to mean voluntary euthanasia, and nonvoluntary practices, such as the thousand cases of "life-terminating acts without explicit request," are not grouped under this term. Nor are the two additional categories of practices, mentioned earlier, which were treated as distinct "medical decisions concerning the end of life" in the Remmelink and van der Wal reports (as they are also in the United States): doses of opiates intended to relieve pain but which, foreseeably, may shorten life; and discontinuations or withholdings of treatment, even when death is likely to be the outcome. But although patient choice is a necessary condition for euthanasia, it is not a sufficient condition; the patient who requests euthanasia is not thereby guaranteed it and does not oblige a physician to perform it. Indeed, according to both empirical studies, the majority of requests for euthanasia (60–67 percent) are turned down.

This situation, however, has led some observers to wonder whether there isn't a set of criteria developing for the performance of euthanasia that could in effect serve as indications. If physicians reject up to two-thirds of the requests for euthanasia, it is argued, they must be entertaining some set of criteria according to which some cases are to be accepted and others rejected—criteria other than patient choice. But if this is so, it is argued, it may invite a certain readiness to perform euthanasia whenever these criteria are met, independent of the patient's choice. The Dutch would reply by arguing that there are no positive criteria for euthanasia, but that there are indeed negative criteria for when it is *inappropriate* to perform euthanasia—for example, when the request is motivated by depression or when suffering can be relieved by other means acceptable to the patient. Without positive criteria, "indications" for euthanasia cannot develop: that is, factors in the presence of which the physician ought to perform euthanasia and hence ought to "see to it" that the patient accepts this recommendation. While some Dutch physicians say they do sometimes introduce the topic of euthanasia if the patient has not raised it, they insist that it be performed only at the patient's *request,* not as the result of consent to a procedure the physician has proposed. However, whether criteria are developing— perhaps under the guise of justifications—for life-terminating acts without explicit request, or LAWER, is another matter, perhaps the central (though not fully articulated) issue in the ongoing debate about how life may best end for incompetent patients, since in these cases patient choice is not possible anymore.

9. *The Dutch see the role of law rather differently.* Not only is Dutch law a civil law system rather than common law one; not only does it contain the distinctive Dutch doctrine involving practices that are statutorily illegal but *gedogen,* or tolerated, by the public prosecutor, the courts, or both; and not only does it involve very little medical malpractice activity, but the Dutch also tend to see law as appropriately formulated at a different point in the evolution of a social practice. Americans, it is sometimes said, *begin* to address a social issue by first making laws and then challenging them in court to fine-tune and adjust them; the Dutch, on the other hand, allow a practice to evolve by "tolerating" but not legalizing it, and only when the practice is adequately controlled—when they've got it right, so to speak—is a law made to regulate the practice as it has evolved. That the Dutch do not yet have a law fully shaped to accommodate their open practice of euthanasia may not show, as some have claimed, that they are ambivalent about the practice, but perhaps rather that they are waiting for the practice to evolve to a point where it is under adequate, acceptable control, at which time it will be appropriate to finally revise the law. Both early and recent attempts to completely legalize euthanasia have failed to satisfy enough parties (especially the Christian Democrats) within the Dutch coalition governments, though the 1993 changes, if passed, will provide much more protection than previously to both physicians and their patients. Some observers still think that there will be greater agreement before long, reflecting the end of the debate and the emergence of a social consensus. Of course, some commentators see the delicate balance in which the practice is technically illegal under Dutch law but also legally protected from prosecution by Dutch court decisions and legal policy as a desirable bulwark against abuse, but others argue for a more comprehensive revision of the statute, amending the penal code and spelling out in the Medical Practice Act the

conditions under which a physician could not be prosecuted. [18] Full legalization, they argue, is crucial to providing legal security for both physicians and patients.

It has also often been suggested that it is not the delicate legal situation of euthanasia—tolerated by the courts, yet still technically prohibited by the law—that accounts for the underreporting of actual cases of euthanasia, but that the unreported cases were different and indefensible. Now, however, we know what the unreported cases are. Both the Remmelink and the van der Wal studies provide extensive detail about such cases, since they explored both reported and unreported cases. According to van der Wal, whose study included police reports among the sources of data, the reported cases and the unreported cases described by doctors in responding to the questionnaries differed with regard to procedural matters; the cases not reported tended to be those not meeting the procedural requirements, but the reported and unreported cases closely resembled each other in satisfying the substantive requirements concerning voluntariness, adequate information, the presence of intolerable suffering, and the absence of any acceptable alternatives for treatment. Thus, the unreported cases are those in which there are only procedural lapses to hide, not cases in which there is any greater frequency of substantive irregularities. The number of cases reported is currently climbing rapidly, partly due to simplified procedures and the requirement being dropped for investigation of the physician and the relatives by the police. In 1992, with simplified procedures, reporting reached almost half: 1,318, or 49 percent of the estimated total cases.

10. *The economic circumstances of euthanasia in the Netherlands are also easily misunderstood.* The Netherlands' national system of mixed public and private health insurance provides extensive care to all patients, including all hospitalization, nursing home care, home care, and the services of physicians, nurses, physical therapists, nutritionists, counselors, and other care providers, both in institutional settings and in the home. Virtually all residents of the Netherlands, 99.4 percent, are comprehensively insured for all medical expenses (those who are not are those who, with incomes above a stipulated level, are wealthy enough to self-insure), and 100 percent are insured for the costs of long-term illness. All insurance, both public and private, has a mandated minimum level that is very ample. Americans who raise the issue of whether some patients' requests for euthanasia are motivated by financial pressures or by fear of the effect of immense medical costs to their families are committing perhaps the most frequent mistake made by American observers: to assume that the choices of patients in the Netherlands are subject to the same pressures that the choices of patients in the United States would be. While there may be some administrative changes in the national health insurance system in the Netherlands in the near future, cost pressures on the system as a whole are met by rationing and queueing (neither currently severe), not by exclusion of individuals from coverage or by increased costs to patients. The costs to oneself or one's family of an extended illness, something that might make euthanasia attractive to a patient in the United States, are something the Dutch patient need not consider.

11. *Differences in social circumstances often go unnoticed.* In American discussions of euthanasia, considerable emphasis is placed on slippery slope arguments, pointing out risks of abuse, particularly with reference to the handicapped, the poor, racial minorities, and others who might seem to be ready targets for involuntary

euthanasia. The Netherlands, however, exhibits much less disparity between rich and poor, has much less racial prejudice, virtually no uninsured people, and very little homelessness. These differences underscore the difficulty both of treating the Netherlands as a model for the United States in advocating the legalization of euthanasia and also of assessing the plausibility of slippery slope arguments opposing legalization in the United States.

12. *The situation isn't getting worse; it's getting better.* Many of the foreign commentators have interpreted those cases of which the Dutch are not proud and do not wish to defend as evidence that the Dutch are indeed sliding down the slippery slope, moving from sympathetic cases of voluntary euthanasia to morally indefensible, broader-scale killing motivated by such matters as impatience, money, or power. They cite several celebrated outlier cases involving gross violations of the guidelines, such as an infamous nursing-home case in which nurses administered euthanasia to a group of terminally ill, mentally disturbed cancer patients when a physician refused to do so, and the cases the Remmelink Commission report identified as falling outside a strict interpretation of the guidelines. The recognition that there are cases of life-terminating acts without explicit request, or LAWER, not counted as euthanasia contributes to this view. Furthermore, several commentators—especially Carlos Gomez[19] and John Keown[20]—have argued that the Netherlands' legal and other protections against future abuse are wholly inadequate.

But the Dutch themselves see things in quite a different way: that bringing euthanasia and related practices out into the open is a way of gaining control. For the Dutch, this is a way of identifying a practice that, in the Netherlands as in every other country (including the United States), has been going on undercover and entirely at the discretion of the physician. It brings the practice into public view, where it can be regulated by guidelines, judicial scrutiny, and the collection of objective data. It is not that the Dutch or anyone else have only recently begun to practice euthanasia for the dying patient, nor is this a new phenomenon in the last decade or so; rather, the Dutch are the first to try to assert formal public control over a previously hidden practice and, hence, to regulate it effectively. Both open public discussion and the development of formal mechanisms such as guidelines, hospital protocols, and reporting requirements are seen as crucial in developing a social consensus, understood and accepted by both physicians and patients, about what can and cannot be permitted.

These dozen caveats are intended to point to differences between the American and Dutch health care climates that are often unnoticed in the discussion of euthanasia, although they are only a few of the principal cautions that should be exercised in entering this discussion. There are a great many other differences between the United States and the Netherlands that pose further risks of misinterpretation and misunderstanding; however, because these two highly sophisticated, industrialized, modern nations resemble each other in so many ways—including the general forms of their economic systems, their common cultural roots in the European Enlightenment, their sophisticated medical systems, and so on—these differences often go unnoticed. It is unlikely that Americans can fully understand why the Dutch support their practice of euthanasia, and conversely, it is unlikely that the Dutch will understand why the Americans are so ambivalent about its legalization or why they are so likely to distort the Dutch practice, until these differences are incorporated into both sides of the debate. In doing this, our principal problem is to detach ourselves from the antecedent biases we Americans bring to this issue, rooted in our own troubled health-care climate, and to examine Dutch practices and the reasons for them with comparatively open minds.

Notes

I'd like to thank Hans van Delden, M.D. and Loes Pijnenberg, M.D. for comments on this expanded version.

1. The maximum sentence for euthanasia is twelve years' imprisonment; for assisted suicide, three years. See the Dutch Penal Code, sections 293 and 294.

2. *Force majeure,* entered as a plea by the physician, appeals to a conflict of duties in which he or she is both obligated to obey the law and, at the same time, to obey the demands of medical ethics and the explicit wishes of the patient who relies on him or her. It is the physician's professional obligations that force him or her to act against the formal provisions of the law. See Robert J. M. Dillmann, Gerrit van der Wal, and Johannes J. M. van Delden, "Euthanasia in the Netherlands: The State of Affairs," manuscript in progress, Royal Dutch Medical Association, P. O. Box 20051, 3502 LB Utrecht, The Netherlands, p. 5.

3. The following are the questions to which the physician must respond after performing a case of euthanasia.

GUIDELINES FOR THE ATTENDING PHYSICIAN IN REPORTING EUTHANASIA TO THE MUNICIPAL CORONER

The following list of points is intended as a guideline in reporting euthanasia or assistance provided to a patient in taking his or her own life to the municipal coroner. A full written report supplying motives for your action is required.

I. CASE HISTORY
   1. What was the nature of the illness and what was the main diagnosis?
   2. How long had the patient been suffering from the illness?
   3. What was the nature of the medical treatment provided (medication, curative, surgical, etc.)?
   4. Please provide the names, addresses, and telephone numbers of the attending physicians. What were their diagnoses?
   5. Was the patient's mental and/or physical suffering so great that he or she perceived it or could have perceived it to be unbearable?
   6. Was the patient in a desperate situation with no prospect of relief and was his/her death inevitable?
      a. Was the situation at the end such that the prognosis was increasing lack of dignity for the patient and/or such as to exacerbate suffering which the patient already experienced as unbearable?
      b. Was there no longer any prospect of the patient being able to die with dignity?
      c. When in your opinion would the patient have died if euthanasia had not been performed?
   7. What measures, if any, did you consider or use to prevent the patient experiencing his/her suffering as unbearable (was there indeed any possibility of alleviating the suffering) and did you discuss these with the patient?

II. REQUEST FOR EUTHANASIA

1. Did the patient of his/her own free will make a very explicit and deliberate request for euthanasia to be performed:

   a. on the basis of adequate information which you had provided on the course of the illness and the method of terminating life, and

   b. after discussion of the measures referred to at 7?

2. If the patient made such a request, when and to whom was it made? Who else was present at the time?

3. Is there a living will? If so, please pass this on to the municipal coroner.

4. At the time of the request was the patient fully aware of the consequences thereof and of his/her physical and mental condition? What evidence of this can you provide?

5. Did the patient consider options other than euthanasia? If so, which options and if not, why not?

6. Could anyone else have influenced either the patient or yourself in the decision? If so, how did this manifest itself?

III. SECOND OPINION

1. Did you consult another doctor? If so, please provide his/her name, address, and telephone number. If you consulted more than one colleague, please supply all the names, addresses, and telephone numbers.

2. What conclusions did the other doctor(s) reach, at least with respect to questions I.6 and I.7?

3. Did this doctor/these doctors see the patient? If so, on what date? If not, on what were his/her/their conclusions based?

IV. EUTHANASIA

1. Who performed the euthanasia and how?

2. Did the person concerned obtain information on the method used in advance? If so, where and from whom?

3. Was it reasonable to expect that the administration of the euthanasia-inducing agent in question would result in death?

4. Who was present when euthanasia was performed? Please supply names, addresses, and telephone numbers.

*   *   *

4. Dillmann, van der Wal, and van Delden, "Euthanasia in the Netherlands," 3.

5. Dillmann, van der Wal, and van Delden, "Euthanasia in the Netherlands," 2.

6. Paul J. van der Maas, Johannes J. M. van Delden, Loes Pijnenborg, "Euthanasia and other Medical Decisions Concerning the End of Life: An Investigation Performed upon Request of the Commission of Inquiry into the Medical Practice Concerning Euthanasia," published in full in English as a special issue of *Health Policy* 22, nos. 1 and 2 (1992), and, with Caspar W. N. Looman, in summary in *The Lancet* 338 (Sept. 14, 1991): 669–674.

7. Gerrit van der Wal, "Euthanasie en hulp bij zelfdoding door huisartsen," Academisch Proefschrift, Vrije Universiteit Amsterdam (Rotterdam: WYT Uitgeefgroep, 1992), English summary available.

8. Loes Pijnenborg, Paul J. van der Maas, Johannes J. M. van Delden, and Caspar W. N. Looman, "Life-Terminating Acts without Explicit Request of Patient," *The Lancet* 341 (May 8, 1993): 1196–99.

9. The study is being conducted by John Poole and John Griffiths.

10. The study is being conducted by Chris Carlucci and Gerrit Kimsma.

11. Richard Fenigsen, "A Case Against Dutch Euthanasia," *Hastings Center Report* 19 (1989): 22–30.

12. Els Borst-Eilers, M.D., paper delivered at the conference "To Treat or Not to Treat? Dilemmas Posed by the Hopelessly Ill," Royal Society of Edinburgh, Feb. 23–24, 1993. The 1989 figure had been 81 percent. Dr. Borst explains that since about 20 percent of the Dutch population is opposed to euthanasia on religious grounds, future polls will probably remain at about 80 percent.

13. Incorporated in the English summary in van der Maas et al., "Euthanasia and Other Medical Decisions," 671.

14. Pijnenborg, van der Maas, van Delden, and Looman, "Life-terminating Acts without Explicit Request of Patient," 1196.

15. Henk A. M. J. ten Have and Jos V. M. Welie, "Euthanasia: Normal Medical Practice?" *The Hastings Center Report* 22 (March–April 1992): 34–38.

16. The most reliable account is Pieter J. J. Sauer, "Ethical Decisions in Neonatal Intensive Care Units: The Dutch Experience," *Pediatrics* 90 (November 1992): 729–732.

17. Van der Wal, English summary, 150.

18. J. K. M. Gevers, "Legislation on Euthanasia: Recent Developments in the Netherlands," *Journal of Medical Ethics* 18 (1992): 138–141.

19. Carlos F. Gomez, *Regulating Death: Euthanasia and the Case of the Netherlands* (New York: Free Press, 1991); also see the objections in a review of his book by Gary Seay, *American Philosophical Association Newsletter on Philosophy and Medicine* 92, no. 1 (Spring 1993): 89–93.

20. John Keown, "On Regulating Death," *The Hastings Center Report* 22 (March–April, 1992): 39–43.

7

Fiction as Forecast: Euthanasia in Alzheimer's Disease?

Should euthanasia be practiced for persons with advanced dementia? Although the issue of euthanasia is a topic of increasingly heated social debate, already tending to polarize those who support it as voluntary "aid-in-dying" and those who reject it as medical "killing," what is said about active euthanasia on *both* sides is severely challenged by the question of euthanasia in Alzheimer's disease. Whether euthanasia may or should be practiced in Alzheimer's is not an easy moral or social-policy question to answer, as I shall try to show, even if one finds the answers to moral and policy questions about euthanasia comparatively simple in other contexts.

The question of euthanasia in Alzheimer's is also a question with very broad consequences. There are an estimated 1.5 million severely demented persons in the United States, so incapacitated that others must care for them continually, and another 1 to 5 million persons with mild or moderate dementia.[1] While there are some seventy conditions that can cause dementia, Alzheimer's is by far the most prevalent, and it is the variety I shall be considering exclusively here. Alzheimer's is a degenerative disorder; its progression cannot be arrested, although improvements in care and coping skills may make a considerable difference in the patient's circumstances, especially early in the course of the disease, and supportive services may also make a considerable difference for the principal caregivers. There is no proven cure for Alzheimer's and no clearly effective treatment for any of its symptoms. The average duration of illness, from first onset of symptoms to death, is about eight years, though Alzheimer's can last up to twenty-five years.[2] While the patient with Alzheimer's may show some fluctuation in symptoms, the dementia is irreversible.

In showing why the question of euthanasia in Alzheimer's is so difficult to answer, I'd like to survey the three most prevalent arguments for euthanasia in general, the arguments from autonomy, from mercy, and from justice,[3] and show what is problematic about each. All three yield indeterminate answers. Although none of these conventional arguments *for* euthanasia seems to be effective in the

From R. Binstock, S. Post, and P. Whitehouse, eds., *Dementia and Aging: Ethics, Values, and Policy Choices* (Johns Hopkins University Press, 1992). Originally titled "Euthanasia in Alzheimer's Disease?" Copyright © 1992 by the Johns Hopkins University Press. Reprinted by permission of the publisher.

specific circumstances of Alzheimer's, the considerations they raise also fail to produce effective arguments *against* euthanasia. But a philosophically indeterminate position of this sort seems a luxury, given the literally millions of people potentially directly affected by social policies that might be formulated on the basis of such discussions. Given these inconclusive results, I then turn to look at what is usually the principal argument against euthanasia—the slippery slope argument—and find that it gives equally disturbing results. Finally, I look briefly at the question this situation poses: How can one formulate social policy in such a sensitive matter as this, when background philosophical considerations do not seem to prove much help?

What I shall be considering here is whether *active* euthanasia may be practiced on persons with advanced Alzheimer's—that is, direct killing, performed in the paradigmatic case by a physician as a medical procedure intended to produce death. It is without question the case that in terminal illness we already often practice what philosophers (but not doctors or the general public) call passive euthanasia: the withholding or withdrawal of treatment that would otherwise prolong life, thus "allowing" the patient to die. We also often practice a form of life curtailment involving the overadministration of morphine; in these cases, it is usually argued, the intention is to relieve pain, and the respiratory suppression that results in death is a foreseen but unintended consequence. While both of these may and do occur in Alzheimer's, I shall be considering neither here: I am concerned with whether directly produced death, produced because of the Alzheimer's rather than for other reasons, is morally warranted. To be sure, any discussion of the moral issues in euthanasia rejects the categorical argument that killing or causing the death of human beings is always wrong; pointing to practices often regarded as morally acceptable, including killing in self-defense, just war, abortion, and capital punishment, such a discussion presupposes that if any of these practices are morally permissible, it must be argued, not assumed, that killing in euthanasia cannot also be so.

The Philosophical Arguments Concerning Euthanasia as Applied to Advanced Dementia

The Argument from Autonomy

In contemporary defenses of active euthanasia, it is often argued that the right to determine the character and timing of one's own death, wherever doing so is possible, is a basic human right, grounded in fundamental rights of self-determination and autonomy generally. Such autonomy rights include all choices that are self-respecting only and do not seriously damage the interests or violate the rights of others, and certainly include, it is argued, rights of choice in matters so profound and intimately personal as deciding whether to continue to live or to die. On this view, a course of action one knowingly and voluntarily chooses, provided it does not harm others, is one to which a person has at least one and perhaps two sorts of rights: the negative right not to be interfered with in the performance of the action and, perhaps in addition, the positive right to be aided in or provided with means for accomplishing the action. Of course, there may be grounds for interference with exercise of this right, either when it is chosen in an irrational, impaired way or when the interests of other parties would be jeopardized (say, those of minor children who would be left unsupported), but these circumstances are typically irrelevant in choices concerning euthanasia in Alzheimer's. On the argument from autonomy, the patient who knowingly and voluntarily elects death in preference to a medical situation such as Alzheimer's ought not be interrupted in any attempt to commit suicide and may even have claim to positive aid in physician-assisted suicide or physician-performed euthanasia. By and large, suicide by the Alzheimer's patient is possible only just after diagnosis or in the comparatively early stages of the disease, when he or she is still able to form and act on a plan and is likely to have access to means of suicide; active euthanasia could of course be performed at any point, although the issue I wish to address here is euthanasia in the late stages of the disease.

But is it meaningful at all to speak of autonomous choice in Alzheimer's? Can euthanasia be voluntary, the product of informed, free choice, in Alzheimer's? Given that Alzheimer's eventually involves complete deterioration of all cognitive skills, including the capacity to conceptualize, predict, understand information, deliberate about a matter, reason, or perform any sort of planning, it would seem that an Alzheimer's patient, at least in the advanced stages of dementia, could hardly *choose* euthanasia. After all, for such a choice to be fully enough informed to count as voluntary, the person must be able to understand not only the medical procedures actually used to produce death, but also the abstract notion of the transition from life to death. But although an advanced Alzheimer's patient may exhibit some behavior that looks like choosing in certain simple contexts—using a red crayon rather than a green one when coloring, for example, or sitting down or getting up from a chair— we do not suppose that these actions involve choice in any robust way or that they are anything more than simple responses to stimuli. We certainly do not think that such actions provide real evidence of abstract choice.

On the other hand, it would seem that choices of euthanasia governing the advanced Alzheimer's patient must be recognized as voluntary if they are made by the person while still competent and recorded in an advance-directive document such as a living will. The living will provides legally valid evidence (in most U.S. states) of a person's choices about treatment after she becomes incompetent. (The feminine pronoun reflects the fact that, because women live longer, most Alzheimer's patients are female.) To be sure, currently in the United States living-will declarations cannot contain provisions concerning active euthanasia; by contrast, in the Netherlands, where euthanasia is legally tolerated, at least one standard living will form does contain a provision permitting the request of active euthanasia, and I can imagine legislation permitting such choices in this country, too. Of course, the living will brings with it various problems, among them that the signer of it may not correctly foresee the range of medical problems to occur in her future, that one may fluctuate in and out of competence and hence in and out of being subject to the provisions of one's own living will, or that one can revoke one's own living will after becoming no longer competent but cannot then later re-execute it. Nevertheless, the living will, which functions by recognizing precedent autonomy, is designed to expand the range of choices a person can make about her own care: It gives legal force to choices that will take effect after that person is no longer currently capable of making any choice at all. If that person knew she might develop Alzheimer's and chose— with full information, and perfectly voluntarily—to request euthanasia should that occur, her choice ought to be respected.

But does the living will actually represent a voluntary choice by the Alzheimer's patient? After all, the person whom this choice now concerns—the one perhaps to be put to death as a result of this choice, if euthanasia has been requested—can no longer understand the choice or reenact making it; indeed, the severely demented person cannot even remember making this profoundly important choice. After all, the choice was made by a long-distant version of herself, whom she no longer even remembers being. Can we actually say that *she* made this choice? Because only choices resulting in earlier death by withholding or withdrawing treatment are currently recognized in the United States, but not choices employing active euthanasia, and because physicians, family members, payors, and others rarely object to choices to withhold or withdraw in severe dementia, the philosophical issue of the legitimacy of advance directives is rarely raised. Nevertheless, the same issue seems to become much more pressing in the case of a highly contentious provision such as a request for active euthanasia. Is it plausible to say that this person, the one who is now severely demented and has no awareness of her previous advance directive, knowingly and voluntarily requests to be killed? If it is not plausible, is there convincing reason for recognizing such a choice?

But then, can we actually say that she did not make this choice? It was her hand that put the pen to the paper, signing it; it was she who discussed it with her lawyer and relatives; it was she who was the legal agent employing a recognized legal instrument for effecting her own choice concerning the very circumstance in which she now finds herself. Choice is *always* choice about one's own future, though the time gap between present and future may be longer or shorter and the conditions more or less different. Only by adopting a Humean or Parfitean account of the self, in which there is no genuine continuity of person over time but only a set of overlapping bundles or person-stages, can we so radically divorce the present patient from her own former self as to say it is not *her* choice. She has changed, and changed dramatically, to be sure, but it is still she, we are inclined to say, who wrote the directive. After all, if it wasn't she who executed the directive, what other person did it?

The difference between these two conceptions is what Ronald Dworkin describes as the difference in conceiving of the Alzheimer's patient as "a demented person" or as "a person who has become demented."[4] If we employ the former view, we give primary weight to current choices, allowing them to supersede prior ones (as, for example, in revoking a living will); on the latter, we give primary weight to the choices of the previously undemented person. Dworkin favors recognizing precedent rather than current autonomy in severe dementia, primarily because the value of autonomy lies in the way "autonomy makes each of us responsible for shaping his own life according to some coherent and distinctive sense of character, conviction, and interests"[5]; what is essential is the integrity of a person's life plan. This may be a reasonable policy proposal, but it does not really answer the philosophical question: Ought we recognize precedent autonomy in these extreme cases where the agent can no longer recognize her former self, or in this situation is autonomy, if possible at all, always necessarily contemporary?

Can euthanasia in advanced Alzheimer's be voluntary? This, as I said, is not an easy question to answer, and even the sophisticated legal device of the living will, intended to cover circumstances of later incompetence precisely such as these, does not decide the philosophical question.

The Argument from Mercy

Even though it is not clear whether euthanasia in advanced Alzheimer's can be voluntary, can it nevertheless be a gesture of mercy? Traditional arguments for euthanasia have often been arguments from mercy: that euthanasia is morally permissible when it is the only effective way to relieve a patient's pain or suffering and to spare the patient an otherwise agonizing death. Thus, regardless of whether euthanasia in advanced Alzheimer's can be voluntary, it is still open to question whether it might be legitimized, or perhaps even morally mandated, on grounds of mercy. This is not a question of the sufferings of others, especially family members who serve as principal caregivers, but of the sufferings of the Alzheimer's victim herself.

After all, although the early Alzheimer's patient can often still function fairly well, it is a long road downhill, and the advanced Alzheimer's patient's sufferings seem to be extreme. She loses her capacities for effective function in the world; she is increasingly bewildered by her circumstances; and she loses her capacity for interaction with family and friends, even those closest to her. She cannot read, think, play any game, or converse with anyone; and she cannot, as the traditional stereotype of benign old age would have it, sit in a rocking chair sifting through her memories of youth. Hers is a world without meaning, without purpose or project, without affectional ties. This is the condition the Dutch call *ontluistering,* the "effacement" or complete eclipse of human personality, and for the Dutch, *ontluistering,* rather than pain, is a primary reason for choices of euthanasia. Worse still, in those forms of Alzheimer's that involve paranoid delusions, the patient's experience may be peopled with creatures and situations of horrendously threatening sorts, but with patterns she cannot predict and with terms she cannot understand well enough to escape or accept. In some cases, dementia may be a kind of ongoing nightmare, full of shadows and threats that do not vanish when one wakes. Thus, it looks as though euthanasia in advanced Alzheimer's might be warranted on grounds of mercy, whether or not it is voluntarily requested, because the mental suffering it involves may be so great.

But does the argument from mercy really succeed in Alzheimer's? We are often reluctant to speak of suffering where there is no self-aware subject of experiences; if this is so, the Alzheimer's victim cannot be said to be suffering. True, as an organism with a nervous system, the Alzheimer's victim, like other persons and also like animals, can of course feel pain, but pain is not to be confused with the distinctive kind of suffering the loss of cognitive function is said to produce. But does it? Does a person whose life is void of meaningful activity or important interpersonal contact thereby *suffer?* Or is it rather that her sensorium merely includes isolated, unconnected, uninterpreted sensory experiences but no cognitive awareness or experience of what she is missing? But if she had no awareness of what she is missing, she cannot suffer, anymore than one's pet dog experiences suffering from being unable to talk or do arithmetic or from being unable to plan for its own future. Even the demented patient with paranoid delusions, if she no longer has any sense of self, cannot suffer, it would seem, because there is no self there to whom these awful experiences happen; they occur, but in a mental void. But if these things are true and we take the having of a sense of self—that self-awareness often counted as distinctively human and as presupposed by the very notion of "person"—as prerequisite for suffering, then as the deterioration of Alzheimer's advances, the potential for suffering decreases. Paradoxically, it might seem, the greater the patient's losses, the weaker her claim to euthanasia on grounds of mercy.

The traditional argument for euthanasia on grounds of mercy points to physical pain and emotional suffering, but the former is irrelevant in the case of Alzheimer's and it is not clear whether the latter can occur. It is of course true that an Alzheimer's patient might have some untreatable coexisting medical condition about which the question of euthanasia because of intractable pain might be raised, but then this is not a question of euthanasia because of Alzheimer's. It would have only tangential bearing on the million persons with severe Alzheimer's; the two to three million more with milder, though progressive, Alzheimer's; and, indeed, the rest of us, who, if we live to age eighty-five, stand a one in four chance of developing it. But this just raises the question all over again: do we not fear developing Alzheimer's because we do not want to suffer from it?

The Issue of Justice

It is also often popularly argued that the expenditure of funds to care for Alzheimer's victims is a "waste." This is a form of distributive argument; it is based on the assumption that there are other more defensible distributions of health care and that it would be more just to allocate these resources to other parties with stronger claims to them than to have them consumed by Alzheimer's patients who are already severely demented and will never recover. While the cruder forms of the popular argument rarely spell out what distributive arrangement ought to be considered more just, what sorts of claims to resources would outweigh those of Alzheimer's patients, or what assurances of actual redistribution would need to be made, this argument nevertheless often seems to exert considerable intuitive pull: there is something unjust, it is said, about committing large amounts of resources to people who are "already gone" while denying help to others in current need.

Although it is usually considered a distinct argument, this appeal to justice nevertheless trades on the claims involved in the issues already discussed, those of autonomy and mercy. After all, justice in the distribution of resources presupposes that potential claimants to these resources would actually wish to have them or that the receipt of them would actually count as a benefit. If a prospective claimant would not want the resources and they would not be a benefit to him or her, then a distributive scheme allocating resources to this party is unjust if there are other claimants who would want the resources and for whom they would be a benefit. Like the proverbial "dog in the manger," there is no justice in allocating scarce resources to a party who cannot use them; similarly, there is no justice in allocating them to a party who does not want them. Yet given the indeterminate results of the preceding sketches of the issues of choice and mercy, it is by no means clear that Alzheimer's patients "want" the resources that might be allocated to them or that these resources would count as a "benefit."

It is important to note that this is not the same as the "useless eaters" argument advanced by the Nazis as grounds for the destruction of mentally retarded persons and others, though it would have been applied in some of the same cases. The "useless eaters" argument does not assert that the use of resources is not of benefit to the person in question; it asserts that this use of resources is not of benefit to others in the sense that the person in question is "useless" to society. There is no issue in the current question about whether the Alzheimer's patient is "useful" to others, but instead about whether the resources are useful to him or her. Although the two arguments are easily confused, in the background of the current discussion about justice in Alzheimer's there is the assumption that whether or not Alzheimer's patients are "useful" to others or to society in general, society is—and should be— willing to provide care that is useful to the patients themselves.

But this then returns us to the problem. Does the Alzheimer's patient want the resources, and are they a benefit to her? Even if claims on her behalf are pressed by a surrogate, can these claims reflect either substituted judgment or any form of best-interests test? Clearly, the more advanced the deteriorative process, the less plausible it is to speak of contemporary choice in wanting resources: the severely demented patient cannot, presumably, understand any other arrangement of things, nor can she conceptualize the distributive schema itself or the allocations it makes to her in competition with others. Nor, presumably, can the severely demented patient in any conscious sense "want" the continuing life that medical treatment and maintenance care make possible, though of course her bodily processes may continue to operate in the normal, life-continuing way; as we said, this person can no longer have any conception of what life is or of the transition from life to death. Of course, the patient may have had a vigorous conception of all these things prior to the onset of serious disease and may have recorded her wishes in a living will or other document; in this sense, the now-demented person still may "want" access to resources chosen earlier. She can also react favorably to situations she experiences as pleasant and react negatively to those that involve discomfort or pain; in this sense, she can "want" allocations of resources that provide her with, say, foods she prefers, a more comfortable bed, better-fitting clothing (but not more stylish clothing, since appreciating style requires cognitive abilities), and so on. But she can neither conceptualize these wants nor, except by expressions of pleasure or displeasure, articulate them.

Can the severely demented patient benefit from the allocation of resources to her care, including medical treatment, maintenance care, and whatever else is necessary to keep her alive? The answer here is clearly dependent on the argument considered earlier about mercy, and hence we cannot arrive at any clearer answer. Does she benefit from remaining alive, or would she be better off dead? There is quite a lively discussion in the philosophic and economic literature about the value of life, and how one can weigh this against death,[6] but it is not a discussion that proves decisive in the present case. Many or most of the features that are usually said to make life worth living are absent in advanced dementia—for example, the possibilities of enjoying human interaction, planning and undertaking projects, serving causes, having religious and aesthetic experience, and perhaps (as Aristotle would identify the highest good) rational contemplation. With no surviving conceptual skills or even sense of self, it is not clear that continuing life is a continuing good, and hence not clear that allocations that make continuing life possible are really a benefit after all. Nor, however, is it clear that they are not.

What, then, is a fair distribution of resources with respect to people with Alzheimer's? It is not clear that we can even begin to answer this question, because we cannot identify either what Alzheimer's patients want or what would benefit them. Furthermore, we cannot identify wants and benefits either on subjective grounds or on objective, quality-of-life ones: we cannot approximate the severely demented person's point of view, and we cannot assess the quality of her life. Of course, to identify what various claimants want and what would be of benefit to them is not all that is involved in settling distributive issues, since many other matters (for instance, desert, prior claims, rectification) are involved; but one cannot even get off the ground in justifying a given distributive scheme without knowing whether the various claimants to the resources involved actually want and/or would benefit from them. Discussions of distributive justice uniformly assume that the various competing claimants involved all want and would benefit from the resource in question— that is, that they are all appropriately considered *claimants*—but in the case of Alzheimer's no such thing is clear. Because the amount of resources involved in the issue of Alzheimer's is immense, the question of justice is an enormous one, and to say that we simply cannot resolve it on adequate philosophical grounds is no trivial matter.

Developing Policy Concerning Euthanasia in Alzheimer's

Of course, positions on the issue of justice are ultimately expressed in social policy, which puts into practice one or another distributive scheme, allocating resources to or away from various claimants or apparent claimants for them. Needless to say, the development of social policy in the matter of allocating resources in Alzheimer's is a matter with such high stakes that it can hardly wait for philosophers to sift through these questions, especially when there is no indication that they will reach a uniform, workable answer. In the absence of firm philosophical justification, then, what form should social policy take in expressing these issues of justice?

To simplify a huge range of possibilities, there are three principal candidates for social policies distributing medical and supportive care in Alzheimer's:

1. do what is possible to maintain and supply medical and supportive treatment for Alzheimer's patients, though without heroics, until the end of their natural lives;

2. practice passive euthanasia on late-stage Alzheimer's patients: provide maintenance and support but not lifesaving medical treatment, and so allow these patients to die when infections or other potential fatal conditions arise; or
3. practice active euthanasia on late-stage Alzheimer's patients.

Current social policy, not at all well defined, wavers between alternatives 1 and 2, although 2 is never termed "euthanasia." It is 3 that raises the question under discussion here. In the absence of firm answers to the questions of choice and mercy, we must still answer the following question: Should we, or should we not, practice active euthanasia for Alzheimer's patients? To refuse to address this question is already to answer it, since current social policy prohibits active euthanasia, though permitting passive euthanasia, and to refuse to raise the question is to accept the current answer. It is not clear, however, that this answer is a defensible one. But perhaps there are still other ways of looking at the issue.

The View down the Slippery Slope

Another, more clearly consequentialist way of approaching the issue of euthanasia in Alzheimer's, or for that matter, any proposed social policy, is to take a look down the "slippery slope," that is, to examine the likely highly negative outcomes of introducing the policy. The slippery slope argument, as usually employed against euthanasia, predicts the spread of medical killing from a few sympathetic cases, genuinely dictated by the wishes of the patient or the demands of mercy, to more problematic medical cases, then to cases of expensive patients, then to politically undesirable cases, and finally to widespread holocaust. Regardless of whether the advanced Alzheimer's patient wants or would benefit from continuing life, it is argued, active euthanasia ought not be employed, for this would risk the spread of this practice to other persons who both want to remain alive and would benefit by doing so.

Slippery slope arguments trade on empirical claims about likely consequences, either direct causal results of a certain policy or consequences resulting from other forces affected by the precedents set by a policy. Much of the continuing argumentation about euthanasia involves trading claims about how far the slide would go and how broad the spread of the increasingly intolerable practice would be, and it very often cites catastrophic events such as the Holocaust as evidence for its claims. When these slippery slope arguments do so, they generally trade on assumptions about the evil motives of human beings and of physicians in particular, often making reference to the Nazi doctors and their increasing callousness about human experimentation and killing.

It is true that the Nazis' early T4 program began with medical "euthanasia" and that medical staff from this program were later transferred to the extermination camps; but this historical transition does not establish that any practice of euthanasia will always lead to holocaust or that human beings generally, or physicians in particular, are evil. There are apparent counterexamples: active euthanasia is practiced in contemporary Holland without evident abuse, and it was also apparently practiced (by recommending the hemlock) in ancient Greece.[7] However, while the empirical issues can hardly be settled here, it is reasonable to suppose that human beings generally—and physicians in particular—rapidly respond to incentives of various kinds, especially legal and financial ones.

If active euthanasia in advanced Alzheimer's were legal or legally tolerated in the United States, I think we can well imagine the rapid development of cost-saving social policies that would offer fairly strong incentives for physicians to recommend euthanasia in Alzheimer's, say, by reducing reimbursement for treating such persons, by limiting bed space for patients with this condition, or by reconceptualizing the practice as a humane, appropriate course of treatment in this condition. On the other hand, because any spread of such policies beyond advanced Alzheimer's would be rapidly challenged by other groups whose own interests might be threatened, I see no reason to assume that even if active euthanasia were permitted in some sympathetic cases in advanced Alzheimer's, involuntary euthanasia would inevitably spread to wholesale slaughter of the handicapped, the racially despised, or the politically rejected. Thus, although I do not think the broad form of slippery slope argument—which predicts the spread of euthanasia into widespread holocaust—is plausible, at least in the contemporary United States, I can nevertheless imagine the spread of active euthanasia in Alzheimer's from some few cases to a more general policy of comparatively routine use of euthanasia in advanced dementia, and will grant this limited version of the slippery slope claim here. Routine use of active euthanasia in advanced Alzheimer's might or might not involve solicitation of consent from family members—no doubt it often would, but in the same perfunctory way that consent for no-code orders is now often solicited. The point is that one can imagine euthanasia as a widespread, medically customary response to severe, irreversible dementia.

Suppose, then, that most or all severely demented, advanced Alzheimer's patients—all million and a half—were routinely euthanized, although this practice did not spread to any other category of patient. This is the view down the slippery slope, but the question is how we should assess the view we see. Would this be a bad thing? How are we to answer this question at all? We might try to assess the effects of such a policy on the persons involved, but given the difficulties already explored in considering issues of autonomy and mercy, it is not at all clear that this will be possible to do. We have no way of approximating a subjective assessment and no way of making an objective one either.[8] Nor can we determine whether this widespread practice would be just or unjust. Nevertheless, there is a way of approaching an answer, by looking down the slippery slope in a rather different way.

Doing so appropriates the Rawlsian device of the original position, in which rational self-interest maximizers who are behind the veil of ignorance and thus do not know their own personal characteristics agree to principles that will govern the society of which they are members.[9] However, while Rawls does not discuss health policy and does not use this device for direct policy formation, specific features of the circumstances allow it to be adopted in a rather natural way. This is made possible by the fact that, with respect to the possibility of becoming a patient with Alzheimer's, we are naturally in a kind of ''original position'' and behind the veil of ignorance: we know the general incidence of severe dementia—about 1 percent between ages sixty-five to seventy-four, rising to 7 percent between seventy-five and eighty-four, and to 25 percent for those eighty-five and over[10]—but as individuals we do not know whether we will be among those affected. This provides us with a natural way of considering what principles we would assent to, in seeking to protect our own self-interests, and hence what policies we would be willing to formulate. Thus, rather than speculate about the effects of such a policy on others, we can ask— that is, each of us can ask—whether our own worlds would be better ones for us if, should we become demented, our lives would be protected or would be terminated in euthanasia?

Clearly all the issues we have considered in reflecting on the arguments from autonomy, mercy, and justice reemerge here. However, because the slippery slope argument is essentially an argument from fear and each potential target of the policy may in principle share this fear, let us look down the slippery slope from the point of view of a single individual who might have such fears. Thus we can ask a more personal form of the question: Would *I* be more afraid, or less so, in a world that practiced active euthanasia on severely demented Alzheimer's patients? To what sort of policy would I, without knowing into which category I will eventually fall, consent?

Exactly what do I fear, then, in fearing euthanasia, if the slippery slope prediction comes true and I, like other Alzheimer's patients, may be killed? Assume that I have not previously executed a living will requesting euthanasia, or even that I have no living will indicating any treatment preferences at all. Euthanasia performed on me will be clearly nonvoluntary. This is the scene I can imagine:

Golden Harbor Nursing Home. Morning. The nurses' station in the hallway, then my room. A young doctor, wearing a standard white coat and stethoscope, but with steel-rimmed glasses and a slightly disordered crop of thick brown hair, flips quickly through my chart. He extracts a little plastic-coated chart labeled "Functional Criteria in Alzheimer's Disease" from his pocket, checks it, flips through the chart a little further. "I think it's time for Mrs. Battin," he says absently to the nurse, then moves to my room.

"Good morning, Mrs. Battin," he says cheerily, though he already knows I will not respond. "What day is it today?" I tell him a few words, though they are not days of the week. "Who is the President?" I tell him a few more words, though I do not name the current fellow, and the doctor makes notes in my chart. He does a variety of other tests, none of which I pass. He, or the other doctors like him, have done these tests every month for the past half year, and I never show any improvement. Now I have failed again. As he goes out I hear him mutter, "Yes, it's time." When the nurse comes in, she is equally cheerful. "So it's time, Mrs. Battin, is it?" She also knows that I do not understand. A phone call will be made to one of my children, explaining the situation and proposing a date; this child will phone the other one, and they will agree.

They will both fly to this city, where the Golden Harbor Nursing Home is; they will come here to see me for the last time. They do this even though they know I will not recognize them, and have not recognized them for some time. They will try once more to make conversation, though they know it is futile, because they do not know what else to do or how to relate to their mother. They will try to help me remember my husband, though I no longer can, and they will try to elicit even the tiniest fragment of memory. In between, they talk about the house and the arrange-

ments with the lawyer about the estate, though they do not seem to have any
particular interest in this—no, they are sad; I see a tear forming in the eyes of one of
them, they both grasp my withered old hands, stroke my cheek. They rub and caress
my hands and cheek as if they were trying to implant them forever in their own
memories. Now they are both crying. After a little while one, then the other, bends
over the bed to kiss me. "Goodbye, Mom," each of them finally says, and then
they stand and leave, looking back once or twice over their shoulders.

  The young doctor is there in the corridor. "Would you like to be with her?" he
asks. He notices their own age and the early symptoms of decline: One of them is
fifty-seven already, and the other almost sixty. One of them wavers a bit, but the
other says no. "She wouldn't know we were there anyway," he explains, but the
doctor understands why: They are not used to death, and it would be a difficult thing
for them to watch. There are a few papers to sign, but that is all; no one objects to
the procedure.

  The nurse has the syringe already filled for the doctor as he returns to the room,
and out of sheer habit she swabs the injection site with alcohol. I say a few more
miscellaneous words, and the nurse puts her hand gently on my forehead as the
doctor positions the syringe. I feel only a little prick, like so many injections I have
had before, and then after that the doctor leans over my chest with his stethoscope to
listen to the silence where the heartbeat had been.

So this is how it might go, in an ordinary nursing home, with an ordinary doctor,
with an ordinary old lady in the later stages of progressive dementia. If the predictions of the slippery slope are correct, this is how it might go in many nursing homes,
all over the country, with all sorts of doctors, with virtually all the 1.5 million
patients in the late, irreversible stages of Alzheimer's.

  And what are my fears, as a likely victim of this spread? Pain? Loss of dignity?
Being constricted by involuntary choice? The cursoriness of the visit from my
children? Having my life ended without my consent by a physician I don't even
know? But of course, I can have experienced none of these things, and indeed my
imagined account of these events is entirely misleading: I experienced no pain, nor
any loss of dignity; I could not make a choice nor know if my choices were being
countervened. I heard the doctor say "it's time," but had no way of understanding
what he meant. Although my children's visit was cursory, I did not recognize them
as my children. That this doctor was different from the previous one could not have
made any difference to me: I could not have known whether I had ever seen him
before. I did not know that I had passed or failed any tests, or even that they were
tests at all. What was my actual, direct experience in euthanasia? Life as usual until
the very end, except for a gentle hand on my forehead and a small needle-prick in my
vein. What we fear, in fearing the kind of widespread practice of euthanasia that the
slippery slope predicts, are all things we can now imagine but would not then
experience; in this sense, our most personal fears are completely unrealistic. This is
not the comparison between subjective and objective views of the events contem-
plated, but between two different forms of subjective view.

  What if, on the other hand, there were no euthanasia for severely demented
patients, and, as in option 1 such patients were provided full maintenance and
medical treatment?

Golden Harbor Nursing Home. Morning. Same year as before, then a year later, then sometime during the following year, then at various intervals after that. The young doctor in the corridor, but a different one each time. In the first episode my activities are reassigned to a group for more demented patients, and I now spend the days sitting vacantly at a table with crayons and coloring books in a continuously monitored dayroom; in the second, I am treated for a pneumonia; in the third, I am put in restraints in a day chair; in the fourth, treated for another pneumonia and also decubiti from prolonged sitting; in the fifth, I am spoon-fed. Perhaps somewhere in the series I develop paranoid delusions or undergo episodes of random aggressive behavior. By the end of the series, some ten or twelve years later, I cannot communicate at all or walk or get out of bed or feed myself or bathe or control my bladder or bowels. My children have still made a dutiful point of coming to visit me from their respective cities at least once a year, and they still pay the bills, but now they do so with a sense of sullen resignation. The end finally comes with a cardiac arrest, probably about 3:00 A.M., but it is not noticed until the first nursing round in the morning.

So this is how it might be in an ordinary nursing home, with an ordinary string of doctors, for an ordinary old lady with Alzheimer's. What is there to fear in this scenario? The deterioration I do not notice, since I cannot remember myself as I was nor compare previous stages to this one, nor do I recognize my children at their many visits. But I do experience some new things: I am feverish with infections, I feel the discomfort of the bedsores and, if they are not treated properly, smell their bad odor; I have foods put into my mouth, some of which I like but some I do not; I cannot move my arms out of the restraints on my day chair; I feel the irritation of sitting sometimes for hours in a diaper soiled with urine or feces. If there is any struggle at the end, I, no doubt like many of the other million and a half Alzheimer's patients in the same condition, and indeed, the rest of the several million who will soon reach this condition, am alone while it happens. But it makes no difference; this nursing home, like most, does not perform resuscitation.

Is this a better scenario or a worse one than the scenario involving active nonvoluntary euthanasia? Clearly the effects on my children are worse, since they have had no genuine contact with me for years but continue to make their annual visits and to pay the bills; they are no longer sad, but resigned and sullen. Is it better for me? I have been alive for all these years; but I can think of no compelling reason to say I would not have been better off dead—that is, without any experience at all. Of course, there have been positive experiences—a shaft of sunlight warming my cheek through the slats of the venetian blind in my window, well-meaning hugs now and then from an indefatigable nursing staff or from visitors I do not recognize—but there are also the diapers, the restraints, the bedsores, and the episodes of illness and infection that I cannot understand but for which I am treated. If my claim to care under distributive scarcity rests on the assumption that I want this continuing life or that it is a benefit to me, is my claim really secure?

But what about the apparent compromise position, 2? This is the position that represents an increasingly pervasive policy today: to take advantage of intercurrent infections or illnesses and, by refraining from providing treatment, let the patient die. This is the compromise position favoring passive euthanasia (though it is rarely called that), which rejects both indefinite extension of life and active termination. What would it be like, and could I fear it? The scene at Golden Harbor will be the same as before, except that various young doctors will not order treatment for various infections or illnesses, and I will survive a few of these, though with difficulty, until finally one of them kills me. My children will be summoned hastily, or perhaps after the fact, but will have had no general sense of where in the overall downhill course of my Alzheimer's disease my death might occur, whether a few years earlier or perhaps a lot of years later. My sensory experiences, though shorter, will have been in one way worse than the second series just outlined—I will have endured at least one or perhaps several episodes of illness without treatment, or with only whatever symptomatic control is possible consistent with letting the disease take its course. The difference between alternative 3 (active euthanasia), and this one, 2 (passive euthanasia), is that in the former the doctor killed me; in the latter, it is a disease that does the killing. When the doctor killed me, my only experience was a gentle hand and a tiny needle-prick; in alternative 2, I am "allowed to die," and this necessarily occurs only at the conclusion of a period in which I am mortally ill.

Why then should I fear the slippery slope, or let it count as a persuasive argument against euthanasia? Even if we grant that the spread that this argument predicts would actually occur and some 1.5 million currently institutionalized Alzheimer's patients would be medically killed, as well as the rest of the several million whose disease eventually progresses and in addition all new cases developing, it is not clear that *from the point of view of each of them* this would be a bad thing. Figures in the millions, of course, recall the appalling butchery of the Holocaust, but that killing, seen from the points of view of each of those victims, was a catastrophically bad thing. After all, the victims of the Holocaust wanted to stay alive, in the sense discussed earlier, and would clearly have benefited from doing so. But the victims of Alzheimer's are different. After all, their points of view will be exactly like my own, accurately and not unrealistically imagined, if I should develop Alzheimer's—a point of view without a sense of self, without cognitive capacities for comparing one's past and present circumstances, without memory, without the ability to understand or predict death, and with only the capacity for current sensation. As a rational self-interest maximizer who does not yet know whether I will or will not develop Alzheimer's, can I fear euthanasia, if this is what my future may hold? Clearly the answer is no.

Of course, there may be aspects of euthanasia I could fear—for instance, that the doctor would be hasty or irresponsible in conducting the tests of functional capacity, that the nurse would be rough, that the nursing home would be callous in contacting my children. To be sure, medical personnel and institutions can be hasty, rough, and callous in all sorts of situations, but there is no special incentive for acting in this way in the case of euthanasia; on the contrary, given special legal protections, the presence of witnesses, and so on, one might expect incentives to run the other way. If I have no reason to fear euthanasia in principle and no reason to think that in practice it would be cruelly conducted, there seems to be no basis for responding to the slippery slope argument at all. Generalizing thus from my own imagined single case behind my current veil of ignorance to that of severely demented persons generally, it looks, on the contrary, as though alternative 3, a world of routine active euthanasia, rather than passive euthanasia or continuing treatment, would better protect my self-interest. Hence, it is the policy to which I would agree.

Developing Social Policy

Philosophical reflection seems to produce no compelling argument against euthanasia in advanced Alzheimer's and no sound reason why we should fear it. Should we then, as a matter of social policy, practice nonvoluntary active euthanasia on advanced Alzheimer's patients, developing a set of guidelines for functional status that would serve to determine the appropriate timing—guidelines that the physician could, like the young doctor in the Golden Harbor Nursing Home, carry around in his pocket on a little laminated card? If this seems a disturbing suggestion, reopening all the fears the slippery slope points to, it is important to be clear about what the problem is.

The problem in developing policy, I think, arises from the difference in the perceptions the public is likely to have of this issue and what philosophic reflection produces. Ordinary—that is, precritical, nonreflective, nonphilosophical—perceptions of the prospect of nonvoluntary euthanasia are likely to take the form in which my little scenarios have been described here; it is the way most of us see this issue most of the time. We tend to see the issue from the point of view of a conscious, self-aware person (ourselves now) capable of remembering and comparing circumstances and engaging in human relationships, not from the point of view of those persons actually affected by the practice, namely, those persons who are severely demented (ourselves in a possible future). In reflecting on the nature of euthanasia and the possibility of the slippery slope, we do not readily assume the perspective of the persons most directly affected, but rather our own *current* view. This is why the little imagined descriptions presented earlier are so misleading: they presuppose the wrong point of view. They are fictions in the fullest sense, even though they purport to describe a possible future. The imaginary account of euthanasia in the Golden Harbor Nursing Home involves a narrated personal experience— the doctor enters *my* room, looks at *my* chart, asks *me* questions that provide a diagnostic test, listens to the garbled answers *I* tell him, prepares to inject the euthanaticum into *my* vein. This little story is narrated in a temporal sequence as seen from an individual point of view, that of the self to whom it would happen; but of course this is a misleading description of the experience of a severely demented person. This is not what will happen to me, not because it will not happen, but because if I am severely demented, it cannot happen *to me*.

Although imaginary narratives of this sort—developed as a way of employing a natural version of the Rawlsian device for selecting principles and at the same time as a way of looking down the slippery slope—are misleading in one way, they are enormously useful in another. For they also provide a way of foreseeing what problems certain social policies might cause. In this sense, fiction serves as forecast. If it is correct that, as ordinary human beings, not philosophers, we are more likely to view the prospect of widespread involuntary euthanasia from our own current perspective than from the perspective of ourselves in the future, a policy permitting involuntary euthanasia of millions of advanced Alzheimer's victims might well produce considerable anxiety, even anguish, for most of us, depending on how these stories are interpreted. Of course, it is anxiety to persons *before,* though not after, they contract Alzheimer's; but it is still a kind of anxiety to be considered in developing social policy. Indeed, anxiety before, rather than after, developing advanced Alzheimer's is the only kind of anxiety that can be experienced, insofar as it is anxiety about what will happen in the future to oneself and hence presupposes the cognitive capacity both to anticipate the future and to entertain a conception of oneself.

However, philosophic reflection can also produce anxiety of another sort for possible future Alzheimer's patients: the anxiety of recognizing that the prevailing policies 1 and 2, favoring continuing treatment or allowing to die, are really much less defensible than they may seem. The anxiety results from knowing that these policies are unlikely to change, and that if one does develop Alzheimer's, these indefensible policies will govern how one is treated. Furthermore, this anxiety is compounded by knowing that once one is in the circumstances in question, one can no longer do anything to change them and can no longer protect oneself from being governed by them, say, by executing a directive stipulating exactly how one wishes to be treated.

Thus, in thinking about social policy and on what basis it is to be formulated, we are faced with two kinds of anxiety: that produced by ordinary, unreflective attitudes about euthanasia in Alzheimer's, and that resulting from considered, philosophical reflection at odds with the ordinary view. These are two forms of subjective view, as I've mentioned earlier, not a subjective and an objective one, and neither has clear pride of place. The real question here is whether social policy ought to be formulated on the basis of one rather than the other, and if so, which one—for they will produce very different policies indeed. Basing policy on the ordinary view will be a vote for the status quo; basing it on the considered, philosophical view will support policies endorsing nonvoluntary active euthanasia in advanced dementia of advanced Alzheimer's patients.

Permitting active euthanasia of advanced Alzheimer's patients only in conjunction with an antecedently executed living will or personal directive voluntarily requesting it might seem to be the best policy compromise—and indeed, realistically speaking, I think it is.[11] Such a compromise might seem to protect against unreflective fears of nonvoluntary euthanasia, but also protect those who make antecedent choices on more philosophical grounds. But a further thought-experiment—another sort of fiction—might persuade us that this compromise is not a fully adequate one.

> Suppose there were a simple medical device, based on triple technology of the timed-release capsule, the subdermal contraceptive implant, and a painless, quick-acting euthanasia drug developed in the Netherlands. The device is called a "delayed-onset euthanatic implant." Anybody newly diagnosed with Alzheimer's disease (or any other long-term, degenerative, ultimately fatal disease), while still lucid and competent, can request one. Positioned painlessly and invisibly just below the surface of the skin inside the upper arm, the implant is designed to release its lethal drug instantaneously after a designated delay—say, two or three years, or whatever the patient requesting the implant stipulates. The implant can be easily

removed and there are full legal guarantees, rigorously observed in practice, that a patient can have it removed at any time, for any reason, with no delay. If it is removed there are no aftereffects. But if the implant is not removed, it will release the euthanaticum after the designated delay—without further warning, without pain or discomfort, and without requiring activation of any sort. It will just go off, and like an instantly fatal but painfree heart attack, that will be the end.

Does this further fiction provide an answer to the question about public policy in a way that the earlier fictions did not? To be sure, it invites worries about surreptitious or forced implantation of such capsules, but coercion aside (let us assume for the sake of this thought-experiment that the fully voluntary character of the patient's original choice can be protected), does this thought-experiment provide insight into what the desiderata of public policy must be, and why proposals like reliance on living wills or other advance directives are an only partly adequate compromise? The delayed-release mechanism succeeds in doing three distinct things, which could not be jointly accomplished in any of the previous scenarios: it permits the autonomously choosing early Alzheimer's patient who wishes to avoid late-stage Alzheimer's to bring about her own death; it avoids having others kill the patient by means of nonvoluntary or involuntary euthanasia after she is no longer competent; and it does not force her to waste "good" life during the phases where there are still lucid intervals by having to commit suicide, if she wishes, while it is still possible to do so. When the patient has the implant put in place, she thus sets in motion the causal train that will bring about her death long before she reaches the feared end-stages of the disease, but in choosing a delayed-release implant, she also provides herself with the entire designated delay—two or three years, in this example—in which to change her mind. Thus, this is a form of euthanasia which, unlike others, is reversible: if she does change her mind after she has had the implant installed, she simply has it removed and it has no further effect; she presumably goes on to live through the full course of the disease. After all, she may have discovered, during the lucid periods interspersed with confusion and memory loss, that Alzheimer's is not so bad, and that she would rather be alive with this condition than avoid it by death. Or, in reflecting on her choice after she has had the capsule implanted, she may have come to feel that it provides her enormous comfort to know that she will not have to endure the end-stages of the diseases, and that, in addition, it is a huge relief to know that she does not have to rely on family, physicians, or caretakers to help her avoid this. If she does not have the implant removed, it will release the euthanaticum after the designated interval, but by this time her Alzheimer's will be so far advanced that she will not only no longer recognize specific persons or be aware of her surroundings, but she will no longer remember about the implant. She cannot worry about oncoming death (nor, for that matter, look forward to it), and her experience will be little different from having, say, a fatal, completely unexpected heart attack, except that it will involve no prodromal symptoms, no current alarm, and no pain. Indeed, her experience is little different than that she would have had in the Golden Harbor Nursing Home, except that it would not involve the physician, the nurse, or her children in any direct, decision-making way. Though she no longer knows it is coming, her death is the result of her own doing, not theirs.

What this thought-experiment illuminates, I think, is the way in which both

living wills and other advance directives (though I think them the only realistic
policy alternatives available), still displace actual decision-making about timing and
implementation onto persons other than the patient, even though what is to be
effected is the *patient's* original choice. They may masquerade as instruments of the
patient's choice, but do not fully serve this purpose. The implant, in contrast,
permits direct choice, antecedently made but which can be revised later on. This
may do a better job than living wills of both taking account of the two sorts of
subjective view we entertain in facing possible futures with Alzheimer's—the fictions we create now in imagining what those futures might be like, and the philosophic reflections that lead us to see what is wrong with our fictions—and at the
same time protecting against the erosions of choice that we fear.

Notes

I'd like to thank Virgil Aldrich, Leslie Francis, and Brooke Hopkins for discussion of this
chapter.

1. Figures from Office of Technology Assessment, *Losing a Million Minds: Confronting
the Tragedy of Alzheimer's Disease and Other Dementias* (Washington, D.C.: Government
Printing Office, 1987).

2. Ibid., Congressional Summary, 20. Dispute currently surrounds the efficacy of Tac-
rine in slowing memory loss; there are now some reports of possibly effective diagnostic skin
tests for Alzheimer's disease.

3. See "Euthanasia: The Fundamental Issues," chapter 5 in this volume, for a discussion
of this typology.

4. Ronald Dworkin, "Autonomy and the Demented Self," *The Milbank Quarterly,* 64,
suppl. 2 (1986): 4.

5. Ibid., 8.

6. For two notable examples, see, for example, Anthony L. Brueckner and John Martin
Fischer, "Why Is Death Bad?" and Dan W. Brock, "The Value of Prolonging Human Life,"
both in *Philosophical Studies* 50 (1986).

7. The Hippocratic Oath objects to what was apparently common practice. For discussion
and references, see M. Pabst Battin, *Ethical Issues in Suicide* (New York: Prentice-Hall,
1982), 22, n. 59.

8. See Thomas Nagel, *The View from Nowhere* (New York: Oxford University Press,
1986), especially chap. 11, for a discussion of subjective and objective views about death.

9. John Rawls, *A Theory of Justice* (Cambridge, Mass.: Harvard University Press, 1971).

10. Office of Technology Assessment, *Losing a Million Minds*, Congressional Summary,
9. The figures are for all forms of severe dementia.

11. See, however, Leslie Pickering Francis, "Advance Directives for Voluntary Euthanasia: A Volatile Combination?" *The Journal of Medicine and Philosophy* 18 (June 1993):
297–322, for a lucid exploration of the ways in which the combination of advance directives
with active euthanasia may exacerbate the difficulties with each.

8

Voluntary Euthanasia
and the Risks of Abuse

In the quite volatile public debates over the legalization of voluntary active euthanasia and physician-assisted suicide in the United States, much has been made of the
risk of abuse. Indeed, it was probably fears of abuse that contributed more than any
other single factor to the 1991 defeat of the United States' first ballot test of legalizing
euthanasia, the state of Washington's Initiative 119 followed a year later by California's Proposition 161—despite prior state and national polls in both cases suggesting
the measures would pass. Opponents of Initiative 119 and Proposition 161, which
would have legalized physician-performed euthanasia or physician-provided aid in
suicide only when voluntarily requested by competent terminally ill patients with
less than six months to live, variously claimed that the legislation would encourage
greedy family members to pressure patients into choosing death, that unscrupulous
physicians would kill patients who became unattractive to treat, that cost-cutting
pressures from hospitals, insurers, and other institutions would force patients into
death, and that race-, age-, and handicap-prejudice would take an especial toll
among vulnerable groups.

These risk-of-abuse arguments, also known as slippery slope or wedge arguments, were often fortified with claims about abuse in the Netherlands, the one
country that currently openly permits active euthanasia.

Nor has the discussion ceased with the defeat of 119 and 161. On the contrary,
many observers are predicting that euthanasia will become *the* social issue of the
next decade. If so, claims about the possibilities of abuse are likely to continue to
play a very major role. Nor are they trivial: most slippery slope arguments predict
abuse on a quite broad scale, and the more flamboyant of them warn against complete moral holocaust.

While these warnings of abuse seem characteristically both alarmist and unclear,
I think we must take them seriously—especially those of us who support legalization
in the United States of both voluntary active euthanasia and physician-assisted
suicide. This requires both the effort to discover what, in fact, is the predicted evil

From *Law, Medicine, and Health Care* 20: 1–2 (Spring/Summer): 133–143. Originally titled "Voluntary
Euthanasia and Risks of Abuse: Can We Learn Anything from the Netherlands?" Copyright © 1992 by
Law, Medicine, and Health Care. Reprinted by permission of the publisher.

against which the warning is being delivered, and what is the likelihood that such an outcome will really come about. Do we fear that greedy family members will maneuver patients into choosing death? Exactly how, and how can we know whether this will really happen? Do we think physicians will lose their scruples and begin to kill their patients? Why might they lose these scruples, exactly, and what were these scruples in the first place? Will wholesale "medical homicide" take place, as former Surgeon General C. Everett Koop warned in television spots broadcast in Washington on the eve of the vote on Initiative 119? Will cost-conscious institutions force patients into euthanasia or into requesting means for suicide, and if so, precisely how? What forms will race-, age- and handicap-prejudice take in exacerbating this problem, and how will it be that members of such groups are especially victimized?

California's Proposition 161 attempted to address concerns about Initiative 119 by imposing additional protections. It required that the patient's request be "enduring," that there be special protections for persons in skilled nursing facilities, that there be prohibitions against intimidation, inducement, and tampering, provisions for psychological consultation and for the independence of physicians, stipulations that the time and place of death be determined solely by the patient, limitations on fees, and record-keeping requirements; furthermore, the patient is encouraged to notify his or her family.[1] There have also been various other proposals in the public media for the addition of protections to legislation legalizing euthanasia and assisted suicide; for example, one such set of suggestions, following 119, would have required that aid-in-dying be performed only in a hospital, that it be performed only within the context of an established doctor-patient relationship, and that it be restricted to residents of the state of Washington.[2] Another recommended that training in pain control and terminal care be made a condition for the renewal of M.D. licenses, implying that euthanasia and assisted suicide could be practiced without abuse only if physicians were fully skilled in techniques of treating patients' pain.[3] A Dutch proposal offered early in that country's discussions of euthanasia would have required an extensive autopsy and mortality review for every patient who died by euthanasia, comparing not only the physician's diagnosis with pathologies found on examination of the cadaver but also reviewing the deliberations leading up to euthanasia.[4] Whatever the various recommendations for the addition of protections to any proposal for legalization, it is important not to treat them too lightly; on the contrary, it is crucial to try to see precisely what fears of abuse they attempt to respond to, and also how effective they might be in preventing or controlling such abuse. In general, I think it is crucial to be as clear and forthright about the issue of abuse as possible, even if one supports, as I do, the legalization of aid-in-dying.

In doing so, one must answer two central questions: (1) Will there be abuse, and if so, precisely what kind? and (2) Can abuse of this sort be prevented? It is to the second of these questions that I will be particularly attentive here. In doing so, I shall consider only the possible effects of legalizing voluntary, active, physician-performed euthanasia and physician-assisted suicide, restricted to cases in which such help is requested by competent, terminally ill patients with less than six months to live—that is, I shall be considering only what Initiative 119 and Proposition 161 would have legalized—but some of the arguments will clearly apply to a wider range of possible legislation as well.

Slippery slope arguments are designed to address the first of the two questions above: *Will there be abuse, and if so, precisely what kind?* Because they are predictive empirical arguments intended to show that permitting a given practice will result in abuse, the principal strategy available to counter these arguments is to show that they fail to specify what causal mechanisms will be involved, what background precedents would permit such erosion, and so on. Thus, opponents of legalization warn of abuse in the future, pointing to alleged current abuse in the Netherlands as evidence; supporters of legalization, on the other hand, reply that claims about abuse in Holland are unsubstantiated or exaggerated and that there is little reason to think abuse would occur in the United States. One cannot fear an analogue of the Holocaust, supporters of the legislation argue, because even though there are local excrescences of anti-Semitic, anti-African-American, and other racially prejudiced political activity, it is inconceivable that a country with such strong guarantees of civil rights could permit a large-scale extermination program. Thus the argument moves back and forth between opponents and supporters, however erratically; but it remains an essentially empirical argument about the potential consequences of legalization.

It is this argument that I would like to join here. As I have said elsewhere in this book, I do not think there is any compelling argument in principle to be made against voluntary active euthanasia or physician-assisted suicide, at least in specific circumstances, and I believe that on the contrary, control of one's own death as far as possible is a matter of fundamental human right. However, I also think that the warnings of potential abuse require much more sensitive and careful examination than either supporters or opponents of such legislation have generally given them. Indeed, I think it is morally responsible to advocate the legalization of euthanasia and assisted suicide *only* if one can conscientiously argue either that abuse would not occur or that it could be prevented, and it is on this project that I would like to embark. Conversely, I also think it is morally responsible to oppose the legalization of euthanasia and assisted suicide, given the importance of the freedom to be suppressed, only if one can show with reasonable likelihood that abuse would occur and that it could not be prevented.

Either way, it is crucial to consider the issue of abuse, and this is an obligation that no party to the discussion, on either side, ought to evade; the burden of proof in establishing what the consequences of the proposed legislation would be falls, in this special case, on both sides. That persons have a basic, fundamental right to control as much as they wish and as much as is possible the timing and circumstances of their own deaths is a claim that I shall assume here,[5] but this assumption does not relieve one of the obligation to consider the risk of abuse. After all, if the risks of abuse are great enough, this may entail that even basic, fundamental rights of persons should be curtailed. If, on the other hand, the risks of abuse turn out to be small or if abuse can be prevented, then it is morally imperative that persons' basic, fundamental rights to control as much as possible the circumstances of their own dying be legally recognized.

Will Abuse Occur?

While euthanasia is presumably practiced clandestinely virtually everywhere else, it is openly practiced only in the Netherlands. Thus, our principal source of empirical information about the potential for abuse where euthanasia is effectively legal must come from the Netherlands. To be sure, euthanasia is not fully legal in the Netherlands; it remains a violation of statutory law, punishable in principle by imprisonment, but the lower and Supreme courts have developed a series of guidelines under which euthanasia is immune from prosecution. Not until February 1993 were these guidelines, protecting physicians who meet the guidelines for euthanasia from prosecution, acknowledged in statutory law. Nevertheless, euthanasia has been effectively legal and openly practiced for a number of years, and it is supported by a substantial majority of public opinion. To prevent inept experimentation, the Royal Dutch Pharmaceutical Association mailed explicit information on how to perform euthanasia to all Dutch physicians. Most Dutch hospitals now have protocols governing euthanasia, and many health-care institutions, including nursing homes and hospitals, also have developed publicly stated policies concerning whether they do or do not permit the practice.

The first nationwide study in Holland on euthanasia and other medical decisions at the end of life, prepared by a commission appointed by the Dutch government (the so-called Remmelink Commission), involved detailed interviews with 405 physicians from different disciplines, a questionnaire mailed to the physicians of 7,000 deceased persons, and a prospective survey in which physicians interviewed in part I gave information concerning every death in their practice (a total of 2,250 deaths) during the six months after the interview.[6] This study found that about 1.8 percent of total deaths per year in the Netherlands are the result of euthanasia with some form of physician involvement and that about 0.3 percent of deaths involve physician-assisted suicide. But it also reported that in 0.8 percent of all deaths "drugs were administered with the explicit intention to shorten the patient's life, without the strict criteria for euthanasia being fulfilled,"[7] and it is this that has been widely interpreted in the United States to mean that a thousand patients were killed against their will. While this is a clear misinterpretation of the data in the Dutch study, fair treatment of the issue of abuse must take account of both actual and conjectural evidence from Holland.

There are several further matters to be remembered in addressing the issue of abuse. First, judgments about abuse should in principle be comparative, weighing influences on choice, adjusted for the severity of outcome, against influences on other alternative choices. Would choices of euthanasia be more or less abused than, say, choices of high-risk surgery or choices to withhold or withdraw life-sustaining treatment? After all, any of these choices can lead to death, not only choices about euthanasia. Furthermore, judgments about abuse ought not to cloak judgments about outcomes: it cannot be assumed, without further argument, that—in the kind of case at issue here—influences on a choice for euthanasia are potentially abusive whereas influences on a choice to stay alive are not. It is also to be remembered that there is little theoretical agreement on just what constitutes abuse: is it a distortion of voluntariness, a violation of a person's interests, or what?

Finally, it is important to remember that the issue of whether abuse would occur is an issue about the outcomes of policy, not about idiosyncratic acts. In every society and with regard to every kind of social policy, unstable, psychopathic, or otherwise deranged individuals commit acts that clearly constitute abuses: nurses who randomly inject patients with fatal drugs, doctors who perform deliberately damaging, unwarranted operations on patients, anaesthetists who have sex with patients on their operating tables. Such outlier cases will occur from time to time, regardless of the type of policies in effect. To be sure, one ought not be sanguine about the occurrence of such cases, but the real issue is not so much whether such outlier cases will occur—they will, in any country, with or without legislation—but whether the legislation itself would permit or encourage such cases on a more frequent, more accepted, more "normal" basis. Thus, the question is whether the policies at issue—the legalization of active euthanasia and of assisted suicide— would engender an abusive pattern of practice, not whether a handful of isolated, marginal cases of abuse would occur from time to time. It is "normal" patterns of abuse that the slippery slope arguments are properly concerned with: Would family members readily and routinely manipulate patients? Would physicians generally become callous about death? Would institutions regularly force patients into euthanasia or suicide in an effort to save costs? Would prejudice against racial minorities, the aged and the handicapped further infect these practices?

Although I have no doubt that some outlier cases of abuse would occur from time to time, I do not think the general answer to these questions is yes. Nor do I think euthanasia choices would be more abused than choices of high-risk surgery or of withholding or withdrawing life-sustaining treatment. Nevertheless, I will assume the contrary for purposes of this essay, since my real concern here is whether—if such abusive patterns might be tolerated or encouraged by legalizing euthanasia and suicide—there are effective ways of preventing abuse. This is not to assume that human nature is evil or that abuse is humanly inevitable; rather, it is to assume that different policies and the incentives and disincentives incorporated in policy can encourage or discourage quite different patterns of practice. Thus, the question is: would the legalization of euthanasia and suicide, with or without safeguards such as those proposed in American legislative proposals like Initiative 119 or Proposition 161, or those already in place in the Netherlands, engender abuse? If so, what sort, and can such abuse be prevented even if it would otherwise occur?

Types of Possible Abuse

Three conceptually distinct types of abuse can be identified among the scenarios that slippery slope arguments portray: what we might call interpersonal abuse, professional abuse, and institutional abuse. Although they are conceptually distinct, it is to be expected that in practice they would often be closely intertwined. Although the parallels are not exact, they also invite three rather different sorts of solutions, that is, three rather different sorts of strategies for preventing such abuses from occurring.

Interpersonal Abuse

Chief among the varieties of interpersonal abuse, one might expect, would be that occurring in familial situations: the resentful or greedy spouse, or other family member, who maneuvers a terminally ill patient now perceived as a burden into requesting euthanasia or assistance in suicide. Such pressures might be malevolent, the product of long years of hostility: or, perhaps more likely, they might be the product of the kind of emotional exhaustion familial caregivers often experience in attending to a patient with a lengthy, deteriorative terminal illness. "All of your suffering could be over soon," such a family member might be expected to say—not seeing that much of the suffering is not so much the patient's but his or her own. Of course, familial messages supporting euthanasia or suicide can be given in an enormous variety of ways, both explicit and inexplicit, verbal and nonverbal, and they can be conveyed by a single individual family member or by a family as a whole.

Familial messages favoring euthanasia or suicide can be comparatively weak, involving suggestion or even the mere raising of the idea; they can be stronger, including what we might variously call recommendation, urging, "talking into," pleading, cajoling, remonstrating, and so on; and they can be a great deal stronger, including such tactics as threats, ultimatums, lies, and so on. Not all family life is harmonious, and underlying pathology can often be exacerbated by the stresses a family member's terminal illness brings. "All right, Granny, it's time to go" is a message we can imagine being conveyed in a large variety of ways, exhibiting an entire range from the faintest suggestion to outright coercion.

Professional Abuse

If family members will manipulate or pressure patients into choosing death in all the usual ways family members control each other's behavior, it can be further argued that physicians will have an even larger range of methods for doing so. For instance, they may give inaccurate diagnoses or unreliable prognoses. They may scare patients with predictions of pain. They may decline to offer adequate pain control, citing, for example, the risks of addiction to narcotic drugs, or offer only pain control that is sporadic or has undesirable side effects. They may refuse to offer other treatment that might produce symptom relief. They may "recommend" premature death in ways that are too persuasive for the patient to resist, or they may recommend it to the family and let the family do the persuasion. Worse still, they may learn to lean on euthanasia as a kind of medical crutch, turning almost automatically to it as the solution for every treatment problem they cannot solve; even worse, they may use it as a cover for their medical mistakes. Perhaps still worse, they will become euthanasia "enthusiasts," employing euthanasia as part of their own political programs for reforming the medical world.

To understand these claims, it is essential first to see what background assumptions make them plausible, given that it is only voluntary euthanasia and assisted suicide that would be legalized, and then only for competent, terminally ill patients with less than six months to live. Yet even given the comparative narrowness of this range of cases, the dire predictions so widely voiced cannot be ignored. For this reason, it is crucial to understand what is distinctive about abuse by doctors, and to some degree by nurses and other care providers as well—that is, what is distinctive about *professional* abuse in contrast to interpersonal (usually familial) abuse of the sort just discussed.

Professional abuse, understood as that range of ways in which professionals, especially physicians, might bring a patient who would not otherwise do so to "voluntarily" request euthanasia or help in suicide, can exhibit most of the features of interpersonal, domestic abuse—suggestion, manipulation, and threats aimed at one person by another—but it incorporates an additional feature: the weight of professional authority. It is the physician who holds the power in the physician/ patient relationship, not only because the physician has greater knowledge of the physiological processes affecting the patient and how to control them, and because the physician's social aura conveys authoritative standing to his or her role, but also because the patient is ill. Especially when it is terminal, illness can place a person in a particularly compromised position: for many patients, illness involves discomfort and pain, anxiety, fear of impending loss of one's relationships, and fear of death. Thus "professional authority" trades on two factors: the greater weight of the physician and the compromised position of the patient. Both factors invite abuse. The nurse may also be regarded as a medical authority, particularly in situations (e.g., home care) where it is the nurse who is the primary or only contact with the patient, but it is the physician whose capacity is greatest for exploiting professional authority.

Given this disparity of power in the physician/patient relationship, physicians are very well aware of their power to influence patient choices—even while preserving the appearance of obtaining informed consent. The Latinate obscurity of medical diagnosis and the overwhelming nature of too much medical information often contribute to this possibility. Thus, many physicians claim they can get patients to agree to nearly anything they propose; it is simply a matter of how the choice is framed. Just as, in the traditional example, the glass of water can be described as half empty or half full, a proposed surgical procedure with a 50/50 predicted outcome, for example, can be described as a probable success or a probable failure; a "good chance" can mean anything from a 10 or 20 percent chance of success to 80 or 90 percent. Information can be orchestrated to emphasize benefits or to emphasize risks, even when information about both benefits and risks is actually provided. Presumably, physicians would thus find is easy to frame choices about euthanasia or suicide in similar ways: unfavorably for patients whom they wanted to discourage, but favorably for those whom they hope to maneuver into this choice. Thus, even under legislation that protects only *voluntary* choice by competent patients, it can be argued, the physician could manipulate the patient into choosing death when the patient would not otherwise have chosen it or when it is actually contrary to his or her own wishes. In all these cases, the fiction that the patient has given informed consent can be preserved; what is problematic is the way in which the physician presents the information on which the patient's choice is based.

There is a second way in which professional authority can play a substantial role in shaping patient choice. Much of the interaction, as well as the legal support, for the relationship between physician and patient is based on assumptions of *informed consent*—that is, that the patient retains the right to give or withhold consent to treatment and that in making these choices the patient is entitled to adequate information about the alternatives involved. Informed consent must be explicitly documented for specific procedures, such as surgery; it is assumed for a wide range of minor tests and procedures involved in medical care. But reliance on informed consent also reinforces power disparities in the physician/patient role and exacerbates the weight of professional authority: in informed consent, it is the physician who proposes the specific course of treatment and the patient who gets to say yes or no. But in this arrangement, it is the physician who identifies the problem, frames any suggested solution to it, and controls how many alternative solutions are proposed. The patient cannot know whether the problem could be seen in some other way or as some different sort of problem, whether other sorts of solutions could be proposed, whether in making the choice to give or withhold consent he or she is making a choice among all the reasonable alternatives, and, sometimes, whether there really is any problem at all. The agenda is, so to speak, entirely in the control of the physician. This of course may be a reasonable arrangement for consent to medical procedures that do not raise values dilemmas, but it is hardly a defensible arrangement in the case of euthanasia. Euthanasia is, after all, a quintessential "values" issue: whether a person prefers a chance of extended life in spite of suffering or pain, or whether he or she perfers an earlier, easier end to life in order to avoid suffering and pain. If consent to euthanasia is treated in the same way as consent to other medical procedures, it will be the physician's agenda, not the patient's, that is on the table for action, and to which the patient's only option is to agree or disagree. But this, of course, is fertile ground for abuse.

Furthermore, the physician's capacity to shape patient choice in euthanasia, both by selective control of information and by initial formulation of both the problem and the solution presented for consent, may be influenced not only by malevolent intentions, but also by paternalistic ones. To be sure, there are physicians motivated by greed, prejudice, fear of malpractice action for a medical mistake, and so on. But there may also be physicians who genuinely believe that euthanasia would be in the best interests of the patient, given the pain and suffering the physician knows otherwise lies in the patient's future, and who thus may seek to influence patient choice in this direction for the patient's own sake. Of course, whether manipulation of the patient in what the physician perceives to be the patient's own interest is to be counted as abuse depends in the end on theoretical issues about the nature of paternalism and whether abuse is defined as violation of voluntary patient choice or as violation of patient interests, but the possibility of paternalistic manipulation of the patient by the physician must at least be considered among the varieties of possible abuse.

Institutional Abuse

Institutional abuse will no doubt include some of the features of both interpersonal and professional abuse, but it is conceptually distinct in its central feature: it operates by narrowing the range of actual choices open to the patient. It may seem to closely resemble those forms of professional abuse in which the physician shapes the patient's choice by selectively providing information or proposing one rather than another possible course of action for consent, but it functions in a distinct way: it erects barriers so that certain choices can be made only with difficulty or cannot be made at all. It is not only that choices are shaped, but, more importantly, that only certain choices are possible, while other choices are closed off. There need be nothing clandestine about this, as there may seem to be when the physician withholds specific information or selectively emphasizes some information in order to promote certain choices; in institutional abuse, in contrast with professional abuse, the policies in question are typically open and sometimes widely known, even though they may have manipulative or coercive consequences.

What are the fears, so vocally and variably expressed in the public discussions of euthanasia? They are fears about various sorts of institutions: hospitals, nursing homes, insurance companies, the government. They are fears primarily of policies that are financially motivated, seeking to cut costs in medicine by offering less care, imposing barriers, and withdrawing certain options. They are fears that hospitals will not provide certain types of care or will provide it only to some patients, that nursing homes will let the quality of care and of institutional life deteriorate to the point where it is unbearable, that insurance companies will exclude from coverage many forms of treatment and palliation that might benefit the patient, or that they will exclude some patients from coverage altogether. They are often fears about the government, usually fears of government intrusion via restrictive policy development.

Furthermore, these fears of what might occur were active euthanasia and assisted suicide to be legalized are rooted, it is evident, in current observations of what is perceived to constitute institutional abuse already, even though such abuse cannot now openly lead to choices of euthanasia and suicide. These are perceptions of institutional abuse in a health-care system that is grossly inequitable and in which costs are out of control: a health-care system in which many persons have no medical insurance; in which medical insurance is often prohibitively expensive; in which some insurance policies are misleadingly and seriously inadequate; in which insurance companies proceed by "cream skimming" and experience-rating for risk avoidance, selecting for coverage persons whose health risks are good and refusing coverage to those whose health risks are not; in which both private and governmental insurers evade payment by delay and by nuisance requirements concerning filing claims; in which coverage for some sorts of patients (e.g., Medicaid) is so low that they become unattractive to providers; in which some sorts of facilities (e.g., rural and ghetto clinics) are closed or never provided; and in which the general degree of evasion and virtual deception in public statements about health care is perceived to be high. Given the chaotic nature of the current U.S. health-care system, in contrast to the well-developed national health-provider and insurance systems in place in other industrialized nations, it is reasonable to suppose that fears of institutional abuse in the legalization of euthanasia will be higher here than in any of these other countries—indeed, with good reason, unless there is sweeping reform..

Fears of institutional abuse are further exacerbated by the fact that a very substantial portion of health-care expenses are spent in the last month, two months, or six months of life. Of course, it is only possible to determine what were the last

month, two months, or six months of life for a given patient retroactively. But these
months in general coincide with the period in which a patient is understood to be
terminal—and in which, under a statute like Initiative 119 or Proposition 161, active
euthanasia or assistance in suicide would be legal. Thus, it is not just that the health-
care system is inequitable and chaotic, with costs spiraling wildly out of control, it is
also that a very substantial portion of these costs are directly associated with precisely those patients for whom euthanasia and assisted suicide would first become
legally available. The shorter and easier a terminal course is, the cheaper it is to
cover; the cheapest patient of all is one who chooses death now. This, of course, is a
particularly inviting occasion for institutional abuse.

To understand the pervasive possibilities of institutional abuse, we must also
understand the various mechanisms by which this abuse operates. There are, I think,
three primary mechanisms that wholly or partially close off choice: direct policy
stipulations, indirect policy agendas, and the use of policies that control preference.
The first of these involves direct, usually overt and publicly announced policy
stipulations or rules: for instance, policies or rules requiring the use of certain forms
of treatment or prohibiting the use of others, covering some but not all care, and so
on. But some seemingly direct policies, overt and public, may also have indirect
agendas; this is the second form of mechanism by which institutional abuse can take
place. Several current examples come to mind, and though they cannot now lead to
legally performed euthanasia or assisted suicide, they represent the kind of indirect-
agenda policy one might also expect to see if euthanasia were legal. These include
the development of diagnosis-related groups or DRGs as a basis for Medicaid and
Medicare reimbursements to hospitals: although DRGs are officially formulated and
were originally announced as "averages" for care costs for specific disease classi-
fications, they have become—quite predictably—ceilings. Similarly, the Patient
Self-Determination Act, which became effective December 1, 1991, requires hospitals, nursing homes, hospices, home health agencies, health maintenance organizations, and other health-care facilities that treat Medicaid or Medicare patients to
inform patients at the time they are admitted of their right to make decisions concerning their own medical care, "including the right to accept or refuse medical or
surgical treatment and the right to formulate advanced directives"[8] by signing a
living will or durable power of attorney. These facilities must also ask incoming
patients if they have already executed an advanced directive. This legislation seems
an impressive acknowledgment of patients' rights to autonomy in health care. But is is
already widely believed—predictably so—that the legislation does not simply require health-care facilities to ask patients *if* they have living wills, but that it requires
health-care facilities to make sure that patients *do* have living wills. To bureaucratic
entities concerned with controlling costs in terminal care, this cannot be an un-
welcome misunderstanding.

Third, some policies have the effect of making only some choices rational ones
for a person in specific circumstances, even if other choices would be permitted. An
example already in place, which might be thought to be particularly coercive if
euthanasia or assisted suicide were legal, is the provision requiring spend-down for
coverage by Medicaid: a person facing an extended period in a nursing home must
exhaust virtually all his or her own funds before public assistance begins. For the

person who is already terminally ill and who faces a choice between exhausting his or her legacy for a comparatively short period of additional life versus leaving earlier but managing to leave one's legacy behind for a spouse or for children, this may not seem to be a choice at all, but a situation in which federal policies make the choice of earlier death the only really rational one. And, of course, policies such as this may trigger various forms of interpersonal abuse as well: the spouse who will be impoverished if the patient chooses to live, but left with a legacy if euthanasia is the choice, may be unable to resist innuendo, manipulation, or open coercion in the matter.

Protections Against Abuse

The picture of possible abuse is a grim one, particularly in a society with a chaotic health-care system, but it is, I think, a real risk. Yet I also think it is possible to erect protections against such abuse that can be both stable and effective. Such protections are not foolproof, and the policies and regulations in which they are incorporated are not likely to stop those who operate outside the law in any case. Nevertheless, these protections are adequate, I believe, to prevent the kind of general, large-scale, "normal" abuse that many forms of the slippery slope argument predict, and thus render unwarranted the large-scale limitation of patient choice that laws prohibiting euthanasia and assisted suicide represent.

These protections fall into three general categories—policies designed to protect the quality of the patient's choice, policies designed to control professional and institutional distortions of a patient's situation, and policies designed to permit the development of objective indices of abuse. Though they are to be described separately here, they will function best, of course, in concert and interactively. Indeed, I think that all or nearly all of the forms of protections described here will need to be in place to provide reliable prevention of abuse.

Protecting the Quality of the Patient's Choice

Policies designed to protect the quality of the patient's choice must attempt to look at two things: how the patient reached that choice, and what the content of that choice is. Both raise enormous theoretical issues, requiring answers to two philosophically difficult questions, drawing on two distinct senses of the term *rational:* what must one have done to have made a "well-chosen" or "rational" choice? and what characteristics must the "right" or "best" choice, that is, the "rational" choice, display? Nevertheless, we can intuitively discern choices that are badly made in the sense that they are the product of irrational thinking, inadequate information, undue outside influence, and so on; we can also discern choices that seem to be, given the interests and values of the individual making them, simply bad choices for him or her to have made, regardless of how carefully they were considered. Of course, this raises enormous issues of paternalism, but we can nevertheless discern at least the broad outlines of "badly made" and "bad" choices. The two mechanisms discussed below attempt to protect the quality of the patient's decision in both these cases.

Psychological Evaluation. Several proposals for amending the proposed aid-in-dying legislation recommended provisions for offering or requiring a psychological evaluation of the patient who requests euthanasia or assistance in suicide. Generally, such evaluations would seek primarily to identify psychopathology or other disturbances of reasoning, especially depression, which might affect the patient's capacity to reach a fully voluntary, autonomous choice; they thus would be designed to protect the patient from choosing badly. Such evaluation might routinely use standard scales of depression, such as the Beck Inventory; it might also involve interviews by the physician involved or by a consulting physician, psychologist, or psychiatrist. Such evaluation should be conducted in private with the patient, away from the influence of family members or other parties who might exert pressures of various subtle sorts. However, it cannot be too easily assumed that any evidence of depression that could be detected in this way is grounds for rejecting a request for euthanasia or assistance in suicide. Depression is a natural accompaniment of terminal illness, though more pronounced in some stages of the dying process than in others, since terminal illness, although it may involve some gains in intimacy with one's loved ones, is also a period of continuing loss. The routine use of psychological evaluation adapted for other situations, especially to detect depression, ought not to impose a higher standard for decision-making than for other important decisions in life; instead, it ought to be used just to identify the clearest cases of transient, *reversible* depression that may be affecting patient choice. Thus, psychological evaluation measures used in these situations—for persons diagnosed as terminally ill, with less than six months to live—must be redesigned so that the expression of thoughts about death, considerations of suicide, or the wish to die is not interpreted as prima facie evidence of depression and so taken to preclude voluntary choice.

Counseling. Until recently, most counseling available in the United States has been committed to the principle of suicide prevention, and would view any expression of a wish or intention to die as grounds for further treatment. In this sense, most counseling has been directive: it has been concerned to direct clients or patients toward life-affirming choices and constructive ways of resolving their problems, away from death. Furthermore, perhaps as a result of the *Tarasoff* decision, in which a University of California psychiatrist was held responsible for failing to warn the prospective victim of her former boyfriend's plan to kill her—which he did[9]— most psychologists have understood themselves to be obligated to report serious potential harm to third parties or to the patient, and hence obligated to take action (for instance by initiating involuntary commitment) with respect to a patient who reports a serious intention to commit suicide. In a large range of cases, these postures are entirely appropriate. But they are not appropriate in the circumstances at issue in terminal illness, especially if the patient has a legally protected right to euthanasia or assistance in suicide; here, what is in order instead is genuinely nondirective counseling, designed to help the patient discover whether his or her request for euthanasia or assistance in suicide is in fact a genuine one, carefully thought through, fully understood, and in keeping with his or her most basic values—that is, whether it is the "right" or "best" or "rational" choice *for this person.* Of course the request might be a "cry for help" or the product of external manipulation or other abuse, but it might also be a genuine product of the person's most considered, reflective choice. Any counseling offered ought to serve solely to differentiate these two, not to close off one set of options; if not, it is useless in these situations. Suicide-prevention centers and crisis hotlines have, I have argued elsewhere, been particularly remiss in failing to serve that proportion of the population who may find their services most valuable: persons considering suicide (or euthanasia) as a way of responding to the prospect of deteriorative terminal illness, as well as those with severe permanent disabilities or advanced old age.[10] Such persons, who take themselves to be considering a rational response to difficult circumstances, cannot avail themselves of services whose announced purpose, "suicide prevention," makes it clear that they will work to preclude such a choice, or of services whose policies require initiating involuntary commitment for persons viewed as likely to commit suicide. Rather, what is needed is counseling designed to help a patient think through the issues in "rational suicide," including requests for assistance or for physician-performed euthanasia. Such suicide-neutral counseling takes the request at face value and seeks to help the patient be sure he or she has considered all consequences, acknowledged his or her own emotions, and recognized all conflicts or affirmations of value such a choice might involve.[11] Indeed, such counseling may well serve to reduce the psychopathology of such situations by allowing more open discussion of them; but it cannot do so if it is committed to pre-shaping choice.

Continuity Requirement or Waiting Period. Some proposals have suggested that a waiting period be required between the initial request for euthanasia or assistance in suicide and the provision of these services. The clear intent behind such proposals is to ensure that the choice is stable and enduring, rather than a fleeting, transitory response to a new setback, and hence that it is an expression of the patient's true, underlying values. Other mechanisms that might be said to provide concrete evidence of the patient's values at earlier periods in life would include such instruments as a living will executed before the onset of the terminal illness or at an earlier point during it; some courts have relied on records of, or testimony about, earlier comments made by the patient concerning other persons in similar circumstances. Although a short waiting period (say, twenty-four or forty-eight hours) may serve as some protection against impetuous decision-making, longer waiting periods (say, a month or two) are not only artificial but have the potential to be cruel, since they postpone that very relief the patient is seeking. Paradoxically, waiting periods may also encourage some patients to make premature requests as a way of getting into the queue early. Living wills and durable power of attorney documents need not be signed under controlled circumstances, and it is sometimes argued that they do not reliably represent a patient's true choices over time, especially as the patient may be unable to correctly anticipate his or her future situation. Despite the deficiencies of waiting periods and advance directives, nevertheless, some form of protective device designed to ensure both the stability of the choice and its consonance with the patient's own values seems appropriate—provided, of course, that it does not completely preclude any possibility for the patient to change his or her mind. Notice what is *not* recommended here as a protective device: the deliberations of a committee. These can only be deliberations about the content of the patient's choice, not the patient's voluntariness in making that choice, and I do not see that a committee decision on whether the patient may or may not end his or her life protects the quality of the patient's choice. More likely, it serves to protect the institution in which the committee is based.

Protecting against Professional and Institutional Distortion of a Patient's Choices

The sorts of policies considered in this section are designed to prevent both intentional and inadvertent distortion of a patient's situation and, hence, a patient's choices by either the physician or other health-care providers or by institutions, including hospitals, nursing homes, home-care agencies, insurance companies, and governmental agencies.

Prohibition of Fees. In remarks made before the vote on Initiative 119, Professor Albert Jonsen warned of a "flood of persons" who would travel to Washington in order to seek euthanasia. Other voices warned of the development of "death houses" or "euthanasia clinics," clearly drawing on the analogy with abortion clinics, and some suggested that unscrupulous physicians would offer inducements to patients to seek such services, perhaps by advertising in the public or medical media. Remote as these predictions might seem to be, there is a simple way to prevent such traffic and the institutional stimulation of such traffic: no physician or other health-care provider should be permitted to charge a fee for performing euthanasia or for providing assistance in suicide, or at least no fee beyond minimal compensation for the time actually involved. Advertising such services, at least in any way more elaborate than announcing their availability, should also be prohibited. Euthanasia is not a complex procedure, if reliable information is available to the physician about methods for performing it (as would presumably be the case if the procedure were legalized), though it may be performed in comparatively slow ways that do involve extended time. Physicians in the Netherlands, where euthanasia is in effect legal and where medical information about methods to be used is widely available, report that they do not accept fees, even though the procedure may be performed in a hospital or in a home, and even though, at the request of the patient, the procedure is often performed in a way that involves a long, slow induction of sleep followed by coma over a period of several hours, usually to make the transition from life to death easier for the family to watch. Dutch physicians report that they expect to remain with the patient (and the family) throughout this time, though they do not take fees for it.[12] Similarly, prohibiting health-care facilities from advertising and from charging fees for euthanasia or any closely related ancillary services, or from charging fees that would provide a profit over expenses, would preclude at least some incentives for euthanasia and for the development of a euthanasia "trade" or market.

Documentation. A second form of protection against abuse involves extensive documentation of any procedure involving euthanasia or the provision of assistance in suicide. Such documentation, presumably to be a part of the patient's medical record, would include the medical history, the prognosis, the nature of the current problem(s), the reasons for the patient's request (both the patient's stated reasons and the physician's perceptions of the patient's reasons, if different), and a record of the physician's discussions with the patient's family, if any. Also to be included in the documentation would be a clear expression of the patient's choice: not merely a signed "informed consent" to the procedure itself, but documentation of the patient's active request. This might take many forms—a letter, a tape recording of the patient's voice, or witnessed statements by observers—but the central element is documentation of the fact that euthanasia or assistance in suicide is the patient's idea, not that of the physician, the family, or the health-care facility.

As a second, equally important component, the documentation should also include a record of treatment alternatives discussed with the patient, including treatment alternatives refused by the patient as well as those accepted, forms of pain relief or symptom control offered the patient, and, also equally important, any forms of treatment potentially effective for the patient's condition but excluded from coverage by insurance policies, by the health-care facility's care priorities, by governmental rationing policies, and so on. These three elements of documentation serve to reflect interpersonal, professional, and institutional abuse, respectively.

Reporting. The performance of euthanasia or the provision of assistance in suicide should also be reportable to an appropriate external agency. At the moment, of course, there is no such designated agency, but a number of possibilities suggest themselves: for instance, the coroner (since presumably the cause of death, euthanasia, perhaps together with the disease causing the terminal condition, would be entered on the death certificate), or the Centers for Disease Control (as a keeper of mortality statistics), or the National Institutes of Health (as a federal research agency), or Health and Human Services (as the highest level of federal bureaucracy for health issues), etc. However, the national analog to the Dutch reporting requirement would not be immediately plausible in the United States; in the Netherlands, because euthanasia is technically a violation of statutory law, and the guidelines developed in lower and supreme court cases and now recognized by law serve as a defense to prosecutions for homicide, the physician is obligated to report any occasion of euthanasia to the Ministry of Justice after the fact, where it is reviewed and prosecution undertaken if the guidelines are not met. (As is well known, only a small proportion of Dutch physicians have been doing so, though this number has been increasing in recent years.) However, if in the United States euthanasia and assistance in suicide were legal under statutory law, reporting to the Department of Justice or state-level judicial authorities would not seem immediately plausible, since technically, no crime would have been committed; perhaps, however, a reporting requirement could be inserted in the authorizing law. Whatever the agency to which the report is made, what is important in preventing abuse is that detailed information about cases of euthanasia be available for review; the effectiveness of this structure would clearly also be enhanced by a substantial penalty for failure to report.

Developing Objective Indices of Abuse

Documentation and reporting of euthanasia cases makes possible what is perhaps the most important mechanism for the control of abuse and the reliable provision of protection to patients. What is central here is the possibility of retroactive inspection on a broad scale of patterns of performance of euthanasia. As in current analyses by John Wennberg at Dartmouth and others of geographical variation in surgical procedures and other statistical assessments of medical practice, the performance of euthanasia and assistance in suicide, if documented and reported, would also be open to objective review. Review, of course, could be made at all levels and for all factors reported: by individual physician, by health-care facility, by insurance carrier, by type of terminal condition, by length of association between patient and physician, by types of pain control and symptom palliation provided, by types of alternative treatment denied, by age, race, gender, handicap status, and so on. Many quite revealing questions thus could readily be answered: Do some doctors provide assistance in suicide more frequently than others? Do the patients of some nursing homes request euthanasia more frequently than the patients of others? Are patients covered by some health insurance plans more frequently denied care for certain sorts of conditions, and are these denials listed among their reasons for choosing euthanasia? How often are spend-down provisions among the reasons for such choices? Do African-American patients ''choose'' euthanasia more often than white? Do patients with poor educations or lower incomes choose euthanasia more often than patients with privileged backgrounds? Although such data might not always be easy to interpret, physicians who had become euthanasia enthusiasts, nursing homes providing deliberately intolerable care, and insurance companies forcing patients into euthanasia choices by refusing to cover certain sorts of care could be initially identified, and further examination of specific situations then conducted by the appropriate review organizations.

Furthermore, not only would analyses of such data reveal patterns of euthanasia practice and hence probable patterns of euthanasia abuse, but there is already some basis for comparative analysis of such data. The Remmelink Commission study from the Netherlands has provided the first objective glimpse of euthanasia practice in a climate in which it is widely accepted and in which it is legally tolerated: it is now known, as discussed earlier, that about 1.8 percent of all deaths in the Netherlands are the product of euthanasia and that about 0.3 percent of all deaths involve physician-assisted suicide. Additional information about these patients is also available: for example, their average age at the time of euthanasia sixty-two for men, sixty-eight for women (interestingly, Dutch physicians report very few requests from older patients); their regional location (more in urban areas); and the approximate amount of life forgone (in 70 percent of cases, more than one week; in 8 percent, more than six months). Information is also available about the reasons for their requests of euthanasia: loss of dignity (mentioned in 57 percent of cases), pain

(46 percent), "unworthy dying" (46 percent), being dependent on others (33 percent), and tiredness of life (23 percent). According to this study, in just over 5 percent of cases was pain the only reason. Furthermore, about two-thirds of initial requests for euthanasia do not end up as a serious and persistent request at a later stage of the disease, and of the serious and persistent requests, about two-thirds do not result in euthanasia or assisted suicide since, according to the study, physicians can often offer alternatives. [13]

Information of this sort would provide an initial basis for comparison of U.S. experience with a country in which two relevant characteristics are different. First, the Netherlands is a country in which the practice of euthanasia is widely and generally accepted, both by patients and by physicians; thus, it is a country in which the incidence of euthanasia is, presumably, not distorted by severe social discouragement. Second, it is a country in which the practice of euthanasia is uncoerced by financial considerations on the part of the patient (the Netherlands has an effective national health insurance system that provides all residents with extensive care in the hospital, nursing home, and at home); it therefore is a country in which patient choice is not constricted in at least one way common in the United States. Thus, the Dutch experience can provide tentative expectations about what our own experience might be were euthanasia accepted and were it not affected by financial considerations; of course, this is a highly conjectural strategy, but examining the practices in the Netherlands can at least initially provide very rough, informal guidelines for scrutinizing our own practice. If we suppose, for example, that, despite differences between Dutch and American culture, somewhere around 1.8 percent is the "normal" percentage of persons dying who would choose to do so by euthanasia when that alternative is socially accepted and when it is not coerced by financial considerations, and that a tiny additional fraction would choose physician-assisted suicide, we then have an easy measure for suspecting abuse in our own society. Are, say, 10 or 20 percent of terminally ill Medicaid patients choosing suicide, but not such a high number of privately insured patients? Thirty or forty percent of the uninsured? Some fifteen to twenty percent of Dutch AIDS patients die by euthanasia; is the proportion higher among AIDS patients here? Is "pain" the reason for which a large proportion of patients are said to have chosen euthanasia? Since this is the sole reason for only 5 percent of Dutch patients choosing euthanasia, we might well suspect foul play—or its medical and bureaucratic variations, such as deliberate neglect or refusal to provide adequate symptom control—if the rates in the United States were much higher. Of course, these figures can hardly be treated as rigid norms, and certainly not as either quotas or ceilings; but they can give us some idea of what we might expect were we to permit the practice here, and what would be wildly out of bounds. This is not to assume that the Dutch have got it right, so to speak, nor that abuse never occurs in the Netherlands; but inasmuch as there is no documented evidence that abuse is occurring (other than very rare outlier cases), it is reasonable to begin with Dutch experience as a guide to what, if all went well, we might expect in the United States. To be sure, these proportions might change as social attitudes change, and would no doubt increase if acceptance for self-determination in dying were to grow; of course they may also change in the Netherlands. And these proportions would change dramatically if Robert Kastenbaum's well-known prediction were to come true, that suicide will become the *preferred* mode of dying because it enables a person to control the time, place, and circumstances of doing so.[14] Thus statistical analysis cannot by itself identify patterns of abuse without some further analysis of social values and trends; nevertheless, it is adapted to identify variations in pattern within a culture and across institutional and geographic lines. What the data from the Netherlands now tell us is that we should expect that euthanasia would be quite infrequent—less than 2 percent of all deaths—and that the reasons for which patients choose it would not have to do only with pain. Of the various mechanisms for protecting against abuse, it is the possibility of potential public exposure, incurring the risk of further legal action, that provides the most secure protection, provided the penalties for not reporting are substantial as well. It is true that many of the slippery slope arguments warn of abuse on a vast scale, but these arguments overlook the fact that we can easily put in place expert methods for detecting and thus preventing it.

As I said earlier, I think it is the moral responsibility of those who favor legislation to show how abuse can be prevented; I also think it is the moral responsibility of those who oppose legalization to try to show that abuse will occur and that it can be prevented in no other way. The burden of proof in this immensely important, sensitive area falls on both sides, and neither side can be certain of its predictions about the future. However, the present does provide us with a good deal of evidence for thinking clearly and specifically about just what sorts of abuse we might expect and what sorts of abuse can be prevented, and I think the weight of the argument falls in favor of recognizing patients' rights to self-determination: even if abuse might otherwise occur, there are sophisticated, effective ways to prevent it, and the right in question is too fundamental to suppress without compelling reason. I have no doubt but that abuse could occur; in fact, all the forms of potential abuse elaborated here already occur in our current choices about death—that is, in choices of withholding and withdrawing treatment, the only forms of control over death legally permitted in the United States. Because these sorts of choices about death are less conspicuous than choices about euthanasia and assisted suicide, they are less subject to review and control via the various mechanisms identified here. Indeed, I think the open, legal practices of voluntary active euthanasia and physician-assisted suicide will have not only the morally important effect of leading to recognition of a wider range of what I believe to be fundamental rights, but, insofar as they will require us to erect protections against abuse, these practices will also prod us to develop much stronger protections for the kinds of choices about death we already make in what are often quite casual, cavalier ways.

Notes

1. *The California Death with Dignity Act,* California Civil Code Title 10.5, Initiative; failed.
2. Edward Larson, "Washington State: The Nevada of Death?" *Seattle Times,* October 1991.

3. Robin Bernhoft, M.D., "Should Aid-in-Dying Be Allowed? No." *Seattle Times,* 27 October 1991, p. A21.

4. The proposal was put forward by F. I. Meijler, a cardiologist at the University of Utrecht, in 1984. See Carlos Gomez, *Regulating Death: Euthanasia and the Case of the Netherlands* (New York: Free Press, 1991), 96, citing Teresa Takken.

5. This does not, however, entail that love-sick teenagers have a fundamental right to suicide or that one ought not intervene to prevent the suicide of a person who is depressed. For an extended discussion of how a right to suicide can be fundamental but not entail these conclusions, see my "Suicide: A *Fundamental* Human Right?" chapter 14 in this volume.

6. Reported in English in Paul J. van der Maas et al., "Euthanasia and Other Medical Decisions Concerning the End of Life," *The Lancet* 338 (September 14, 1991): 669–674.

7. Ibid., 671.

8. Public Health and Welfare, *The Patient Self-Determination Act,* 42 section 1395cc(f)(I)(A)(i).

9. Tarasoff v. Regents of the University of California, 551 P. 2d 334, 17 Cal. 3d 425, Supreme Court of California, July 1, 1976.

10. See M. Pabst Battin, "Suicide Prevention Centres Fail the Elderly," *Current Awareness Bulletin* of the Suicide Information and Education Centre (Calgary, Canada) 3:3 (Summer 1988), p. 1.

11. For specific recommendations concerning how to conduct such counseling, see "Assisting in Suicide: Seventeen Questioms Physicians and Mental-Health Professionals Should Ask," chapter 13 in this volume.

12. Source: personal interviews in the Netherlands, September–October 1988, 1989, 1990.

13. Van der Maas et al., "Euthanasia," 673.

14. Robert Kastenbaum, "Suicide as the Preferred Way of Death," in *Suicidology: Contemporary Developments,* ed. Edwin S. Shneidman (New York: Grune & Stratton, 1976), 425–441.

III

Suicide

9

Suicide: The Basic Issues

Philosophical issues concerning suicide—most broadly understood as the question of what role the individual may play in bringing about his or her own death—arise in a wide range of end-of-life contemporary bioethics dilemmas: the withdrawal or withholding of medical treatment, involuntary treatment, high-risk, experimental, and unconventional treatment, euthanasia, assistance and physician assistance in suicide, requests for maximal treatment, and many others. Two focal issues concerning suicide are evident in these dilemmas. First, and centrally, should suicide be recognized as a right, and if so, under what (medical?) conditions? On this first question rest the foundations for various applications of the "right to die," as well as a variety of other issues in high-risk and self-sacrificial behavior. Second, what should be the role of other persons toward those intending suicide? On this second question rest practical, legal, and public policy issues in suicide prevention and suicide assistance. Both focal issues raise larger questions concerning the nature of choices about dying and the relevance of mental illness, about the role of the state, about conceptual issues in determining what actions are to be counted as suicide, about the role of religious beliefs concerning suicide, about the possibility of autonomy, and about the moral status of suicide.

The Incidence of Suicide

The United States exhibits a reported suicide rate of 12.4 per 100,000 population per year (1990 figures), which falls approximately into mid-range between societies in which reported suicide rates are extremely low, such as the Islamic countries, and those in which reported rates are extremely high, for example, Hungary. In the United States, there are over 30,000 reported suicides per year and about eight to twenty times that many reported attempts; the worldwide suicide rate is about 13 per 100,000 population, or about 715,000 deaths per year in a world population of 5.5 billion. In the United States, suicide is the third leading cause of death for the young, behind accidents and homicide; for the population as a whole, it is eighth. Suicide

From *Encyclopedia of Bioethics*, ed. Warner T. Reich (New York: Free Press, forthcoming). Based on "Suicide," from *Encyclopedia of Ethics*, ed. Lawrence E. Becker (New York: Garland Publishing Co., 1992). Reprinted by permission of the publisher.

rates are approximately equivalent across socioeconomic groups. Completed suicide rates are higher for males, but attempted suicide rates are higher for females. Attempt rates for whites and blacks are equivalent; rates of death by suicide are lower for blacks, although climbing. For white males, suicide rates increase with age, rising to a peak of 72.6 per 100,000 population at the age range of eighty to eighty-four; for women, suicide rates peak in mid-life, declining thereafter, and black women in the age range of eighty to eighty-four have the lowest rate of all adult groups, 1.2 per 100,000 population. In the United States, on average, one person kills him- or herself every seventeen minutes.[1] There are no reliable estimates of the number of unreported suicides, particularly in medical situations involving terminal illness. Although suicide rates are typically low among married persons, in recent years joint suicides involving terminal illness among married couples have achieved some publicity, as have cases of suicide openly assisted by physicians.

Scientific Models of Suicide

Contemporary scientific understandings of the nature of suicide tend to fall into one of three groups; the medical model; the "cry for help," "suicidal career," or strategic model; and the sociogenic model.

The Medical Model

On this model, heavily influential throughout most of the twentieth century, suicide has been understood on the model of *disease:* if suicide is not itself a disease, then it is the product of disease, usually mental illness. Thus, suicide is understood as involuntary and nondeliberative, the outcome of factors over which the individual has no control: it is something that *happens* to the victim. Studies of the incidence of mental illness in suicide often tacitly appeal to this model by attempting to show that mental illness—usually depression, less frequently other mental disorders—is always or almost always present in suicide; this invites the inference that the mental illness or depression *caused* the suicide.

The "Cry for Help" Model

A second model, developed in the pioneering work of Edwin Shneidman and Norman Farberow,[2] understands suicide as a communicative strategy: it is a "cry for help," intended to seek aid in altering one's social environment. Thus it is primarily "dyadic," making reference to some second person (or less frequently, an institution or other entity) central in the suiciding person's life. On this view, it is the suicidal gesture that is clinically central; the completed suicide is an attempt that is (often unintentionally) fatal. Although the "cry for help" is manipulative in character, it is also often quite effective in mobilizing family, community, or medical resources to assist in helping change the circumstances of the attempter's life, at least temporarily. Later theorists, expecially Ronald Maris, have developed a related model also interpreting suicide attempts as strategic in character: this is a notion of "suicidal careers,"[3] in which an individual uses repeated suicide threats and attempts as a method of negotiating the world, until—as for Sylvia Plath[4]—such an attempt proves fatal.

The Sociogenic Model

Originally developed by sociologist Emile Durkheim (1858–1917) in his landmark work, *Suicide*,[5] the sociogenic model sees suicide as the product of social forces varying with the type of social organization within which the individual lives. "Each human society," Durkheim wrote, "has a greater or lesser aptitude for suicide . . . a collective inclination for the act, quite its own, and the source of all individual inclination, rather than their result." In societies in which the individual is very highly integrated into the society and his or her behavior is rigorously governed by social codes and customs, suicide tends to occur just when it is institutionalized and required by the society (as, e.g., in the Hindu practice of *suttee*, or voluntary widow-burning); these are termed "altruistic" suicides. In societies in which the individual is very loosely integrated, suicide is "egoistic," almost entirely self-referential. In still other societies, Durkheim claimed, the individual is neither over nor underintegrated, but the society itself fails to provide adequate regulation of its members: this situation results in "anomic" suicide, typical of modern industrial society. In Western societies of this sort, institutionalized suicide has been extremely rare but not unknown, confining itself to highly structured situations: the sea captain has been expected to "go down with his ship," and the Prussian army officer was expected to kill himself if he was unable to pay his gambling debts.

Like the medical model, the sociogenic model understands suicide as "caused," but it identifies the causes as social forces rather than individual psychopathology. Like the "cry for help" model, the sociogenic model sees suicide as a responsive strategy, but the responses are not so much matters of individual communication as conformity to social structures.

Prediction and Prevention

Two principal strategies are employed for recognition of the prospective suicide *before* the attempt: the identification of verbal and behavioral clues, and the description of social, psychological, and other variables associated with suicide. Suicide prevention strategies then include alerting families, professionals (especially those likely to have contact with suicidal individuals, such as schoolteachers), and the public generally to the symptoms of a potential suicide attempt: they are trained to recognize (and take seriously) both direct warnings (e.g., "I feel like killing myself") and indirect warnings (e.g., "I probably won't be seeing you anymore") and behavior (e.g., giving away one's favorite possessions). They are also encouraged to be especially sensitive to such symptoms in individuals at highest risk: those who are older, who live alone, who are alcoholic, who have negative interactions with important others, or who are isolated, and, especially, those with a history of previous suicide attempts. Prevention strategies take a vast range of forms, from the "befriending" techniques developed by the Samaritans in England and the crisis "hotlines" widely used in the United States to involuntary commitment to a mental institution. Prevention strategies also include "postvention" for the survivors—spouse, parent, child, or important other—of a person whose suicide attempt was fatal, since such survivors are themselves at much higher risk of suicide, especially during the first year.

These models of suicide and the associated forms of prediction and prevention are ubiquitous in contemporary medical and psychiatric practice. All three models have been influential in twentieth-century scientific views of suicide; however, although suicide has largely been treated as a medical or psychiatric matter, the conceptual, epistemological, and ethical problems it raises have reemerged as right-to-die issues in bioethics. These issues redirect attention to the individual's role in his or her own death, questioning whether the current views of suicide are appropriate in situations of terminal illness and other serious medical conditions.

Conceptual Issues

The term "suicide" carries extremely negative connotations. However, there is little agreement on a formal definition. Some authors count all cases of voluntary, intentional self-killing as suicide; others include only cases in which the individual's *primary* intention is to end his or her life. Still others recognize that much of what is usually termed suicide is neither wholly voluntary nor involves a genuine intention to die: suicides associated with depression or other mental illness, for example. Many writers exclude cases of self-inflicted death that, while voluntary and intentional, appear aimed to benefit others or to serve some purpose or principle—for instance, Socrates' drinking of the hemlock, Captain Oates' walking out into the Arctic blizzard to allow his fellow explorers to continue without him, or the self-immolation of war protesters. These cases are usually not called suicide, but "self-sacrifice" or "martyrdom," terms with strongly positive connotations. However, attempts to differentiate these positive cases often seem to reflect moral judgments, not genuine conceptual differences. Cases of death from self-caused accident, self-neglect, chronic self-destructive behavior, victim-precipitated homicide, high-risk adventure, and self-administered euthanasia—which all share many features with suicide but are not usually termed as such—cause still further conceptual difficulty. Consequently, some authors claim that it is not possible to reach a rigorous formal definition of suicide, and that only a criterial or operational approach to characterizing uses of the term can be successful. Nevertheless, conceptual issues surrounding the definition of suicide are of considerable practical importance in policy formation, as, for instance, in coroners' practices in identifying causes of death, insurance disclaimers, psychiatric protocols, religious prohibitions, and laws prohibiting or permitting assistance in suicide.

Suicide in the Western Tradition

Much of the extraordinarily diverse discussion of suicide in the history of Western thought has been directed to ethical issues. Plato (c. 430–347 B.C.) acknowledged Athenian burial restrictions (the suicide was to be buried apart from other citizens, with the hand severed and buried separately), and in the *Phaedo,* he also reported the Pythagorean view that suicide is categorically wrong. But Plato also accepted suicide under various conditions, including shame, extreme distress, poverty, unavoidable misfortune, and "external compulsions" of the sort imposed on Socrates by the Athenian court. In the *Republic* and the *Laws,* respectively, Plato obliquely insisted that the person suffering from chronic incapacitating illness or uncontrollable criminal impulses *ought* to allow his or her life to end or cause it to do so. Aristotle (384–322 B.C.) held more generally that suicide was wrong, claiming that it is "cowardly" and "treats the state unjustly." The Greek and Roman Stoics, in contrast, recommended suicide as the responsible, appropriate act of the wise man, not to be undertaken in emotional distress but as an expression of principle, duty, or responsible control of the end of one's own life, as exemplified by Cato (95–46 B.C.), Lucretia (sixth cent. B.C.), and Seneca (c. 4 B.C.–A.D. 65).

Although Old Testament texts described individual cases of suicide (Abimilech, Samson, Saul and his armor-bearer, Ahithophel, Zimri), nowhere do they express general disapproval of suicide. However, the Greek-influenced Jewish general Josephus (A.D. 37–100) rejected it as an option for his defeated army, and clear prohibitions of suicide appeared in Judaism by the time of the Talmud, often appealing to *Genesis* 9:5, "For your lifeblood I will demand satisfaction." Nor does the New Testament condemn suicide, and it mentions only one case: the self-hanging of Judas Iscariot after the betrayal of Jesus. There is evident disagreement among the early church fathers about the permissibility of suicide, especially in one specific circumstance: although some disapproved, Eusebius (c. A.D. 264–340), Ambrose (d. A.D. 397), and Jerome (c. A.D. 342–420) all held that a virgin might kill herself in order to avoid violation. Although Christian values clearly include patience, endurance, hope, and submission to the sovereignty of God, values that militate against suicide, they also stress willingness to sacrifice one's life, especially in martyrdom, and absence of the fear of death. Some early Christians (e.g., the Circumcellions, a subsect of the rigorist Donatists) apparently practiced suicide as an act of religious zeal: suicide committed immediately after confession and absolution, they believed, permitted earlier entrance to heaven. In any case, with the assertion by Augustine (A.D. 354–430) that suicide violated the commandment "Thou shalt not kill" and was a greater sin than any that could be avoided by suicide, the Christian opposition to suicide became unanimous and absolute.

This view of suicide as morally and religiously wrong intensified during the Christian Middle Ages. Thomas Aquinas (1225?–1274) argued that suicide was contrary to the natural law of self-preservation, injured the community, and usurped God's judgment "over the passage from this life to a more blessed one." By the High Middle Ages the suicide of Judas, often viewed earlier as appropriate atonement for the betrayal of Jesus, was seen as a sin worse than the betrayal itself.

During the Enlightenment, some individuals began to question these views: Thomas More (1478–1535) incorporated euthanatic suicide in his *Utopia* (1516); John Donne (1572–1631) treated suicide as morally praiseworthy when done for the glory of God (as he claimed in *Biathanatos* [1608, published posthumously 1647] was the case for Christ); David Hume (1711–1776) mocked the medieval arguments, justifying suicide on both autonomist and beneficent grounds; and later thinkers such as Mme. de Staël (1766–1817) (though she subsequently reversed her position) and Arthur Schopenhauer (1788–1860) construed suicide as a matter of human right. Throughout this period other writers insisted that suicide was morally, legally, and religiously wrong: for instance, John Wesley (1703–1791) said that suicide attempters should be hanged, and Sir William Blackstone (1723–1780) described suicide as an offense against both God and the King. Immanuel Kant (1724–1804) used the wrongness of suicide as a specimen of the moral conclusions the categorical imperative could demonstrate. In contrast, the Romantics tended to glorify suicide, and Friedrich Nietzsche (1844–1900) insisted that "suicide is man's right and privilege."

In Western thought, the volatile discussion of the moral issues in suicide ended fairly abruptly at the close of the nineteenth century. This was due in part to Durkheim's insistence that suicide is a function of social organization, and also to the views of psychological and psychiatric theorists, developing from Esquirol (1772–1840) to Freud (1856–1939), that suicide is a product of mental illness. These new "scientific" views reinterpreted suicide as the product of nonvoluntary conditions for which the individual could not be held morally responsible. The ethical issues, which presuppose choice, have reemerged only in the later part of the twentieth century, stimulated primarily by discussions in bioethics of dilemmas at the end of life.

Nonwestern Religious and Cultural Views of Suicide

Among religious moralists, Christian thinkers variously assert that divine commandment categorically prohibits suicide, that suicide repudiates God's gift of life, that suicide ruptures covenantal relationships with other persons, or that suicide defeats the believer's obligation to endure suffering in the image of Christ. But the prohibition of suicide has been absolute only in Christianity and Islam. Many other world religions hold the view that suicide is for the most part wrong, but that there are certain exceptions. Judaism, for example, prohibits suicide, but venerates the suicides at Masada and accepts *kiddush hashem* (self-destruction to avoid spiritual defilement). (To be sure, martyrdom to avoid apostasy, accepted and venerated by Christianity, may seem to very closely resemble this practice, but since the time of Augustine, Christianity has uniformly rejected self-caused death, as distinct from allowing oneself to be killed.) Many traditional societies exhibit insitutionalized suicide practices, such as the *suttee* of a Hindu widow, who is expected to immolate herself on her husband's funeral pyre, the *seppuku* or *hara-kiri* of traditional Japanese nobility out of loyalty to a leader or in infractions of honor; and, in cultures as diverse as Sumer and China, the apparently voluntary submission to sacrifice at the time of his funeral by the retainers of a newly dead king in order to accompany him into the next world. Eskimo, American Indian, and some traditional Japanese cultures have practiced voluntary abandonment of the elderly, a practice closely related to suicide.

In addition, some religious cultures have held comparatively positive views of suicide, at least in certain circumstances. The Vikings recognized suicide as a form of violent death that guaranteed entrance to Valhalla. The Jains, and perhaps other groups within traditional Hinduism, honored deliberate self-starvation as the ultimate asceticism, and also recognized religiously motivated suicide by throwing oneself down from a cliff. The Maya held that a special place in heaven was reserved for those who killed themselves by hanging (though other methods of suicide were considered disgraceful), and recognized a goddess of suicide, Ixtab. Many other pre-Columbian peoples in the Western Hemisphere engaged in ritual self-sacrifice, especially the Aztec practice of heart sacrifice, which was characterized, at least in historical periods in which it was voluntary, by enhanced status and social approval. The view that suicide is intrinsically and without exception wrong is associated most strongly with post-Augustinian, especially medieval, Christianity, surviving into the present; this absolutist view by and large is not characteristic of other cultures.

Contemporary Ethical Issues

Is suicide *morally* wrong? Both the historical and contemporary discussions exhibit certain central features. Consequentialist arguments tend to focus on the damaging effects a person's suicide can have on family, friends, coworkers, or society as a whole. But, as a few earlier thinkers saw, such consequentialist views would also recommend or require suicide when the interests of the individual or others would be served by suicide. Deontological theorists have tended to treat suicide as intrinsically wrong, but are typically unable to produce support for such claims that is independent of religious assumptions. Contemporary ethical argument has focused on such issues as whether the individual hedonic calculus of self-interest—where others are not affected—provides an adequate basis for choices about suicide; whether life has intrinsic value sufficient to preclude choices of suicide; and whether it is possible, on any ethical theory, to show that it would be *wrong,* rather than merely imprudent, for the ordinary, nonsuicidal person, not driven by circumstances or acting on principle, to end his or her life.[6]

Epistemological Issues

Closely tied to conceptual issues, the central epistemological issues raised by suicide involve the kinds of knowledge available to those who contemplate killing themselves. The issue of what, if anything, can be known to occur after death has, in the West, generally been regarded as a religious issue, answerable only as a matter of faith; few philosophical writers have discussed it directly, despite its clear relation to theory of mind. Some writers have argued that since we cannot have antecedent knowledge of what death involves, we cannot knowingly and voluntarily choose our own deaths; suicide is therefore always irrational.[7] Others reject this move, instead attempting to establish conditions for the rationality of suicide.[8] Still other writers examine psychological and situational constraints on decision-making concerning suicide. For instance, the depressed suicidal individual is described as seeing only a narrowed range of possible future outcomes in the current dilemma, the victim of a kind of "tunnel vision" constricted by depression;[9] and the possibility of preemptive suicide in the face of deteriorative mental conditions such as Alzheimer's disease is characterized as a problem of having to use the very mind that may already be deteriorating to decide whether to bear deterioration or die to avoid it.[10]

Public Policy Issues

It is often, though uncritically, assumed that if a person's suicide were "rational," other individuals ought not interfere with it and the state ought not prohibit it. However, this raises policy issues about the role of the state and other institutions in the prevention of suicide.

Rights and the Prevention of Suicide

In the West, both church and state have historically assumed roles in the control of suicide. In most European countries, ecclesiastic and civil law imposed burial restrictions on the suicide and additional penalties, including forfeiture of property, on the suicide's family. In England, suicide remained a felony until 1961. Suicide is now decriminalized in most of the United States and in England, primarily to facilitate psychiatric treatment of suicide attempters and to mitigate the impact on surviving family members, although in slightly more than half of U.S. states, assisting another person's suicide is a violation of statutory law. In Germany, assisting a suicide is not illegal, provided the person is competent and acting voluntarily; in the Netherlands, physician-assisted suicide is legally tolerated under the same guidelines as active voluntary euthanasia.

In recent years, suicide prevention strategies have been enhanced by considerable advances in the epidemiological study of suicide, in the identification of risk factors, and in forms of clinical treatment. Suicide prevention professionals welcome increased funding for education and prevention measures targeted at youth and other populations at high risk. Nevertheless, philosophers are increasingly alert to the more general theoretical issues these strategies raise. Because of their potentially substantial false positive rate, suicide prevention strategies raise significant public policy issues in any society that rejects unjustified coercion. Preventive restrictions—such as involuntary incarceration in a mental hospital or suicide precautions in an institutional setting—typically limit liberty, but because those predictive measures available are neither perfectly reliable nor perfectly sensitive, they will identify some fraction of persons as potential suicides who in fact would not kill themselves, and fail to identify others who will.[11] There are two distinct issues here: how great an infringement of the liberty of those erroneously identified is to be permitted in the interests of preventing suicide by those correctly identified, and, second and more generally, whether restrictive measures for preventing suicide can be justified at all, even for those who will actually go on to do so. Civil rights theorists are generally disturbed by the first of these problems; libertarians by the second.

Although U.S. law does not prohibit suicide, it is not usually interpreted to recognize suicide as a right. There is considerable pressure from right-to-die groups in favor of recognizing a right to self-determination or "self-deliverance" in termi- nal illness, usually by means of statutes that would legalize physician-assisted sui- cide and voluntary active euthanasia. Other rights issues are also raised by suicide and the question of prevention: when Hemlock Society president Derek Humphry's *Final Exit* (a book addressed to the terminally ill that provided explicit instructions for committing suicide, including lethal drug dosages) was published in 1991, it rose rapidly to the top of *The New York Times* how-to bestseller list, selling over 500,000 copies. Not protected by the same rights of freedom of expression, however, *Final Exit* was banned in several other countries, including France and Australia.

Physician-Assisted Suicide

Although issues about the permissibility of suicide generally have been the focus of sustained historical discussion, contemporary public policy debate tends to focus on a narrower, specific issue: that of physician-assisted suicide, usually coupled with the question of voluntary active euthanasia. Two principal arguments are advanced for the legalization of these practices. The first is based on claims about autonomy, an appeal to a conception of the individual as entitled to control, as much as possible, the course of his or her own dying. To restrict the "right to die" to the mere right to refuse unwanted medical treatment and so be "allowed" to die, this argument holds, is an indefensible truncation of the more basic right to choose one's death in accordance with one's own values; thus, advance directives such as living wills or durable powers of attorney, do-not-resuscitate orders, and other mechanisms for withholding or withdrawing treatment are inadequate to protect fundamental rights. The second principal argument for legalization of physician-assisted suicide, usually together with euthanasia, involves an appeal to what is variously understood as mercy or nonmaleficence; because not all terminal pain can be controlled and because suffering encompasses an even broader, less controllable range than pain, it is argued, it is defensible for a person who is in irremediable pain or suffering to choose death if there is no other way to avoid them.

Two principal arguments form the basis of the opposition to legalization of these practices: first, the claim that killing (in both suicide and euthanasia) is simply morally wrong (and hence wrong for doctors to facilitate or perform), and second, that legalization would invite a slippery slope leading to involuntary killing. The slippery slope argument contends, among other things, that permitting assistance in suicide or the performance of euthanasia would make killing "too easy," so that doctors would turn to it for reasons of bias, greed, impatience, or frustration with a patient not doing well; that it would set a dangerous model for disturbed younger persons not terminally ill; and that in a society marked by prejudice against the elderly, the disabled, racial minorities, and many others, and motivated by cost considerations in a system that does not guarantee equitable care, "choices" of death that are not really voluntary would be imposed on vulnerable persons: suicide in these circumstances would become a matter of social expectation or imperative. The counterargument for legalization replies that more open attitudes toward suicide would reduce psychopathology by allowing more effective counseling, and that, by bringing out into the open, and hence under adequate control, practices that have always gone on in secrecy, legalization would provide the most substantial protection for genuine patient choice. Particularly relevant to public policy discussions is the contention of some contemporary writers that suicide will become "the preferred way of death,"[12] since it allows control over the time, place, and circumstances of dying, and that it will grow increasingly acceptable and appropriate as the likelihood of otherwise dying of prolonged deteriorative illness in advanced age continues to increase.

Notes

1. Data prepared for the American Association of Suicidology by John L. McIntosh, February 1993, based on National Center for Health Statistics, advance report of final mortality statistics, 1990. *NCHS Monthly Vital Statistics Report* 41 (7, Suppl.), 1993; and on U.S. Bureau of the Census, *Current Population Reports*, Series P-25, No. 1095 (1992).

2. Edwin S. Shneidman and Norman L. Farberow, eds., *Clues to Suicide* (New York: McGraw-Hill, 1957). Anthology assembled by the founders of contemporary suicidology.

3. Ronald W. Maris, *Pathways to Suicide* (Baltimore: John Hopkins Univ. Press, 1981); also see Ronald W. Maris, Alan L. Berman, John T. Maltsberger, and Robert I. Yufit, *Assessment and Prediction of Suicide* (New York: Guilford Press, 1992).

4. See the account of Sylvia Plath's death, together with an extended historical essay, in A. Alvarez, *The Savage God: A Study of Suicide* (London: Weidenfeld and Nicolson, 1971).

5. Emile Durkheim, *Suicide: A Study in Sociology* [1897], tr. J. A. Spaulding and G. Simpson (New York: Free Press, 1951).

6. These issues are discussed by Jan Narveson in "Self-Ownership and the Ethics of Suicide," by Thomas E. Hill, Jr. in "Self-Regarding Suicide: A Modified Kantian View," and by Donald H. Regan in "Suicide and the Failure of Modern Moral Theory," all in Margaret P. Battin and Ronald W. Maris, eds., *Suicide and Ethics* (a special issue of *Suicide and Life-Threatening Behavior*) (New York: Human Sciences Press, 1983).

7. Philip E. Devine, "On Choosing Death," in M. Pabst Battin and David J. Mayo, eds., *Suicide: The Philosophical Issues* (New York: St. Martin's Press, 1980), pp. 138–143.

8. Margaret P. Battin, *Ethical Issues in Suicide* (Englewood Cliffs, N.J.: Prentice-Hall, 1982), chapter 4, pp. 131–153; and comments by Richard Momeyer, *Confronting Death* (Bloomington: Indiana University Press, 1988), pp. 112–121.

9. Richard B. Brandt, "The Morality and Rationality of Suicide," in Seymour Perlin, ed., *A Handbook for the Study of Suicide* (Oxford: Oxford University Press, 1975).

10. C. J. Prado, *The Last Choice: Preemptive Suicide in Advanced Age* (Westport, Conn.; Greenwood Press, 1990).

11. Rolf Sartorius, "Coercive Suicide Prevention: A Libertarian Perspective," in Battin and Maris, *Suicide and Ethics*, pp. 293–303.

12. Robert Kastenbaum, "Suicide as the Preferred Way of Death," in Edwin S. Shneidman, ed., *Suicidology: Contemporary Developments* (New York: Grune & Stratton, 1976), pp. 425–441.

10

Manipulated Suicide

Resuscitating an issue once quite widely explored by the Greeks, many contemporary bioethicists are now reexamining the notion of *rational* suicide, and are suggesting that death can, in some unfortunate cases (for instance, painful terminal illness), be a choice that is as reasonable, or more reasonable, than remaining alive. This is often accompanied by a call for more than merely intellectual assent and a demand for its recognition in religion, custom, medicine, psychiatry, and law. Indeed, a relaxation of traditional impermissive attitudes about suicide is already—albeit slowly—beginning to take place.

Reservations about the notion of rational suicide may be based on the dangers of erroneous choice: the risk that acceptance of rational suicide might on some occasions encourage impulsive or irrational suicide among those whose choices are not reasoned or clear. However, this risk, it may be argued, is countered by the moral imperative of allowing individuals to exercise what is clearly their right to die. On this view, the moral issue in suicide centers on a weighing of the interests of two groups: the "irrational" suicides, who are now thwarted in their attempts, but in the absence of social, legal, and psychological barriers to suicide might succeed at something they do not really want, and the "rational" suicides, who, by these same barriers, are dissuaded from that to which they have a right.

The benefits that most advocates of rational suicide have in mind seem to be based on a scenario something like this. Consider the cancer victim who suffers his illness in a society (like ours) that rejects suicide on religious, legal, social, and psychological grounds: he is, in effect, forced to endure the disease until it kills him, watching it rob his family of financial security and emotional health, rather than perform an act that he and his family are led to believe would make him a coward, a sociopath, a deviant, a lunatic, and an apostate. "Hang on a little longer," he and they urge each other, for to do otherwise would on all counts be wrong.

But the same individual, suffering the same disease in a society that offers no barriers to self-administered death in the face of terminal illness, will be very much more able to choose suicide, since if he does he, and his family, may take him to be acting decently and rationally, to be making a socially responsible choice, and to be doing what is sane, moral, and devout. To make such choices possible, and to give

From *Bioethics Quarterly* 2:2 (Summer 1980), 169–182. Copyright © 1980 by Human Sciences Press. Reprinted by permission of the publisher.

them social support, it is held, would be a great gain for human welfare, by allowing us to forgo suffering for ourselves and ruin for others when they can in no other way be avoided. As David Hume once put this point:

> . . . both prudence and courage should engage us to rid ourselves at once of existence when it becomes a burden. This is the only way that we can then be useful to society, by setting an example which, if imitated, would preserve to every one his chance for happiness in life, and would effectually free him from all danger or misery.[1]

But this is not the only outcome we might expect from the adoption of the notion of rational suicide. For, as I shall try to show, I think this notion—seemingly paradoxically—first gives rise to the possibility of large-scale manipulation of suicide, and the maneuvering of persons into choosing suicide when they would not otherwise have done so. This is the other, darker side of the future coin.

The Mechanisms of Manipulation

Let me try to describe manipulation in suicide by sorting out its cases: I think we can distinguish two principal mechanisms at work.

Circumstantial Manipulation

The rationality or irrationality of a given choice of suicide is in part a function of the individual's circumstances: his or her health, living conditions, degree of comfort or discomfort that daily life involves, political environment, opportunities for enjoyable or fulfilling activities and work, and so forth. Thus, when a person's circumstances change, so does the rationality or irrationality of his or her committing suicide: what may have been an unsound choice becomes, in the face of permanently worsened circumstances (say, a confirmed diagnosis of painful and incurable deteriorative illness) a reasonable one. But it is just this feature of suicide—that its rationality may change with changing circumstances—that makes one form of manipulation possible. What the manipulator does is alter the victim's immediate and/or long-range circumstances in such a way that the victim chooses death as preferable to continued life.

Manipulation of this sort may happen in a glaring way, as, for instance, in sustained torture; where blatant circumstantial manipulation of this sort is intended to result in suicide, it is called coercion, and counted as a form of murder. No doubt much more frequent, however, is the small, not very visible, often even inadvertent kind of manipulation that occurs in domestic situations, where what the manipulator does is to "arrange things" so that suicide becomes—given the other alternatives— the reasonable, even attractive choice for the victim.[2] For instance, negligent family members may fail to change the bed sheets of an incontinent bedridden patient, and in other ways provide poor or hostile nursing care; abusive parents may so thoroughly restrict and distort the circumstances of an adolescent child that suicide seems the only sensible way out. Perhaps only because it is so often invisible, we do not always recognize this kind of "domestic" manipulation as coercion and thus do not always call it murder.

Of course, suicide will not be the rational choice in such circumstances if these circumstances are likely to change or if they can be altered in some way. Where adverse circumstances are the result of coercion or manipulation by some other person or group, the obvious *rational* response would be to resist or attack the perpetrator in an effort to stop the manipulation and improve the circumstances. Thus, the incontinent bedridden patient's rational move is to complain to friends or authorities that her bed sheets are unchanged and that the care she is given is cruel; the beleaguered adolescent's may be to fight back or to run away.

In some cases, however, resistance may not be possible: the victim may be unable to elude her torturers, and suicide may *in fact* be the only way of escape. Perhaps such cases are rare. But if we recognize the notion of rational suicide, we must also recognize that in such cases, suicide may be the only rational choice for the victim, whether she is coerced or not and whether her circumstances have been deliberately worsened or not. Where the victim can identify the perpetrator and retaliate in some effective way, to do so is clearly the more rational choice, but manipulation is not always easy to detect, and even when it is, its perpetrators are not always easy to stop.

Ideological Manipulation

The rationality of suicide is also in part a function of one's beliefs and values, and these, like circumstances, can also change. Suicide can be said to be irrational not only if it is chosen in a hasty, unthinking way, or on the basis of inadequate information, but also if it violates one's fundamental beliefs and values. For instance, suicide can be said to be an irrational choice for someone who believes that it will bring unwanted, eternal damnation, or for someone who believes that active, this-world caring for another is his or her primary goal.

But of course, suicide may also be in accord with one's most fundamental beliefs and values. For instance, Stoic thinkers held slavery to be a condition so degrading that death was to be preferred to it, and those who took their lives to avoid slavery (Cato, for instance) regarded themselves and were regarded by others as having made a fully rational choice.[3] These fundamental beliefs vary from one society and era to another: though loss of virginity and chastity was a basis for rational suicide in early Christian times,[4] the contemporary rape victim does not typically consider sexual assault reason to kill herself, even though it may cause very severe emotional distress. Nor does contemporary Western society countenance suicide in bereavement, for honor, or to avoid poverty, insanity, or disgrace, although all these have been recognized in various cultures at earlier times.[5]

Once we see that the beliefs and values on which the rationality of suicide in part depends can vary from one individual or historical era to another, we also recognize that such ideology can change. Ideological change may occur as part of the natural evolution of a culture; however, such changes can also be engineered. The contemporary world is already well familiar with deliberate attitude and values manipulation, from the gentle impress of advertising to the intensive programming and conditioning associated with various religious and political groups. If our attitudes and values in other areas can be deliberately changed, it is not at all unreasonable to think that our conceptions of the conditions under which suicide would be the rational choice can be changed too.

Current Circumstantial and Ideological Change

If we look at contemporary society, we can already see considerable evidence of change in areas relevant to the practice of rational suicide. To detect such change, of course, is not to find evidence of deliberate manipulation, but it is to show the kinds of change in association with which we might expect manipulation—deliberate or otherwise—to occur. These changes are all of a sort in which someone might be brought to choose suicide who would not otherwise have done so.

In the first place, we may note various kinds of circumstantial change relevant to the practice of rational suicide. Some are changes that might work to decrease the incidence of suicide: the development of more effective methods of pain relief, for instance, or institutions like Hospice.[6] But others tend on the whole to worsen the conditions of certain individuals or groups: here one might cite our increasing tendency to confine elderly persons in nursing homes, the increasing expense of such institutional care, the loss of social roles for the elderly, and the increasingly difficult financial circumstances of those living on marginal or fixed incomes. One might also mention increasing loss of autonomy in the seriously ill, as "heroic" practices in medicine become increasingly mechanized; new abilities to maintain seriously in-jured or birth-defective persons in marginal states, and so forth. Gerontologists and patients' rights advocates have been pointing to the inhumane consequences of such circumstantial changes for some time, and such observations are hardly new; what is new, however, is alertness to their role with respect to rational suicide. Increasingly poor conditions, in a society that is coming to accept a notion of rational suicide, may mean an increasing likelihood that suicide will be the individual's choice.

Second, we can also diagnose several significant ideological changes in contem-porary society. For instance, there has been a profusion of recent literary accounts favorable to suicide and assisted suicide in terminal illness cases—real-life stories of one partner assisting the other in obtaining and taking a lethal drug to avoid the ravages of cancer.[7] There are increasingly frequent court decisions favoring pa-tients' rights to refuse medical treatment, even when refusal will mean death.[8] There have appeared some public accounts of suicides conceived of and conducted as rational: the cases of Henry and Elizabeth Van Dusen, Wallace Proctor, and Jo Roman, to mention a few.[9] And some religious groups have begun to devote atten-tion to the issue of whether suicide may be, in certain kinds of terminal circum-stances, an act of religious conscience, even though Western Christianity in general has not allowed it for the past fifteen hundred years, since Augustine.[10] Almost all these cases involve suicide in the face of painful terminal illness, and that illness is very often cancer. If we were to diagnose our own ideological changes with regard to suicide, we would probably say that they involve a very recent move—by no means universal, but already clearly and widely evident—from the recently predominant view that there is *no* good reason for suicide (and hence that all suicide is irrational or insane) to the view that there is after all one adequate reason for suicide: extreme and irremediable pain in terminal illness.

The transition may not seem to be a very large one. But there is no reason to think it is complete, and one may perhaps predict the direction in which it will continue by noticing the kinds of reasons that are typically given to justify killing and nonprolongation of life in several closely associated phenomena: euthanasia, abortion, infanticide of defective newborns, and noninitiation or withdrawal of treatment in chronic or terminal illness cases. Extreme pain is one such reason. So is extreme physical dependence, sometimes called degradation; this is often cited as a reason for discontinuing long-term tube feeding or maintenance on life support systems, nonresuscitation, and hospital no-code procedures.[11] Financial burdens are now also sometimes mentioned, even by the Catholic church: the expense of a protracted chronic or terminal illness may count among the reasons to withhold heroic treatment, even when the patient will die instead.[12] Expense is also often a consideration in decisions to withhold or terminate *ordinary* treatment, especially in the elderly and in defective newborns.[13] Still another consideration coming to the fore in current life-versus-death decisions is that of impact on the immediate family: one now hears as a justification for passive and active euthanasia, abortion, infanticide, and withdrawal of treatment in the chronically or terminally ill the claim that this will ''spare the family'' the agony of watching someone die a protracted and painful death or enter a seriously deficient life. Considerations regarding scarce medical resources are also sometimes heard, together with those involving the care burden placed on medical personnel and family members by someone suffering a lengthy difficult illness or with a severe birth defect. Finally, we now also recognize religious reasons for voluntary death when life could be continued: the Jehovah's Witnesses blood transfusion cases appear to establish the right of an individual to relinquish his or her life in order to protect his or her basic religious beliefs, at least where this does not infringe on the rights of others.[14]

Except for pain, none of these considerations is now generally recognized as a reason for *suicide*. But they are already recognized as reasons that may justify the killing of others and the nonprolongation of one's own life, and it is highly plausible to expect that they will soon be recognized as relevant in suicide decisions too.

The kinds of alterations in the ideology and circumstances of rational suicide diagnosed here as now in progress all involve medical and quasi-medical situations. They would begin to allow what might be called euthanatic suicide, or a choice of death in preference to prolonged and painful death. As the circumstantial changes mentioned earlier—increasing displacement of the elderly and increasing loss of autonomy for the ill—operate to make the conditions of those who are faced with dying increasingly difficult, there is reason to think the attractiveness or euthanatic suicide as an alternative will increase. But there are no a priori checks on the breadth of such extensions of the concept of rational suicide, and no reason why future extensions must be limited to euthanatic medical situations. As I have said, such conditions as dishonor, slavery, and loss of chastity have sometimes been considered suicide-warranting conditions in Western culture in the past: widowhood and public dishonor have assumed such roles in the East, and it seems merely naive to assume that these conditions, or others we now find equally implausible reasons for suicide, could not come to be regarded so in the future. This is particularly obvious if we keep in mind the possibility of circumstantial manipulation and of both inadvertent and deliberate ideological engineering. The motivation for such manipulation and engineering, in a society confronted with scarcities and fearful of an increasingly large "nonproductive" population, may be very strong. Old age, insanity, poverty, and criminality have also sometimes been regarded as grounds for rational suicide in the past; given a society afraid of demands from increasingly large geriatric, ghetto, and institutional populations, one can see how interest in producing circumstantial and ideological changes, in order to encourage such people to choose the "reasonable" way out, might be very strong.

Not all manipulation toward suicide need be malevolent or self-interested on the part of the manipulator. Such manipulation can also be paternalistic, where one pleads with a victim to "consider yourself" and end a life the paternalist perceives as hopelessly burdensome.[15] And, of course, such pressures may be both paternalistic and other-interested at once: one imagines a counselor advising an old or ill person to spare both himself and his family the agony of an extended decline,[16] even though this person would not have considered or attempted suicide on his own and would have been willing to suffer the physical distress. Can he resist such pressures? Not, perhaps, in a climate in which suicide is "the rational thing to do" in circumstances such as these. To resist, indeed, might earn him the epithets now applied to the individual who does choose suicide: coward, sociopath, deviant, lunatic, apostate. He has, after all, refused to do what is rational and what is believed to be not only in his own interests but in those of people he loves.

It is important to understand that such choices of suicide can be manipulated only under a prevailing notion of *rational* suicide. Manipulation of this sort does not involve driving one's victims into insanity or torturing them into irrationality; rather, it consists in providing a basis for the making of a *reasonable* decision about the ending of one's life and in providing the criteria upon which that decision is to be made. The choice remains crucially and essentially voluntary, and the decision between alternatives free. Furthermore, in a suicide-permissive society, the choice of suicide would be protected by law, religion, and custom, and would be recognized as evidence of sound mental health. But the circumstances of the choice have been restructured so that choosing now involves weighing not only one's own interests but those of others. Where, on balance, the costs of death will be less for oneself and for others than the costs of remaining alive, suicide will be the rational—and socially favored—choice. Indeed, perhaps the choice is not so free after all.

As I have said, there is no reason to think that such questions must remain confined to medical situations or what might be called euthanatic suicide. Not only do these considerations apply to nonterminal as well as terminal illness cases (consider, for instance, the pain, dependence, expense, impact on the family, and use of scarce medical resources in connection with nonterminal conditions such as renal failure, quadriplegia, or severe arthritis), but they will also apply to conditions where there is no *illness* as such at all: retardation, genetic anomaly, abnormal personality, and old age. One can even imagine that continuing ideological redefinition might invite us to regard life as not worth living and the interests of others as critical in a much wider variety of nonmedical situations: chronic unemployment, widowhood, poverty, social isolation, criminal conviction, and so forth. Such claims may seem absurd. But all these conditions have been promoted as suicide-warranting at some time in the past, and they are all also very often associated with social dependence. After Hitler, we are, I trust, beyond extermination of unwanted or dependent groups. But we may not be beyond encouraging *as rational* the self-elimination of those whom we perceive to constitute a burden to themselves and to others, and I think that this is where the risk in manipulated suicide lies.

Responses to Manipulation: A Moral Dilemma

But there is a problem. Manipulated suicide is morally repugnant, and we recognize that families, social groups, and societies should encourage respect and care for ill or disadvantaged members instead. But suicide may be both manipulated *and* rational, and herein lies the philosophical problem. Once we grant that it may be rational for an individual to choose death rather than to live in circumstances that for her are unacceptably or intolerably painful, physically or emotionally, or that are destructive of her most deeply held values, then we cannot object to her choice of death—even though she may be choosing to die because her circumstances have been deliberately or inadvertently worsened, because she has been brought to see her life as worthless, or because she believes she has an obligation to benefit her family by doing so. Certainly we can object to the manipulation of a person's circumstances or the distortion of her ideology. And we can attempt to point out to the victim what has happened. But we cannot object to her choice of suicide, if that remains her choice. To insist that we could not allow suicide that results from manipulation would be to insist that the victim remain alive in what to her have become intolerable circumstances or with her values destroyed; this would be to inflict a double misery—precisely what the notion of rational suicide is intended to prevent. Yet, we must see that the very concept that allows this person escape is what first makes possible manipulation of these kinds, since it is the very notion of *rational* suicide that stipulates that under certain conditions one may reasonably seek to end one's life.

If we refuse to adopt the notion of rational suicide, we fail to honor the moral imperative of allowing individuals in intolerable and irremediable circumstances their fundamental right to die. If we do adopt it, we fail to honor a moral imperative of a different kind: protecting vulnerable individuals from being manipulated into choices they otherwise might not make. Nevertheless, I think that this second imperative is not so strong as the first, and that it is not as strong as the imperative to protect individuals from outright coercion. Indeed, a rational person may be willing to accept the possibility of manipulation that is engendered by the notion of rational suicide in exchange for the social freedom to control one's own dying as one wishes—even knowing that he or she may eventually also succumb to that risk and be "encouraged" to choose death sooner than might otherwise have been the case. This, after all, will be experienced as a free, rational, voluntary choice. Most of us, in the end, will grow ill or old or both, and so become candidates for manipulation of this kind. But the alternative—to maintain or reestablish rigid suicide prohibitions—

is not attractive either, and is particularly cruel to precisely those people for whom death is or may become the rational choice—that is, those persons in the most unfortunate circumstances of all. After all, these prohibitions also serve to manipulate choice, though in the direction of choosing to stay alive. I myself believe that on moral grounds we must accept, not reject, the notion of rational suicide. But I think we must do so with a clear-sighted view of the moral quicksand into which this notion threatens to lead us; perhaps then we may discover a path around.

Notes

1. David Hume, "On Suicide," in *The Philosophical Works of David Hume,* vol. 4 (Edinburgh: Printed for Adam Black and William Tait, 1826), 567. Hume's essay, in modernized spelling, is to be found in a number of contemporary collections, including Raziel Abelson and Marie-Louise Friquegnon, eds., *Ethics for Modern Life* (New York: St. Martin's Press, 1975); in an abridged version, Samuel Gorovitz, ed., *Moral Problems in Medicine* (Englewood Cliffs, N.J.: Prentice-Hall, 1976); and abridged but with a commentary in Tom L. Beauchamp and Seymour Perlin, *Ethical Issues in Death and Dying* (Englewood Cliffs, N.J.: Prentice-Hall, 1978).

2. It is Virgil Aldrich who suggests the use of the phrase "arrange things" in connection with manipulation into suicide. It is good to notice, however, that terms such as "arrange things" and "manipulation" suggest conscious intentionality on the part of the "arranger" or "manipulator," though conscious intentionality need not always be a feature in these cases.

3. See, for example, Seneca, *Letters* 70, 77, and 78 on preferring death to slavery, and Plutarch's *Lives of the Noble Greeks and Romans* on the death of Cato the Younger. This view is not confined to Stoicism; see Josephus, *The Jewish War,* vol. 7, 320–419, on the mass suicide of the 960 defenders of Masada.

4. See, for example, St. Ambrose, *On Virgins,* and St. Eusebius, *Ecclesiastical History,* chap. 12, for accounts of Christian women who committed suicide rather than be violated by the Romans. Support for this view ends, however, with St. Augustine's repudiation of suicide as an alternative to sexual defilement, *City of God,* bk. 1, chaps. 16–28.

5. See H. Romilly Fedden, *Suicide: A Social and Historical Study* (London: Peter Davies Ltd., 1938), for an account of suicides for bereavement, insanity, dishonor, poverty, and disgrace in Western and non-Western cultures. Note also that bereavement suicides are familiar to us in the Hindu practice of *suttee,* and honor suicides in the Japanese practices of *seppuku* or *harakiri* and in *junshi.* See also the group of articles on suicide in various cultures in the James Hastings, *Encyclopaedia of Religion and Ethics,* vol. 12 (New York: Charles Scribner's Sons, 1925), and in chapter 9 of this volume.

6. Hospice, devoted to providing palliative but medically nonaggressive care for terminal illness patients by means of prophylactic pain control, makes equally significant attention to the emotional needs of the patient's family. Hospice is not, however, a panacea, and is not designed to approach many of the sorts of social and physical problems that confront the chronically ill, the elderly, the seriously disabled, and others for whom suicide might be seen as a rational choice. An account of the theory and methodology of Hospice can be found in a number of the publications by Cicely Saunders, including "The Treatment of Intractable Pain in Terminal Cancer," *Proceedings of the Royal Society of Medicine* 56 (1963): 195, and "Terminal Care in Medical Oncology," in *Medical Oncology* ed. K. D. Bagshawe (Oxford: Blackwell, 1975), 563–576. A careful assessment of potentials for abuse of the Hospice

system may be found in John F. Potter, ''A Challenge for the Hospice Movement,'' *The New England Journal of Medicine* 302, no. 1 (Jan. 3, 1980): 53–55.

7. Jessamyn West, *The Woman Said Yes* (New York: Harcourt Brace Jovanovich, 1976); Lael Tucker Wertenbacker, *Death of a Man* (Boston: Beacon Press, 1974); Derek Humphrey with Ann Wickett, *Jean's Way* (New York: Quartet Books, 1978).

8. See accounts of a number of these cases, including *In re Yetter, Saikewicz,* and *Perlmutter,* in Alan Sullivan's ''A Constitutional Right to Suicide,'' in M. Pabst Battin and David Mayo, eds., *Suicide: The Philosophical Issues* (New York: St. Martin's, 1980), 229.

9. For an account of the deaths of Henry P. Van Dusen, former president of Union Theological Seminary, and his wife Elizabeth, leaders in American theological life; see *The New York Times,* February 26, 1975, p. 1. The Van Dusens left a note explaining the motivation for their suicide (he, at age seventy-seven, had had a disabling stroke five years before, and she, age eighty, had severe arthritis), and saying ''we still feel this is the best way and the right way to go.''

An account of the suicide of Wallace Proctor, a retired dermatologist with Parkinson's disease, is reported in *The New York Times,* December 11, 1977; that of Jo Roman, an artist with cancer who ended her life in a much-publicized gathering of intimates, is reported in *The New York Times,* June 17, 1979.

10. See, for example, a pastoral letter of the Presbytery of New York City. March 9, 1976, which concludes that ''it is clear that for some Christians, as a last resort in the gravest of situations, suicide may be an act of their Christian conscience.''

11. Decisions that support the assertions made here are difficult to document in detail. However, the court in the Karen Ann Quinlan case observes: ''. . . it is perfectly apparent from the testimony we have quoted . . . , and indeed so clear as almost to be judicially noticeable, that humane decisions against resuscitative or maintenance therapy are frequently a recognized *de facto* response in the medical world to the irreversible, terminal, pain-ridden patient, especially with familial consent. And these cases, of course, are far short of 'brain death''' (*Matter of Quinlan* 355A.2d 647 at 667).

12. The text of Pope Pius XII's 1958 statement on medical resuscitation, ''The Prolongation of Life,'' is available in Stanley Joel Reiser, Arthur J. Dyck, and William J. Curran, eds., *Ethics in Medicine* (Cambridge, Mass.: MIT Press, 1977), 501–504. The physician is not obligated to use ''extraordinary means'' (including, e.g., respirators) to sustain the biological life of someone who is ''virtually dead.'' Considerations to be made in individual cases include whether an attempt at resuscitation is ''such a burden for the family that one cannot in all conscience impose it upon them,'' and is usually interpreted to include both financial and emotional burdens.

13. Again, although particular decisions on such bases are difficult to document, see the symposia ''Spina Bifida'' and ''Infants and Ethics'' (in *The Hastings Center Report,* 7 [No. 4, August 1977] and 8 [No. 1, February 1978], respectively) and many other articles in this and other bioethics and medico-legal journals for a sense of kinds of considerations that are made with respect to life versus death choices.

14. *Erickson v. Dilgard* (252 N.Y.S.2d 705) held that an adult patient had the right to refuse a blood transfusion even if medical opinion was to the effect that the patient's decision not to accept blood was tantamount to the taking of the patient's own life; *Application of President and Directors of Georgetown College* (331 F.2d 1000 [1964]) authorized an unwanted transfusion to a patient who objected on religious grounds, but apparently because she was the mother of a seven-month-old child.

15. Diogenes Laertius relates that when Antisthenes was mortally ill, Diogenes brought him a dagger, offering it to Antisthenes to release himself from his pains. Antisthenes declined, saying he wanted release from his pains, not from his life; Diogenes Laertius

observes "it was thought that he showed some weakness in bearing his malady through love of life." (*Lives of Eminent Philosophers,* vol. 6, 18–19, on Antisthenes, tr. R. D. Hicks [Cambridge, Mass.: Harvard University Press, 1965]. vol. 2, 21.) Tales of paternalistic assistance in suicide are common in Stoic Greece and Rome.

16. In Thomas More's *Utopia,* the state priests and magistrates go to a person suffering from painful incurable illness and "urge him to make the decision not to nourish such a painful disease any longer. He is now unequal to all the duties of life, a burden to himself and to others . . ." (Book II: "Their Care of the Sick and Euthanasia," tr. H.V.S. Ogden [Northbrook, Ill: AHM Publishing Corp., 1949], 57).

11

Prohibition and Invitation:
The Paradox of Religious
Views about Suicide

In an increasingly secular age, it may seem curious to attend to views of suicide based on explicitly religious assumptions. In part, this reflects the fact that arguments against suicide originated within religious contexts, and that present legal and social practices in the Western tradition arose from medieval religious law. We in the West tend, correctly, to assume that it is Christianity's opposition to suicide that is the basis of much of our cultural and legal disapprobation of suicide, but we do not stop to examine whether the scriptural and theological foundations of this tradition provide adequate support for its absolute prohibition. On what basis is the Christian religious tradition opposed to suicide, and why is its opposition so strong—indeed, so much stronger than that of other major religious traditions?

Quite independent of matters of personal religious belief, it is important to understand Christianity's view of suicide for two principal reasons. First, it is Western, Christian-influenced attitudes toward suicide that have historically led to the development of modern psychological, sociological, and legal views of suicide; these now form the basis for the "scientific" and professional study and treatment of suicide throughout the world, even in culturally quite diverse areas. Second, it is only Christianity (and, derivatively, Judaism and Islam[1]) that has promulgated a strict, thoroughgoing doctrine prohibiting suicide. Other religious cultures do have teachings concerning the permissibility and impermissibility of suicide, but these are nowhere as strict as the traditional Christian doctrine, and do permit or encourage self-killing in various circumstances. Other religious cultures have not developed an elaborate theological, argumentative machinery like Christianity's for defending strict prohibitions; but Christian-influenced cultures are often insufficiently sensitive to the nuances of the kinds of situations in which the issue of suicide might arise. If this study of religious views about suicide is primarily oriented toward Christianity, this is because it is Christian theology that yields the paradox of both prohibition and invitation, and consequently provides a basis for the attitudes toward suicide taken

Based on M. Pabst Battin, "Religious Views of Suicide," in *Ethical Issues in Suicide* (Englewood Cliffs, N.J.: Prentice-Hall, 1982). Copyright © 1982 by Prentice-Hall. Reprinted by permission of the publisher.

by the scientific and professional community throughout the contemporary world—a basis we have not adequately recognized as unstable.

Almost all of the traditional and contemporary religious arguments concerning suicide to be examined here presuppose the existence of a divine being, as well as the meaningfulness of such concepts as salvation, retribution, and sin; and almost all of these arguments could be defeated by denying these beliefs. In a secular society, this is often the approach taken: the argument that suicide is wrong because life is a gift from God, for instance, is often said to be unsound because there is no God. But to discard the religious arguments in this summary way is to ignore what is interesting and significant about them, and to fail to see why they remain so strongly influential in supporting prohibitions and in forming public attitudes about suicide. My goal in this chapter will be to see what is paradoxical in the modern world about these religious views of suicide, even if one grants these traditional theological beliefs.

The Religious Arguments against Suicide

I shall begin by examining those arguments explicit within the Christian tradition that lead to conclusions denouncing or prohibiting suicide. These arguments fall into four main groups: those based on biblical texts; those based on analogies to everyday objects and relations, or the so-called religious analogies; the natural-law arguments; and arguments concerning the role of suffering in Christian life. In examining these arguments, we shall be acquainting ourselves with the central aspects of the Christian case against suicide, which culminates in the claim made by some members of that tradition that suicide is a greater sin than any other; these are the arguments that have served as the theoretical basis for strict ecclesiastical penalties for suicide and the corresponding civil penalties in medieval and modern law.

But the religious arguments against suicide are only half the story; in exploring the positions Christianity takes against suicide, we also begin to observe the remarkable way in which Christian theology lends itself to arguments *in favor of* suicide. These arguments favoring suicide, of course, have almost never been explicitly stated; in the second part of this chapter I will attempt to formulate them. It is the persuasiveness of these covert arguments favoring suicide, one may suspect, that has led to the energetic formulation of explicit, theologically based arguments against and prohibitions of suicide, which survive in contemporary society under the protection of a virtual taboo. Christianity *invites* suicide in a way in which other major religions do not; it is for this reason, we may suppose, that Christianity has been forced to erect stringent prohibitions against it.

The nonreligious reader may wish to skip this essay and move directly on to other selections in which other moral arguments concerning suicide are discussed. But I do not think it will be possible to fully understand contemporary Western attitudes toward suicide without understanding something of the religious climate from which they arise, and, more important, without understanding something of the way in which Christian theology necessitates development of a case against it. It is this that may provide insight into contemporary moral views.

Suicide as a Violation of Biblical Commandment

It is one of the more prevalent assumptions of Western religious culture that the Bible prohibits suicide; inspection of the biblical texts, however, shows that this is by no means clearly the case. To begin with, there is no explicit prohibition of suicide in the Bible. There is no word anywhere in the Bible, either in Aramaic, Hebrew, or Greek, that is equivalent to the English term suicide, either in its nominal or verbal form, nor is there any idiomatic way of referring to this act that suggests that it is a distinct type of death.[2] Nor is there any passage in either the Old or New Testament that can be directly understood as an explicit prohibition of suicide; those passages that are often taken to support such a prohibition require, as we shall see, a considerable amount of interpretation and qualification.

However, the biblical texts do describe a number of cases—eight in the Old Testament, two of which are in the Apocrypha, and one in the New Testament[3]—of the phenomenon most contemporary English-speakers would call suicide. None of these passages offers explicit comment on the morality of suicide, nor is there anywhere in the Bible an explicit discussion of the ethical issues. Nevertheless, these passages are of considerable importance in establishing the moral stance of the scriptural texts toward suicide.

Consider, for instance, the passage in I Samuel that describes the deaths of Saul and his armor-bearer in battle against the Philistines:

> The Philistines fought a battle against Israel, and the men of Israel were routed, leaving their dead on Mount Gilboa. The Philistines hotly pursued Saul and his sons and killed the three sons, Jonathan, Abinadab, and Malchishua. The battle went hard for Saul, for some archers came upon him and he was wounded in the belly by the archers. So he said to his armour-bearer, ''Draw your sword and run me through, so that these uncircumcised brutes may not come and taunt me and make sport of me.'' But the armour-bearer refused, he dared not; whereupon Saul took his own sword and fell on it. When the armour-bearer saw that Saul was dead, he too fell on his sword and died with him. Thus they all died together on that day, Saul, his three sons, and his armour-bearer, as well as his men.[4]

It is clear that Saul kills himself only after all hope of victory is lost, after his sons are dead and his army destroyed, and after it is certain that he will be captured, tortured, and will die either of torture or the wounds in his belly. Saul's act could be interpreted as one of cowardice. Yet it could equally well be maintained that Saul killed himself in order to avoid degradation at the hands of the enemy, since the treatment to which these ''uncircumcised brutes'' would subject him would not befit the Lord's anointed; to avoid this would be to defend the honor of Israel. In either case, however, it is clear that the biblical narrator makes no overt condemnation of Saul's act. Futhermore, the populace of the surrounding area is said to have accorded both Saul, a suicide, and his sons, who were not suicides, identical anointment, burial, and fasting rites; this further suggests that no moral disapprobation attached to suicide.

Other Old Testament suicides include Ahithophel, the wise counselor of Absalom, who hanged himself not so much because his pride was wounded when Absalom refused to follow his advice, but because he recognized that Absalom's cause was therefore lost; the usurper Zimri, who burned the royal citadel over him in what is apparently viewed by the redactor as a self-imposed judgment for the sins he had committed; Abimilech, whose suicide also appears to be viewed as a punishment for sins; and Samson, who in destroying the Philistines pulled the temple down upon himself. The only completed New Testament suicide is that of Judas, who hanged himself;[5] the Matthean narrator implies that the motive is remorse over the betrayal of Jesus, and seems to see Judas' death as appropriate in the context. Again, there is nowhere, in either the Old or New Testament, an explicit discussion of the moral status of suicide. There are cases in which a biblical figure expresses despair or weariness of life, often from persecution or physical affliction—for example, Elijah, Job, Jonah, Sarah (the daughter of Raguel), and possibly Jesus at Gethsemane—but although these figures all recover an earlier enthusiasm for life, there is no condemnation of any consideration of suicide they may have made.[6] On the whole, however, suicide is a comparatively rare phenomenon in biblical texts.

An explanation frequently offered in the secondary literature for the paucity of reference to suicide in early Hebrew sources is that because the Jews were "joyously fond of life" and believed that human life was sacred, suicide virtually never occurred; hence, explicit discussions of its morality and injunctions against its practice were unnecessary.[7] This is said to explain the fact, for instance, that there is no mention of suicide in the 613 Precepts, although this code attempted to regulate all aspects of the Jews' everyday and religious lives in minute detail. However, there is no independent evidence to substantiate the claim that suicide was virtually unknown, and we do not know whether suicide prohibitions are absent from early Hebrew literature because suicide did not occur, or because suicide was not prohibited. What we do know is that those few suicides that do occur in the Old Testament literature are not subject to obvious moral censure.

Scholarly views have been expectably diverse. L. D. Hankoff, although acknowledging that no explicit biblical prohibition exists, argues that independent evidence concerning the notions of blood ties, sacrifice, and other elements of early Hebrew culture "suggest that suicide would have been strongly opposed because it represented a dangerous form of the spilling of blood, a loss of community control over the blood of a tribal member, and the possibility of an unattended corpse in the wilderness."[8] In the view of another commentator, however, the Hebrews, at least until late post-Exilic times, "must be counted among those races to whom suicide is simply one of the various possible forms of death and calls for no special comment."[9]

The earliest explicit negative moral evaluation of suicide in the Jewish tradition is to be found in the first century A.D. Josephus, attempting to dissuade his own army from a mass suicide in which he would be forced to include himself,[10] argues that suicide is cowardly, repugnant to nature, and an act of impiety to God; he says that it violates the will to live, that it rejects God's gift, that it misuses God's entrustment of an immortal soul, and that it would be to "fly from the best of masters." He further asserts that the souls of suicides go to the darker regions of the nether world, and that one's descendants will be punished for this act. But this is probably not authentically Hebrew; much of Judaism had become quite hellenized, and Josephus himself had Greek assistants and was familiar with Greek literature. Many of the arguments he presents against suicide can be discovered in Plato and other Greek sources. [11]

With the development of the Talmud in the first several centuries A.D., later rabbinic tradition begins to make explicit a prohibition of suicide, both in stories condemning suicide and by means of mourning and funeral restrictions. The Talmud, unlike earlier Hebrew sources, contains numerous stories of suicide and suicidal martyrdom, and in many of these disapproval of the act is clearly indicated by the narrator or author. The major Talmudic discussion of rules governing suicide appears in the tractate *Semakhot;* this text forbids one to rend one's garments or bare one's shoulders as signs of mourning for a suicide or to say a eulogy at the funeral. [12]

In the developing Talmud, the Old Testament passage at Genesis 9:5 begins to be cited as the fundamental basis of Judaism's prohibition of suicide. What follows is the text, in which the verse considered relevant is emphasized:

> And God blessed Noah and his sons, and said to them, ''Be fruitful and multiply and fill the earth. The fear of you and the dread of you shall be upon every beast of the earth, and upon every bird of the air, upon everything that creeps on the ground and all the fish of the sea; into your hand they are delivered. Every moving thing that lives shall be food for you; and as I gave you the green plants, I give you everything. Only you shall not eat flesh with its life, that is, its blood. *For your lifeblood I will surely require a reckoning;* of every beast I will require it and of man; of every man's brother I will require the life of man. Whoever sheds the blood of man, by man shall his blood be shed; for God made man in his own image. And you, be fruitful and multiply, bring forth abundantly on the earth and multiply on it.''

The Talmudic reading of the emphasized phrase as a prohibition of suicide, however, is much later than the original text, and it is possible to read the original text in several ways. Most plausibly, it is read as a prohibition of the wrongful killing of other human beings, [13] and not as a prohibition of suicide per se.

Whatever the scriptural basis, however, medieval Judaism maintained very strong prohibitions of suicide, and contemporary Judaism continues these. Sanctions are not applied for suicides of children, for those under extreme physical or mental stress, for those not in full possession of their faculties, or for those who kill themselves in order to atone for past sins. [14] However, Judaism, unlike Christianity, also recognizes the sanctity of self-destruction—not only the acceptance of martyrdom at the hands of another—to avoid spiritual defilement; this is known as *Kiddush Hashem.* [15] And, again unlike Christianity, the Jewish tradition cites several mass suicides, notably the suicide of 960 Jews at Masada, who are still very much venerated.

Much like Judaism, Christianity does not rely on particular stories of suicide told in the Bible to justify its assertion that the Bible prohibits suicide; rather, it points to a passage that is held to provide the basis for a general, law-like prohibition. For Christians, this text is Exodus 20:13, the Sixth (Fifth)[16] Commandment, ''Thou shalt not kill.'' Christian authorities do not in general take Genesis 9:5, which serves the Jewish tradition as the central passage, to provide a prohibition of suicide, nor do Jewish authorities locate a prohibition of suicide in the Sixth Commandment; this is particularly odd considering that the Old Testament is scriptural for both traditions and that each tradition claims its scripture to provide a direct and unmistakable condemnation of suicide. Both traditions cite many other biblical passages in support of their anti-suicide claims, although selection and interpretation of these passages also often differs.

The Christian use of the Sixth Commandment as the basis for the prohibition of suicide originates with St. Augustine[17]; prior to the early fifth century A.D., the church had no unified position on the moral status of suicide, and was widely divided on whether various forms of self-killing, including deliberate martyrdom and religiously motivated suicide, were to be allowed. Like the Genesis passage, the Sixth Commandment also presents severe interpretational problems; these involve both the meanings of the words employed, and the scope of the prohibition stated.

First, the semantic difficulties. The term usually translated "kill" actually means "wrongful killing"; the commandment is best translated "Thou shalt do no wrongful killing," or perhaps "Thou shalt do no murder."[18] Nowhere in the Old Testament does the term "wrongful killing" appear in connection with suicide, and there is no philological reason to think that suicide is included under this term. The commandment thus does not serve as a general prohibition of self-killing, since self-killing may not always be wrongful killing. That suicide is *wrongful* killing would need to be established independently; only then could the Sixth Commandment be used to confirm the centrality of a suicide prohibition in the Christian scriptures.

Second, the scope problems. Augustine claims that "Thou shalt not kill" means not only that one should not kill others, but that one ought not kill oneself. But Augustine's conclusion is not immediately evident. For one thing, not only is "Thou shalt not kill" almost universally relaxed to permit the killing of plants and animals, it is usually also interpreted to allow the killing of human beings in self-defense, capital punishment, and war. However, one might argue, if under this commandment the killing of human beings is permitted in these situations, it is hard to see way it should not also be permitted in the case of suicide. Indeed, suicide would seem to have a stronger claim to morality, since suicide alone does not violate the wishes of the individual killed.

To meet such an objection, Augustine draws a distinction between "private killing" and killing that is carried out at the orders of a divine or divinely constituted authority.[19] Private killing, or killing undertaken "on one's own authority," is never right; it is wrong whether one kills oneself or someone else, and it is wrong whether the victim is innocent or guilty of crime in any degree. Consequently, private killing of oneself—that is, self-initiated suicide—is wrong whether one kills oneself in order to declare one's innocence (like Lucretia), or to punish oneself for a crime (like Judas).

However, according to Augustine, not all killing is private. God may command a killing, and when this is the case, full obedience is required. The command may take either of two principal forms: it may be a direct command from God, such as the commandment to Abraham to sacrifice Isaac, or it may be required by a just law. In these two cases, the individual who performs the killing does not do it "on his own authority" and is not morally accountable for it; he is "an instrument, a sword in its user's hand."[20] This accounts for the permissibility of both killing in war and in capital punishment, since both types of killing are performed by persons acting under law. Augustine appears not to permit killing in self-defense, though present-day Catholic moral theology does permit it for persons not capable of attaining the "higher way" of self-sacrifice.

Although suicide is almost always a matter of private killing, in Augustine's view there can be cases in which it is not: an individual may be ordered to kill himself by law (as Socrates was ordered to drink the hemlock by the Athenian court), or he may be directly commanded to do so by God. Just as Abraham's sacrifice of Isaac would not have been wrong, had not God supplied the ram instead, Samson's causing his own death by pulling the temple down does not violate the commandment against suicide because—at least so Augustine conjectures—it was required by God: "And when Samson destroyed himself, with his enemies, by the demolition of the building, this can only be excused on the ground that the Spirit, which performed miracles through him, secretly ordered him to do so."[21] Suicide is permitted under divine command; otherwise, it is not.

Indeed, to say that suicide under divine command is *permitted* is itself short of the truth; suicide in these circumstances is not merely optional or supererogatory but *required*. Inasmuch as most discussion of the religious view of suicide has centered on whether suicide can ever be allowed within the Christian faith, it is crucial to see that the kind of account of suicide adopted by Augustine and followed by virtually all later Catholic writers, at least until recently, holds suicide to be obligatory in specific situations. Killings of oneself or of others committed at the orders of God, whether by direct divine command or under law, may not be avoided. When a soldier kills in war, says Augustine, "he is punished if he did it without orders," but it is also the case that "he will be punished if he refuses when ordered. . . . And so one who accepts the prohibition against suicide may kill himself when commanded by one whose orders must not be slighted."[22] Because since God is "one whose orders must not be slighted," the individual does not have an option to kill himself, but *must* do so if he is to remain religiously devout.

Augustine's explanation of the legitimacy of Samson's suicide has seemed to some entirely ad hoc. In the seventeenth century, John Donne points out that the traditional view was clearly embarrassed by the need to accommodate biblical suicides and those of the later saints—for instance, St. Pelagia—who are portrayed without condemnation and are believed to have attained salvation. Augustine had acknowledged that external observers cannot tell with certainty whether any given suicide, biblical or otherwise, is commanded by God, since the issuance of divine command is not always a public event;[23] Donne disputes the likelihood of such mechanisms altogether. He agrees with Augustine that it is permissible to commit suicide only upon the command of God: "Whensoever I may justly depart with this life," he says, "it is by a summons from God."[24] But Donne supplies a different interpretation of how that command may occur: "Yet I expect not ever a particular inspiration, or a new commission such as they are forced to purchase for Samson and the rest, but that resident and inherent grace of God, by which He excites us to works of moral, or higher, virtues."[25] What Donne was referring to is *conscience,* that faculty in human beings by which, according to seventeenth-century thinkers, the promptings and admonishments of divinity are known. Since conscience, according to these thinkers, is the voice of primary reason, and so provides direct access to the will of God, if one's rectified conscience permits or recommends suicide, then suicide is in accord with the will of God. If one's conscience is troubled or repelled by the idea, then no matter how difficult the circumstances in which one finds oneself, the act would count as disobedience to the will of God. For Donne too, as for Augustine, suicide was not merely permissible, but obligatory at the divine command—though for Augustine this occurred in vision, for Donne, at the prompting of conscience. Donne writes:

> And this obligation which our conscience casts upon us is of stronger hold and of straiter band than the precept of any superior, whether law or person . . . If then, a man, after convenient and requisite diligence, despoiled of all human affections and self-interest . . . do in his conscience believe that he is invited by the spirit of God to do such an act as Jonas, Abraham, and perchance Samson was, who can by these rules condemn this to be sin?[26]

Despite Donne's reinterpretation, Augustine's original reading of the Sixth Commandment remained the basis of the prohibition of suicide not only in Catholicism, but also in much of Protestant Christianity, and the notion of obligation in suicide has been barely examined. The twentieth-century Catholic writer J. Eliot Ross, for instance, admits that it may be "lawful" for a person who is a condemned criminal to act as the state's executioner and take his own life;[27] but he does not recognize that, if ordered by the appropriate authority, self-execution would be not merely "lawful" but obligatory. Nor does Ross consider the possibility that God might directly order self-killing in nonjudicial contexts. Similarly, Joseph V. Sullivan, also defending a contemporary Catholic position, claims: "For a man to take the life of an innocent person directly, even his own life, for any reason whatsoever, apart from a divine command, has always been against the conscience of the West."[28] But what is not explored in recent religious writing is the obligation of the individual to kill himself under divine command. No doubt this has a great deal to do with the frequency of psychotic delusions and imaginings of "divine command"; a feeling of being "ordered to kill myself" is a very frequent concomitant of suicide and attempted suicide in those who suffer from delusional psychoses. Assertions of divine command have also accompanied both individual and mass suicide in contemporary religious cults. But, for the religious, these facts merely underscore the difficulty of distinguishing genuine divine command from hallucination or cult coercion; they do not alter the principle that genuine divine command is always to be obeyed. However, Augustine's distinction between private and divinely ordered suicide has given way in recent Catholic literature to distinctions made on the basis of the doctrine of the double effect (to be discussed later in this chapter), and the notion of suicide as the possible product of divine command is rejected: if suicide is intrinsically evil, it is argued, God could not command it, and suicide can be excused only by attributing it to inculpable ignorance[29] such as that which occurs in mental illness.

In addition to the Sixth Commandment, numerous other biblical passages are also cited as authority for the Christian prohibition of suicide. These include Deuteronomy 33:39, "I kill and I give life"; I Samuel 2:6, "The Lord killeth and maketh alive"; and a number of similar passages that assert God's power over life and death.[30] Some biblical episodes are said to show awareness of the prohibition of suicide: Paul prevented the suicide of his jailor (Acts 16:27–28); Elijah and Job considered suicide and rejected it; wicked figures like Judas do not respect the prohibition. The evidence for such a prohibition, however, is far from compelling.

A number of later interpreters have agreed that the Bible does not prohibit suicide, either in the central Genesis 9:5 and Exodus 20:13 passages, or at other loci throughout the Old and New Testaments. John Donne, for instance, after a meticulous analysis of both the biblical texts and the then-current secondary interpretations, concluded that "in all the judicial and ceremonial law, there was no abomination of self-homicide."[31] A century and a half later, in 1773, Caleb Fleming also admitted that the scriptures did not expressly prohibit suicide, but offered as an explanation the suggestion that suicide was "too deformed" to be mentioned in the Bible.[32] In recent years, a committee of the New York Presbytery has concluded that the Bible does not prohibit suicide; rather, "it is clear that for some Christians, as a last resort in the gravest of situations, suicide may be an act of their Christian conscience."[33] With increasing popular attention to voluntary euthanasia and the "right to die," the issue of whether the Bible does contain an implicit prohibition of suicide is of increasing importance to those with traditional religious commitments. Numerous scholars suggest that renewed examination of the texts will not support the view held by both Judaism and Christianity that the Bible prohibits suicide; but results of such investigations are still forthcoming. In the interim, one interpreter reads the texts in this way: "The Bible tends to be life oriented, life protecting and life affirming. Even in trial and adversity, life is good, and one awaits God's will in the taking of a life, including one's own. But there are times and circumstances when biblical tradition views suicide as within the divine will: when it guards, protects, or allows a larger good; when it constitutes a divine judgment for human sin; and when it prevents a greater evil."[34]

The Religious Analogies

In addition to the claim that suicide is prohibited by the Scriptures, the Judaeo-Christian religious tradition also brings several other kinds of argument against the permissibility of suicide. The most informal and casually propounded among these, though nonetheless interesting, is a loose group of arguments I shall call the religious analogies, or the analogy-based arguments, to denote the fact that they all depend on analogies drawn between the person who commits suicide and some particular everyday circumstance or object. But despite the apparent informality of these arguments and the often superficial way in which they are put forth, they are among the most influential of the religious arguments against suicide, and probably much more operative in the thought and behavior of ordinary persons—both the religiously inclined and the nonreligious—than are more sophisticated arguments developed by Christian theologians. Although these analogy-based arguments are one of the oldest forms of argument against suicide in the Western tradition, many of them considerably antedating the scriptural and natural-law arguments, most of them are still quite alive in popular thought.

In practice, religious analogies are often found intermixed with more formal

natural-law arguments; Thomas Aquinas, for instance, uses one religious analogy—
the gift argument—together with two natural-law arguments in his central statement
against suicide. Also, in practice, we find that the religious analogies are often
propounded by thinkers not generally associated with religious thought, although
these arguments do all depend on the belief in the existence of God. Indeed, some of
these arguments are given their classic formulations by thinkers not primarily concerned with religious matters, including Plato, Josephus, Locke, and Kant.

The analogy-based religious arguments against suicide may be very roughly
divided into two major groups: those that rest on analogies to *property* relationships
between man and God, or that have reference to concrete objects for use or possession, and those in which the central analogy is drawn to a particular kind of *personal*
or occupational relationship between God and man. The argument based on the root
analogy of life as a "gift" from God, for instance, is probably best classed among
the property relationships, since (at least initially) it concerns the treatment and
disposal of the gift object; the argument based on the root analogy of man as a
"sentinel" stationed by God trades on a particular kind of interpersonal relationship.
However, the distinction between property and personal analogies is rarely sharp. In
some arguments, such as Plato's claim that man is slave to God and hence ought not
run away, both property and personal relationships are involved. In others, an
argument that begins with one kind of relationship may conclude with another, as
when the initially property-related gift argument becomes an argument concerning
the personal relationship of gratitude.

The following list presents the central analogy-based arguments in the Christian
religious tradition. A brief statement of the argument is accompanied, whenever
possible, by its *locus classicus* in the history of thought; this is usually its most
explicit or extended statement, though not necessarily the earliest, and not always
from authors whose interests were primarily religious.

A. The Property Analogies

Life is a gift from God, and so should not be destroyed.	. . . life is a gift made to man by God, and it is subject to Him who is master of death and life. Therefore a person who takes his own life sins against God . . . Thomas Aquinas[35]
Life [or, the soul] is loaned or entrusted to the individual by God, and so should not be destroyed.	Know you not that they who depart this life in accordance with the law of nature and repay the loan which they received from God, when he who lent is pleased to reclaim it, win eternal renown . . . Josephus[36]
	Humanity in one's own person . . . is a holy trust. Kant[37]
The human being is made in the image of God [and should not destroy God's likeness].	So God created man in His own image; in the image of God He created him . . . Genesis 1:27

The body is the temple of God, and should not be destroyed.	Surely you know that you are God's temple, where the Spirit of God dwells. Anyone who destroy's God's temple will himself be destroyed by God, because the temple of God is holy; and that temple you are. I Corinthians 3:16–17
The human being is the handiwork of God, and should not destroy what God has created.	For men being all the workmanship of one omnipotent, and infinitely wise maker . . . they are His property, whose workmanship they are, made to last during His, not one another's pleasure. Locke[38]

B. The Personal Relationship Analogies

The human being is God's possession [i.e., slave], and should not destroy himself because he is his owner's property.	I believe that this much is true; that the gods are our keepers and we men are one of their possessions. . . . Then take your own case; if one of your possessions were to destroy itself without intimation from you that you wanted it to die, wouldn't you be angry with it and punish it, if you had any means of doing so? Certainly. So if you look at it in this way I suppose it is not unreasonable to say that we must not put an end to ourselves until God sends some compulsion like the one which we are facing now. Plato[39]
The human being is imprisoned by God [or, the body is the prison of the soul], and should not escape.	. . . we men are in a kind of prison and must not set ourselves free or run away . . . Plato, quoting Orphic doctrine[40]
The human being is the servant of God, and should do his master's bidding.	For men being . . . all the servants of one sovereign master, sent into the world by His order, and about His business . . . Locke[41]
The human being is stationed as a sentinel on earth by God, and should not desert his post.	So the aged ought neither to cling too greedily to their small remnants of life nor, conversely, to abandon them before they need. Pythagoras forbids us desert life's sentry-post till God, our commander, has given the word. Cicero[42]

> This duty [of self-preservation] is
> upon us until the time comes when
> God expressly commands us to leave
> this life. Human beings are sentinels
> on earth and may not leave their posts
> until relieved by another beneficent
> hand.   Kant[43]

The human being is the child of God,   "Your heavenly father [says] 'Thou
and should trust and obey his father in   shalt not kill' [yourself]."
all things.

All of these arguments make reference to concrete, everyday objects, such as gifts, loans, images, temples, and the objects fashioned by craftsmen, or to particular human relationships, such as that between master and slave, prisoner and jailer, master and servant, military superior and subordinate, or parent and child. Since these are familiar objects and relationships, we tend to have a fairly well-developed set of ordinary moral beliefs and practices surrounding them: we believe that gifts ought to be preserved, loans repaid, temples respected, commanders obeyed, and parents loved. It is on these ordinary moral beliefs and practices that the analogy-based arguments rely.

If we isolate these tacit premises, however, we discover that the arguments may not after all succeed in supporting the general Christian prohibition of suicide. First, many of these arguments produce trivial and sometimes rather amusing surface difficulties in interpretation. For instance, it is often claimed that life is a gift from God, and therefore ought not be destroyed. But this invites us to ask who it is who receives God's gift, if that individual does not yet have life; mainstream Christian theology does not assert the antecedent existence of nonliving individuals upon whom such gifts might be bestowed. Or, if life is construed as a "loan" from God to man, one might suggest that suicide can be no more wrong than ordinary death: in either case, life is ended, and is not "repaid" to God. On the other hand, if it is the soul that is said to be loaned, it cannot *not* be returned: since in standard Christian theology the soul is immortal, it will thus be "repaid" whether death occurs by suicide or in some other way.

But these are trivial objections, and should not distract us from the central concern in each of these analogy-based arguments, since it is on this central concern that the analogy actually rides. The analogy to life as a loan, for instance, though indeed subject to surface difficulties, is centrally concerned with what might be called the "entrustment" feature of loans—the notion that the borrower of an object assumes an obligation to protect and care for the loaned object while it is in his or her possession—and it is on this feature that the serious argument against suicide is based. In analyzing this and other analogy-based arguments against suicide, then, we must be careful not to discredit them on the basis of superficial objections: serious attention to these arguments requires a careful search for the central concern beneath its surface. Even so, as we shall see, the analogy-based arguments do not seem to succeed in supporting the traditional blanket prohibition of suicide.

Unfortunately, we have space here to examine only one of these arguments in detail; our specimen will be the argument that suicide is wrong "because life is a gift from God, and ought therefore not be destroyed." There are several reasons for selecting this argument from among the others. It is as complex as any, and very clearly displays the way in which deeper issues emerge from trivial surface difficulties. It involves both property and personal-relationship notions. And because it is used by Thomas Aquinas as one of three central reasons why suicide is wrong, it occupies an influential place among the analogy-based arguments in the history of dispute concerning suicide.

The Gift Argument. The argument that because life is a gift of God, one ought not destroy it by suicide is open to a very simple objection, first formulated by the eighteenth-century Swedish philosopher, Johann Robeck.[44] Robeck, who composed a lengthy treatise defending suicide and later drowned himself, argued that if life is a gift, then it becomes the property of the recipient, who may therefore do with it as he or she wishes. In giving a gift, the donor relinquishes his or her rights and control over the gift item; if he or she does not, then the item is not a genuine gift. Thus, if life is really a *gift* from God to the individual, it is that a person's to do with as he or she chooses.

The tacit premise involved in this first part of the gift argument, that based on notions of property, holds that it is wrong to reject or destroy a gift; thus, to assess the argument, we must examine this premise. Is it wrong to reject or destroy a gift? Generally, we think not. We are, of course, aware of circumstances in which it would indeed be wrong to destroy a gift—for instance, if it is an object like a peck of wheat, a warm coat, or a fifty-dollar bill, which could be useful to others. However, although we might find it wrong to *destroy* such items, we would not think it wrong to decline such gifts if they were then to be given to others instead. Similarly, although we are aware that some gift objects may have intrinsic aesthetic or historical value—a painting or a rare book, for instance—and that it would therefore be wrong to destroy these gifts, we need not also hold that it would be wrong to reject them.

Since to decline or reject the gift of life by suicide is tantamount to destroying it, these counterarguments may seem to support the initial thesis that suicide is wrong. Even so, these counterarguments show only that it is wrong to destroy an item if it is useful to someone else, or if it has intrinsic value of its own; they do not show that it is wrong to destroy something *because it is a gift*. Suicide may be wrong because one's life is or could be useful to someone else, or because life is of intrinsic value; but this is not to say that suicide is wrong *because* life is a gift.

There is another, deeper aspect to this analogy. Though our ordinary conventions may suggest that it is permissible to destroy a gift when it is not of intrinsic value or value to others, there is an additional component of gift-giving that is not recognized either in the original statement of the argument or in Robeck's initial reply. The receiving of a gift usually, though not invariably, involves *gratitude:* gratitude felt toward the donor, which can be expressed in a variety of ways. Sincerely felt and appropriately expressed gratitude we take to be commendable; we often evaluate people morally on the basis of their capacity to feel and express gratitude. It is this feature of ordinary gift-giving to which the central analogy in the gift argument is drawn, involving now a personal rather than property relationship, and it is here that the anti-suicide argument has a foothold. The wrongness of failure to feel gratitude is not, of course, logically entailed by the commendableness of succeeding in doing so, but we nevertheless do make this assumption in our every-day practices: since we recognize gratitude as good, we consider lack of gratitude bad. On this basis, it could be argued, if life is a gift, the expression of gratitude for life—perhaps in prayer, perhaps in euthusiastic living—is morally commendable, whereas the individual who displays lack of gratitude or outright ingratitude by destroying the gift by suicide is morally reprehensible. R. F. Holland suggests that this is the root of our horror of suicide: like parricide, we see it as an act of extreme, ultimate ingratitude for the gift of life.[45]

Gratitude is, of course, a moral, not a legal obligation. For example, the estab-lished patron who helps a struggling student initiate a career has no legal basis to expect later support from his protégé if he himself falls from fame—but as moral obligations go, it may be a fairly strong one. The level of expectation of gratitude is related to the magnitude of the gifts and the size of the sacrifice it requires on the part of the donor: the greater the gift on the part of the donor, the greater the obligation on the part of the recipient, and the more morally appalling we would find ingratitude, particularly for major gifts like a transplantable kidney or an entire estate. If life is the greatest gift of all—and because life is a prerequisite to any further gifts or any human experience whatsoever, it is often said to be the greatest gift—then the greatest gratitude is owed to the giver of life.

However, there are situations in ordinary gift-giving in which the recipient of a gift may be less strongly obligated to gratitude, or not obligated at all. A gift may be unattractive, ill-fitting, or spoiled. It may be damaging to one's health or one's values. It may be unnecessary, burdensome, or embarrassing. We customarily feign gratitude even in situations in which we are not actually grateful, but careful inspec-tion of our beliefs and canons with regard to gratitude and truth-telling will reveal, I think, that we do not consider ourselves obligated to feel or express gratitude in these situations at all. If parallel reasoning applies in the case of suicide, we might want to say that our obligation to be grateful for the gift of life depends on the nature and characteristics of the particular gift. If it is a good life—say, one involving a healthy, handsome body, an intelligent and sane mind, reasonable financial security, a peace-ful political environment, deep human relationships, and so forth—we might well consider ourselves obliged to express gratitude (whether in prayer or in enthusiastic living) to the giver of this gift. But if the life one is given is an unsatisfactory one—involving a diseased or deformed body, severe poverty, desperate political repres-sion, terrifying insanity, unbearable grief or deprivation—we would be very much less likely, if the analogy with ordinary gift-giving situations holds, to claim that one is obliged to be *grateful* for it. Gratitude, in such a circumstance, might seem impossible or perverse.

Nevertheless, there are circumstances in which we do find gratitude morally appropriate, even for unsatisfactory or defective gifts. A perceptive recipient, although she sees a particular gift to be unsatisfactory, knows something about the intentions with which it was given. For instance, although the gift itself may be crude or ungainly, it may have involved a great deal of effort or expense on the part of the giver, and it may be appropriate for the recipient to acknowledge these. Even the strength of the giver's intention to please may itself be an appropriate object of gratitude. If your small child glues together three acorns and a rock as the gift for your birthday, your pleasure in it is not primarily a function of the characteristics of the object itself, but of your child's affectionate intentions in presenting it to you. If the analogy holds for suicide cases, then while the individual who ends his or her painful, misery-filled life might not be held accountable for failing to appreciate the gift-object as such, he or she ought nevertheless to appreciate the affection with which God has bestowed this gift.

But gratitude for the intentions and affections of a giver despite the unsatisfactoriness of the gift can be expected only in a situation where the giver is subject to limitations. The acorn-rock is welcome from a child, but not from an accomplished artist. Life, however, is the gift of a giver who has no limitations: it is the gift of an omnipotent, omniscient being, one who has, presumably, the ability to fashion for any individual a pleasant and attractive life, including a healthy body, a sane mind, and comfortable circumstances. God is not a giver limited to the creative equivalent of acorn-rocks. Furthermore, God's gift is assumed to be freely given; God, presumably, is under no compulsion to bestow any gifts at all. Given these assumptions, the individual who receives from God a life disfigured by pain or deformity cannot excuse the donor on grounds of limitations, and may begin to suspect that the donor's intentions are not the best. Similarly, the individual who does receive an acorn-rock from a skilled artist may suspect hastiness, lack of interest, lack of understanding, jokesterism, or even malevolence behind the gift.

Thus, the potential suicide who, because his or her life is so excruciatingly painful to live, considers discarding the "gift" that an omniscient and omnipotent God has given him or her, in effect asserts that it is the donor's and not his or her own intentions that are subject to moral question.[46] If he or she does commit suicide, it is God who is at fault and not the person: God clearly is not a benevolent God, and one has no obligations to be grateful to the uncaring or even malevolent donor of a horrid and painful "gift." Read in this way, the original gift argument against suicide seems to backfire, and to legitimize suicide wherever life involves unfortunate, deeply unwanted circumstances.

One might reply that what is crucial is not that life is a gift, but that it is a gift *from God.* Because God is not just any ordinary donor, and because God is worthy of utmost reverence, one cannot trifle with His gifts as one might with those of another. But this compounds rather than resolves the problem; we now see clearly that it is part of the problem of evil. Why would God, who is not only omniscient and omnipotent but perfectly good, give to some individuals the gift of good lives, and to some others desperate or painful ones?

Three principal strategies are traditionally used to answer the problem of evil: (1) *The "ultimate harmonies" defense,* according to which there must be some evil in the world in order that the goodness of the whole be apparent, just as there must be shadow in the painting or a pause in the chant, in order that their beauty be appreciated; (2) *The free will defense,* according to which the evil that occurs in the world is the product of the human being's misuse of the free will God has granted him or her;

Suicide

and (3) *The "soul-making" defense,* according to which God permits evil to occur so that it will develop, test, and strengthen souls in their quest for salvation. There are other theodicies, of course, but it is these three that have been central in the traditional discussions of philosophy of religion.

The answer to the question raised here, whether one is morally obligated to retain a deficient or defective life, and to feel or express gratitude to God for it, depends on the type of theodicy with which one attempts to explain the occurrence of evil in the world. Suppose one, for instance, relies on a "soul-making" theodicy: then one explains the evil and pain that occur in Jones' life as a benevolent measure, enabling Jones to develop and perfect his soul in a way that is not possible for individuals not granted an opportunity to suffer. For this opportunity, painful though it may be, Jones is perhaps obligated to be grateful: he, unlike others, may hope for human nobility and higher celestial rewards. But while Jones clearly has a duty of gratitude for this opportunity, this still does not entail that he also has a duty to exercise it, or that he is obligated to retain his life. If, on the other hand, one uses the "ultimate-harmonies" defense, one may argue that though there must be some evil in the world, Jones has no reason to be grateful that it was assigned to him. Finally, if the evil and suffering that occur in Jones' life and that incline him to suicide are seen as the result of his own misuse of free will, then again, one may wish to argue that Jones has no obligation to be grateful for his life. Just as the donor of a penknife is culpable for giving it to a three-year-old child who he knows will cut herself with it, so a God who bestows life on a being who He knows will misuse and thus suffer for it is not to be praised.

The general point is this: the answer to the overriding question of whether gratitude to God is appropriate or morally required, even when the life He has bestowed is unsatisfactory, depends on the type of theodicy we employ. But there is no easy agreement among philosophers of religion or theologians as to which, if any, of these theodicies is successful; all of them are open to considerable objection. If none of them is sound, we may be led to conclude either that God does not exist, or that He does not have all three attributes of omnipotence, omniscience, and perfect benevolence. Of course, if God does not exist, then the "life-as-a-gift-from-God" argument against suicide has no substance. But if God is assumed to exist, but lacks one or more of the three properties traditionally attributed to Him, then the success of this argument may rest on the matter of which property or properties it is that God is said to lack. I pointed out earlier that in ordinary cases of gift-giving, we are sometimes led to question the motivation of the giver of an extremely inappropriate or unsatisfactory gift; it would seem here that it is benevolence, rather than omnipotence or omniscience, that would come into question. But a further question then arises: if the God from whom one receives one's gift of life is not, after all, benevolent, does one continue to owe Him duties of obedience and gratitude; or, rather, does one begin to regard Him as an adversary, from whom any route of escape, including suicide, is justified? On the other hand, suppose it is omniscience or omipotence that God lacks: His bestowing dismal, defective gifts of life upon some unfortunate individuals is the result of His being able to do no better, and the defectiveness of the lives in question serves as a measure of His lack of power and wisdom. One may discover an obligation to be grateful to such a God for His benevolent intentions and well-meaning efforts, but certainly not an obligation to express it by keeping the sorry products of His unsuccessful attempts. Indeed, a God who would insist that you do so would be the one to fault, not the individual affected by those efforts.

We see, then, that if we construe life as a gift from God, we may find gratitude for life and a consequent refraining from suicide an appropriate response for lives that are good ones. But these are not, by and large, the circumstances in which suicide is considered. In cases in which an individual's life is deeply unsatisfactory, and where suicide seems preferable to continued life, gratitude is inappropriate. Thus, the gift argument against suicide backfires: it leads to the conclusion that suicide, at least in certain kinds of cases, is not on these grounds morally wrong.

Other Analogy-based Arguments. Glancing very briefly at the other analogy-based arguments, we see that many of the same issues begin to emerge. Josephus, for instance, argued that suicide was wrong because God's "loan" of life ought not be returned until "he who lent is pleased to reclaim it," yet we recognize a variety of circumstances in which a borrowed object may or should be returned early: when the borrower cannot protect or care for it, for instance, or cannot keep it from damage by outside influences. If life is construed as a loan, which the lendee may keep only as long as he or she can adequately care for it, then by analogy, suicide may seem appropriate in those cases in which the condition of the loaned life is threatened: the beginnings of deteriorative illness, the onset of insanity, the symptoms of degenerating character.

Similarly, if it is argued that suicide is wrong because, according to the biblical text, man is made in the image of God, we can point out that while destruction of an image—a portrait, a photograph—may be an insult to the model when the likeness is a good one, it may be an act of respect when the likeness has become distorted. We can imagine that an individual would find him- or herself, because of sinfulness, criminality, illness, or physical disability, a comparatively poor likeness of God, and our ordinary beliefs concerning image-destruction might suggest that he or she would be justified in ending that life. (This, of course, is independent of the question of whether these self-perceptions are correct.) If, on the other hand, the "likeness" is interpreted, as is customary in Catholic theology, as the conformity of the human will to the will of God, then the tacit premise of the underlying analogy—that one ought not destroy an image or likeness of someone—no longer exerts its initial precritical pull.

There are still other analogies. Considering the body as the "temple of God": although in general we hold it right to respect temples and wrong to desecrate or destroy them, we also recognize cases when for reasons of safety or cost temples are properly deconsecrated and razed. Similarly, considering Locke's notion of man as the "workmanship" of God, analogous to the products of the craftsman, we readily grant that in general it is wrong to destroy such things; but we recognize cases in which it would be morally correct or even praiseworthy to do so: for instance, when a particular piece of craftsmanship is defective, broken, or uncharacteristically clumsy. If, when contrasted with the lives of other human beings, one's own life

seems to be an example of a good craftsman's uncharacteristically bad worksman-
ship, ordinary practices suggest that it would not be wrong or disloyal to destroy it.

The analogies that trade on personal relationships between man and God present
similar issues. Take, for instance, Plato's conception of man as the bondsman or
slave of God: while the Greeks held that a slave had no right to leave his master even
if seriously mistreated, contemporary moral thought—if it were to recognize the
institution of slavery at all—would surely hold that even if a well-treated slave has
some obligation to remain, a mistreated slave certainly does not. Analogously, the
person who escapes from an unusually cruel servitude in life cannot be said to have
done wrong. The Orphic argument that the body is the prison of the soul, from which
one ought not escape until one's sentence is done, is challenged by the popular
(although non-Socratic) conviction that a prisoner has no obligation to remain imprisoned if his conviction is unjust. Or consider Locke's description of people as
"all the servants of one sovereign master, sent into the world by His order, and
about His business": though our ordinary moral beliefs honor the faithful servant of
the trusted master, they also recognize cases in which the servant ought to escape:
when the master is gratuitously cruel, or demands some morally repugnant task.
Similarly, if we conceive of man as a sentinel, as did Cicero (apparently mistranslat-
ing Plato[47]) and Kant, we may recognize that in general, sentinels are obligated to
remain at their posts—except when rendered incompetent by wounds, blindness, or
perhaps pathological fear: in these cases, we hold, it is fitting that they should yield
the post to somebody else. Finally, in perhaps the most contemporary of these
analogies, we may conceive of God as father, man as child, and hold that man's
obligation is to trust and obey; but contemporary ferment surrounding children's
rights and child abuse show that we are beginning to think children ought not always
trust and obey, but in some cases ought to hide, run, or rebel. In this last case, we see
that a traditional moral assumption—the duty of unquestioning filial obedience—is
now undergoing widespread public examination and criticism, and we might expect
its use in analogy-based arguments against suicide to decline. After all, if a person is
God's child, then in circumstances in which that person's life is analogous to that of
the abused child, escape by suicide is not morally wrong.

All of these circumstances involve what we might generally call evil: threat to a
loaned object, poorness of an image or likeness, the crumbling safety of a temple,
the defectiveness of a craftsman's products, mistreatment by the master of the slave,
unjust sentencing by the court, perversity in the orders of the master to the servant,
incapacitation of the sentinel, or the father's abuse of the child. Thus, although we
cannot here give full consideration to these additional analogy-based arguments, we
may nevertheless suspect that many of them will display the same structure as that of
the gift argument just examined: serious consideration of each analogy and its
central concerns will lead directly to the problem of evil, and assessment of the
argument as a whole then rests upon the adoption of one or another theodicy. One
may assume, of course, that we do not always understand God's ways, and that God,
despite appearances, always acts in the best interests of each individual in the world;
but this is to assume, not to provide, an answer to the problem of evil. One may also
hold that the occasions upon which the problem of evil seems to loom largest are
precisely the occasions when the believer is called to *faith*, an absolute trust in God's

ultimate justice and mercy, and that to choose to end one's life would be the act of ultimate despair. As the Anglican theologian P. R. Baelz puts it, suicide would be "a refusal to trust in God, an embracing of death for its own sake, a form of self-justification, a desertion to the enemy. A final act of despair is substituted for a waiting in hope."[48] But again, this is to dictate a stance, not to show that it is the right one in circumstances such as these. Without an answer to the problem of evil or an examination of the best response to its demands, however, the analogy-based arguments used in the Christian tradition to prohibit suicide all seem to defend it instead, at least in the kinds of circumstances in which suicide (as distinct from manipulative suicide attempts) is most likely to occur.

Of course, it is always open to the defender of the analogy-based arguments to observe that this analysis has treated these analogies in a wholly literal way, and to claim that they are not in fact meant literally but "metaphorically" or in some other way. God's gift of life is not like any ordinary gift, one might claim, and so not subject to the same considerations as those operative in ordinary gift-giving; underlying considerations regarding gratitude will presumably be different as well. Similarly, one could maintain that man is not the same kind of sentinel as the military watchman, or that the individual's relation to God is not like that of a child to an ordinary father. These are important objections. But the defender of such positions must then, if he or she is to maintain that these traditional analogy-based arguments provide any reason for thinking one should not commit suicide, supply some new metaphorical or other interpretation of these arguments that can then be examined. It is simply inadequate to claim that the notion of "gift" in the thesis that life is a gift from God ought not to be taken literally when one cannot supply any other interpretation of this term on which an argument might be based. In the history of religious argumentation concerning suicide, these analogies have not been given careful, sympathetic and yet nonliteral interpretations. Perhaps it can be done. The examination here shows only that these analogies do not provide a secure basis for arguments against suicide *when taken literally;* obviously, this finding should not suggest that the religiously committed thinker scrap these arguments altogether, but may rather encourage an attempt to formulate more subtle and substantial versions of these arguments.

It is equally open to the defender of the analogy-based arguments against suicide to claim that although the analogies may be taken literally, our ordinary practices and beliefs regarding everyday things, relationships, and situations are morally incorrect. Ordinary gift-giving beliefs and practices, we have seen, suggest that it is not always wrong to reject the gift of life; yet, one might argue, they are mistaken, and we ought *never* reject a gift or fail to show gratitude. But just as an objection to literal interpretation of the analogies obliges the objector to produce an intelligible nonliteral interpretation, an objection to our ordinary moral practices obliges the objector to provide a thoroughgoing critique of ordinary morality, and replace it with a coherent alternative moral system.

Either defense—that the analogies are not to be taken literally, or that our everyday practices are wrong—would prove an adequate rebuttal to the argument pursued in this section that the life-is-a-gift and other religious analogies are not adequate as arguments against suicide. But neither of these defenses is an easy one to make. In the meantime, we must remember that these analogy-based religious arguments, however they were intended by the historical figures who formulated and publicized them, are very frequently understood by persons within or influenced by the religious tradition quite literally, and are understood with reference to ordinary moral practice. However these arguments may have been presented, this is the way in which they are received, and it is this common, literal, ordinary understanding of these arguments that still lies behind the Western suicide taboo.

Suicide as a Violation of Natural Law

The religious analogies serve to provide easily grasped, popular arguments that suicide is wrong, and the biblical commandments are held to provide fundamental evidence that suicide is contrary to God's will. But the *explanation* of the wrongness of suicide traditionally favored within the medieval and later Christian tradition has involved the assertion that suicide is a violation of natural law.

The concept of natural law has been understood in quite varied ways; when applied to the issue of suicide, it has given rise to at least three distinct types of interpretation. Some authors claim that suicide is contrary to the natural physical laws governing the universe, including those that facilitate God's domination over life and death; others that it defeats the normal, basic biological will to live; still others that suicide perverts humankind's natural ends, or the purposes humans fulfill in the universe.

Suicide and Natural Physical Law. That suicide is a violation of natural law is sometimes interpreted to mean that suicide disrupts the natural physical laws with which God rules the universe or that God has established to ensure the orderly functioning of the universe. As David Hume, the principal critic of this view, describes it, suicide offends God "by encroaching on the office of divine providence and disturbing the order of the universe."[49]

If suicide is a disruption of the established order of the universe, Hume claims, so is any other action that alters the normal outcomes of natural physical or psychological processes. However, we interfere with the operations of nature in many of our everyday activities, and if we did not, we would not long survive.

> All animals are entrusted to their own prudence and skill for their conduct in the world and have full authority, as far as their power extends, to alter all the operations of nature. Without the exercise of this authority they could not subsist a moment; every action, every motion of a man, innovates on the order of some parts of matter and diverts from their ordinary course the general laws of motion.[50]

To bring about an earlier death by suicide is no more, and no less, a disturbance of the operations of nature than to postpone death by attempting to cure oneself of a disease, by bracing oneself against a fall, or by protecting oneself against an enemy. Hume writes: "If I turn aside a stone which is falling upon my head, I disturb the course of nature, and I invade the peculiar province of the Almighty by lengthening out my life beyond the period which by the natural laws of matter and motion he had assigned it."[51] According to this stance, it is no more wrong to shorten one's life than to extend it. Hence, this argument against suicide is wholly ineffective; in order to make the case against suicide succeed, we would have to explain why some but not others among the laws of nature ought not be disturbed. But, Hume claims, there are no relevant differences with regard to human life: "The life of man is of no greater importance to the universe than that of an oyster."[52] Consequently, if disturbing some of the laws of nature is permissible, then it is—unless some further evidence should arise—permissible to disturb any of them, and suicide cannot be held to be wrong because it is such a disturbance. He puts the point in this way: "It would be no crime in me to divert the Nile or Danube from its course, were I able to effect such purposes. Where then is the crime of turning a few ounces of blood from their natural channel?"[53]

Of course, Hume's argument cannot be used as a *justification* of suicide; it merely succeeds in undermining one version of the natural-law argument against it. For if Hume's argument were taken to justify suicide, it would also justify every sort of genuine moral evil that occurs in the world: murder, theft, cruelty, and so forth. These, of course, are not to be justified, but not because they are not disturbances of the universe: they are deemed wrong on other, independent grounds.

A related argument holds that because God has "dominion over life and death," it is wrong to bring about not only the death of others, but one's own death as well. The emphasis here is on God's normal causal role in creating and destroying human life; one must not interfere with it. Thomas Aquinas, for instance, refers to God as "master of life and death," and says: "And God alone has authority to decide about life and death, as he declares in *Deuteronomy, I kill and I make alive*,"[54] This notion, that an individual must not usurp God's power to create and terminate life, is also embedded in the civil law; Sir William Blackstone, in his *Commentaries* of 1775, remarks: "And also the law of England wisely and religiously considers, that no man hath a power to destroy life, but by commission from God, the author of it . . ."[55] And it appears to be central in the anti-abortion, anti-contraception positions of some contemporary groups, both within Catholicism and in various other pro-life groups.

However, this argument may appear flatly wrong in holding that God alone has the power to create *and* destroy life. Even if one grants that God is somehow involved in or responsible for the inception of life, it may seem obvious that God is not the cause of the termination of life: wars, murders, falling rocks, diseases, explosions, and old age are what destroy life. To claim that God creates and destroys the human soul would not answer this objection; in Christian theology the soul is eternal, whether damned or saved, and is not destroyed even by God.[56]

But one might claim that wars, falling rocks, and diseases are the instruments by which God, as agent, indirectly brings about the deaths of human beings. Although this sort of theory is generally associated with the Christian Middle Ages, it is characteristic of classical Greek and other theologies as well. It may occur in a general determinist form, according to which God has at the beginning of time predetermined what natural events will befall each individual in the world, so that these events simply occur as the result of causal laws designed by God. It may also take the so-called interventionist form (the form often used in naturalistic explanations of miracles): God on some particular occasion uses a particular circumstance or item from the natural world—whether a war, a falling rock, or a disease—to bring about designs of His own. In both versions, it is God, operating through natural objects and circumstances and by means of ordinary causal laws, who brings about events that occur to human beings, including their deaths. Suicide is wrong, it would then be claimed, because it preempts God's operations in this manner, and so "encroaches on God's order for the universe."

But, it may be objected, if God is able to use wars, falling rocks, or diseases as His agents to bring about the death of an individual, He is also able to use that individual to bring about his own demise. John Donne pursues this counterargument: "Death, therefore, is an act of God's justice, and when He is pleased to inflict it, He may choose His officer, and constitute myself as well as any other."[57] Under these general theological assumptions, even those deaths we label "suicides" may very well have been brought about by God—with or without the kind of direct command envisioned by Augustine. Thus, we have no basis for assuming that the suicide has acted contrary to God's plans, when he well may have been the agent, witting or unwitting, of God's designs. Hume puts the point this way:

> Do you not teach that when any ill befalls me, though by the malice of my enemies, I ought to be resigned to providence, and that the actions of men are the operations of the Almighty as much as the actions of inanimate beings? When I fall upon my own sword, therefore, I receive my death equally from the hands of the Deity as if it had proceeded from a lion, a precipice, or a fever.[58]

The claim that God has dominion over life and death may, alternatively, be understood to make a normative point about how human beings should behave with regard to life and death. One might formulate this by granting that, as a matter of fact, human beings do have "dominion" or physical control over death, since they are able to end their own or others' lives at any time; whether they *ought* ever to do so is now the issue. Obviously, this version of the question is strongly associated with the general issue of the use of free will. Some writers argue that, although one is granted the freedom to end his or her life, he or she ought never to do so. But others reply that the very fact that one is granted free will in this matter shows that the divine imperative is for the "responsible exercise of our freedom of choice" in bringing to an end our own lives.[59] Because suicide can be moral or immoral, godly or ungodly, it is in this view the responsibility of the individual in his or her own particular circumstances to make the moral, devout choice.

As with the religious analogies, there are a great many additional arguments similar to or based on this first group of natural-law claims, which have been traditionally presented against suicide. Just two need be mentioned here, both originating with St. Thomas: (1) that suicide is forbidden because it attempts to usurp God's judgment over "the passage from this life to a more blessed one"; and (2) the warning that suicide is "very perilous" because it leaves no time for repentance.[60] In reply to the first of these arguments, we might point out that in Christian theology no human act fully determines God's disposition of a soul, and hence the individual cannot force his or her own "passage" from earthly life to that in heaven. The second argument is primarily prudential; it holds that suicide jeopardizes the individual's salvation, so that suicide is not only wrong but foolish. This latter view, that suicide leaves no time for repentance, has been extremely influential as the basis of the Church's traditional denial of Christian burial to suicides (in recent years seldom enforced, on the grounds that most suicides are mentally ill): suicides were assumed to have died unrepentant and therefore in a state of sin. However, Robert Burton claims, even the most rapid forms of suicide cannot be said to preclude repentance: in his landmark psychology, *The Anatomy of Melancholy* (1621), he says that repentance can be instantaneous, and that God's mercy may come "betwixt the bridge and the brook, the knife and the throat."[61] One might reply that the Catholic's examination of conscience does take time, and so Burton's claim can hardly be considered sound prudential advice.

Suicide and Biological Law: The Will to Live. A second major type of natural-law argument against suicide appeals to the *will to live,* or an individual's fundamental, natural tendency to preserve his or her life. Josephus, for instance, claims that: "suicide is alike repugnant to that nature which all creatures share . . . among the animals there is not one that deliberately seeks death or kills itself; so firmly rooted in all is nature's law—the will to live."[62] Also often interpreted in a biological way is St. Thomas' argument that suicide is wrong because ". . . everything naturally loves itself, and it is for this reason that everything naturally seeks to keep itself in being and to resist hostile forces. So suicide runs counter to one's natural inclination . . . Suicide is, therefore, always a mortal sin in so far as it stultifies the law of nature . . ."[63] A failure of the will to live, it is held, is not natural, and therefore wrong.

Biological observations concerning the absence of suicide among animals have been widely accepted by traditional writers, though with specific exceptions. St. Ambrose, for instance, believed that bees kill themselves; in the seventeenth century, it was widely believed that pelicans commit suicide; and the myth of mass suicides among lemmings has persisted in Scandinavia and other northern areas for a number of centuries.[64] Some twentieth-century accounts also hold that suicide is frequent among horses and dogs.[65] Popular beliefs exist that many species stop eating when they are mortally ill or wounded, and so accelerate their own deaths. Nevertheless, despite these exceptions, it is assumed that animals in general do not kill themselves: suicide is a distinctively *human* act.

If it is true, however, that human beings do kill themselves (and although a few human societies report very low rates of suicide, there are very few or none where suicide is unknown[66]) then it is false that "everything naturally seeks to keep itself in being," and that human suicide runs counter to "nature's law" at least in any biological sense. A single case of suicide is sufficient to defeat such claims.

Of course, it is still possible to treat suicide as an exception, although acting in accordance with one's innate will to live is the rule. But even this weakened claim can be disputed. For instance, John Donne, surveying widespread suicide and voluntary martyrdom practices among the early Christians, claims that while people do have a natural will to live, they are also possessed of an ardent natural desire to die. So strong is this desire to die, says Donne, that it has necessitated ecclesiastical and civil laws prohibiting suicide, for otherwise the human population would be destroyed. "Since, therefore, to my understanding it [the prohibition of suicide] hath no foundation in natural nor imperial law, nor receives much strength from those reasons, but having by custom only put on the nature of law, as most of our law hath, I believe it was first induced amongst us, because we exceeded in that natural desire of dying so."[67] Similarly, Freud posits the existence of a natural destructive urge in the human psyche, which may either be displaced onto others in interpersonal aggression, or—though he regards these cases as abnormal—directed toward oneself, often resulting in suicide.[68] For Donne, the desire to kill oneself is not at all abnormal, but a natural feature of the human constitution; for Freud, the impulse that gives rise to suicide is also a natural feature of humankind, though it is usually deflected in outward directions.

An even more recent scientific development has challenged the thesis that suicide "runs counter to one's natural inclinations." New biological data, particularly that assembled under the theoretical construct known as sociobiology,[69] suggests that suicidal behavior is not uncommon among animal species, and is genetically selected for wherever the death of an individual confers upon its nearest kin benefits sufficiently outweighing the genetic value of its own survival. For instance, a given prairie dog, spotting a predator, may issue a warning cry; though this behavior markedly reduces that individual's chance of survival (because it is the individual most likely to be captured by the predator), it markedly increases the survival chances of the individual's near kin, who escape into their burrows at the warning. But these kin share a determinate number of genes with the self-sacrificing dog, including the genes that determine this behavior; thus, in future generations such behavior in similar circumstances will occur with increasing frequency, since it is these kin who survive. Similar altruistic phenomena include broken-wing distraction displays in birds, nest defense by soldier termites and ants, and defensive but fatal stings in social bees and wasps; all of these are suicidal behaviors in that they involve substantial risk to the individual's own life or actually result in death when it could be avoided.

Of course, one may object that kin-benefiting behavior in animals is not properly termed "suicide," since it involves no conscious intention to end one's life. But the issue that concerns us is not whether animals do commit suicide; the issue, rather is whether *human* suicide—especially those forms usually called heroism and self-sacrifice—can be accounted for by the same natural-selection mechanisms. Inspection of earlier and non-Western human societies shows widespread practice of self-initiated or acquiescent suicide, altruism, and self-sacrificial behavior, much of it occurring in various institutional practices like suttee, self-senicide, self-regicide, and voluntary euthanasia associated with serious illness and insanity. Of course, it may not be that such practices in fact serve to promote the survival of one's near kin (though suttee and self-senicide are often explained as practices conferring economic and hence survival benefits upon one's family or immediate community, especially in times of scarcity). Then, too, there is a tremendous amount of cultural variation in the rates and types of suicide practices; this, too, might seem to undermine the sociobiological thesis. Yet the central suggestion of the sociobiological view in its strongest form is an important one: that suicide practices, though they may seem to be only a product of cultural expectation, are in fact genetically based, and merely find more or less free expression in various cultures. Seen from this point of view, some cultures, such as Greek and Roman Stoicism or traditional Chinese culture, can be said to encourage expression of the genetically encoded tendency to voluntary death in certain sorts of situations; others, specifically post-Augustinian Christian culture and Islam, attempt to suppress it. This is not to say that the sociobiological thesis is correct; if it should prove to be so, however, a disposition to self-death behavior in certain types of kin-benefiting circumstances could be said to be natural, in that it has become part of the genetic heritage of the human species.

Whether suicide or suicidal behavior is "natural" in the sense that it arises from central urges in the human psyche or is genetically favored, however, may have little bearing on the moral status of the act. There is some "natural" behavior that our moral systems do not permit, and some "unnatural" behavior that those systems recommend. Celibacy, for example, is hardly a matter of natural inclination, and yet highly prized within some branches of the Christian tradition.[70] Similarly, truth-telling rather than lying, sharing in scarcity situations, monogamy, and so forth are not always matters of biologically natural inclination, and yet are morally recommended in Western culture. On the other hand, stealing, intimidation, and outright aggression may be "natural" behaviors, and yet are severely discouraged. Arguments against suicide that hold that it is "unnatural" because it runs counter to ordinary human inclinations are inadequate as moral arguments against suicide; such arguments move from "is" to "ought," arguing that because human beings do generally attempt to remain alive rather than kill themselves, they ought always to do so.

Suicide as the Perversion of Humankind's Natural End. The previous arguments that suicide violates natural physical or biological law depend on interpreting their natural-law claims as *descriptive* natural laws, and for this reason fail as moral arguments. Another way of interpreting these claims, frequently used in reading St. Thomas, is to argue that although suicide does occur and so is not counter to any descriptive physical or biological law, nevertheless suicide is counter to *prescriptive* natural law, which describes not the way things are but the way things ought to be. To term suicide "contrary to nature" is not to say that suicide cannot or does not occur, just as to term certain sexual acts "unnatural" is not to say that they are not practiced, but rather to say that these "unnatural acts" ought not occur.

This argument holds that certain kinds of activity are "natural" to humankind, and so ought to occur; other acts, like suicide, are not. This version of the natural-law argument has served as the basis of much of traditional and contemporary Catholic thinking on the issue of suicide. Just as it is "natural for the sun to light and heat the earth, for flowers to grow and bloom, for fish to swim and birds to fly,"[71] as one author in this tradition puts it, so it is natural for humans to live and to engage in specifically human activities: thought, communication, the performance of morally good acts, and other actions that promote the fulfillment of humankind's highest potential. Suicide is wrong because it precludes these activities.

Other authors have described this natural-law view in similar ways. In *Julie, or the New Heloise,* Jean-Jacques Rousseau's fictional character Lord Bomston identifies the central human function as "doing good," and uses a concrete statement of the natural-law principle as an explicit argument against suicide.[72] When Saint-Preux, the lovelorn young man who is the central figure of the novel, proposes to kill himself, his mentor Bomston raises this question:

> Is it lawful for you, therefore, to quit life? I should be glad to know whether you have yet begun to live? What! were you placed here on earth to do nothing in this world? Did not Heaven when it gave you existence give you some task or employment? If you have accomplished your day's work before evening, rest yourself for the remainder of the day; you have a right to do it; but let us see your work. What answer are you prepared to make the Supreme Judge when he demands an account of your time? Tell me, what can you say to him?[73]

Lord Bomston also supplies an answer:

> Whenever you are tempted to quit [life], say to yourself, "Let me at least do one good action before I die." Then go in search for one in a state of indigence, whom you can relieve; for one under misfortunes, whom you can comfort; for one under oppression, whom you can defend . . . If this consideration restrains you today, it will restrain you tomorrow; if tomorrow, it will restrain you all your life. If it has no power to restrain you, die! you are below my care.[74]

As a recent writer within the natural-law tradition summarizes the point on which Bomston is relying, "the suicide uses or neglects to use his powers to achieve an object, viz., his death, the very contrary of that for which they are naturally disposed."[75] They are naturally disposed, Bomston supposes, for doing good.

But even if we accept this premise, the argument still will not yield a firm case against suicide. This is because this argument is directed, so to speak, only to the able-bodied and to those of sound temperament; it does not say how persons ought to act who are, for any of a variety of reasons, unable to perform the "natural" functions of human beings. Even if we were to grant that it is "natural" and therefore morally obligatory for human beings to think, communicate, and perform morally good acts for one another, there can be circumstances for individual human beings in which they are not able to do these things. People in severe and unremitting pain or subject to severe mental disturbance, for instance, may be unable to reason or think in any coherent way. Patients who have suffered an aphasia-producing stroke or find themselves in a medical situation involving continuous intubation may be unable to communicate. And some persons may be unable to do good for others, either because of physical disability or because of (as in Plato's recidivist temple-robber) permanent defect of character. The natural-law argument does not make clear what obligations are imposed upon individuals whose capacities to function have been seriously diminished by disease or disability; these, however, are often the situations in which suicide, or prearranged euthanasia, may be considered. Aquinas would hold, surely, that one ought to live the life of reason *as far as one is capable of it,* and to this degree is committed to remaining in being, but does not consider whether suicide might be permissible in cases where this condition cannot be met.

The religious tradition, however, has sometimes maintained that even the human "near-vegetable," although unable to think or communicate or do good for others in any sustained way, nevertheless performs a morally good action by undergoing suffering; we shall examine this claim later. It is tied to the larger issue of the significance of suffering for the Christian believer and the belief that suffering is of value.

Suicide as Avoidance of Suffering

Unlike the earlier religious arguments considered here, the claim that suffering is in itself valuable, and therefore ought not be avoided by suicide, does not depend wholly on claims concerning the nature or properties of God. The theological version does involve a religious framework in which the notion of salvation is intelligible, but an important secular version, emphasizing cowardice, is also possible. Most of the earlier theological arguments we have considered do not survive dismissal of the standard theological assumptions; this one may.

Suicide as Cowardice. Although later strongly associated with the Christian religious tradition, the claim that suicide is wrong because it is cowardly seems to arise from secular roots. Central among these sources is Aristotle; he says that ". . . to die to escape from poverty or love or anything painful is not the mark of a brave man, but rather of a coward; for it is softness to fly from what is troublesome, and such a man endures death not because it is noble but to fly from evil."[76] One finds in many Greek and Roman writers the related notion that true fortitude consists in the heroic endurance of suffering, and a number of these writers point out that this precludes at least hasty suicide. This notion is adopted by Christian writers as well. Augustine, for instance, says that

> . . . greatness of spirit is not the right term to apply to one who has killed himself because he lacked strength to endure hardships, or another's wrongdoing. In fact we detect weakness in a mind which cannot bear physical oppression, or the stupid opinion of the mob; we rightly ascribe greatness to a spirit that has the strength to endure a life of misery instead of running away from it, and to despise the judgment of men . . .[77]

Thomas Aquinas says that suicide is "the inability to bear penal afflictions."[78] Religious authors frequently cite the biblical example of Job, who endured extraordinary misfortunes without seeking to escape. They also frequently compare the suicide of Cato with the death of Regulus: whereas Cato killed himself to avoid becoming Caesar's slave, Regulus, though undefeated, returned to keep his promise to the enemy Carthaginians, although he knew he would be tortured to death in an exceedingly cruel fashion.[79] The notion that suicide is cowardly survives today: an observer commenting on the August 1977 suicide of Wallace Proctor, a seventy-five-year-old dermatologist afflicted with Parkinson's disease, said that it was "unfair" because Proctor "got out of what the rest of us have to go through," namely death due to a long and debilitating illness.[80]

One might point out that not all suicide is "avoidance-motivated"; self-sacrificial, altruistic suicide typically does not involve flight from personally painful circumstances, but commitment to other persons or causes. Furthermore, not all suicide that is avoidance-motivated is necessarily cowardly: some evils are quite reasonably avoided. Besides, suicide itself may be a supremely difficult task. Paul-Louis Landsberg writes:

> It is very customary to find all suicides condemned as cowards. This is a typically bourgeois argument which I find ridiculous. How can we describe as cowardly the way of dying chosen by Cato, or Hannibal, or Brutus, or Mithridates, or Seneca or Napoleon? There are certainly far more people who do not kill themselves because they are too cowardly to do so, than those who kill themselves out of cowardice.[81]

The Stoics claimed that real cowardice lay in fearing death, true bravery in the courage to take it upon oneself. And many contemporary first-person accounts of comtemplated or attempted but not completed suicide admit a lack of courage at the last moment.

In part, those who emphasize the cowardice of suicide stress its relationship to those painful circumstances that are to be avoided, including illness, disgrace, poverty, and loss; those who emphasize its courageousness are attending to certain painful features of the performance of the act, particularly evident in suicides that involve cutting, piercing, burning, falling from heights, and other violent means. But suicide can be seen as courageous in another way: it involves entering death, a state of which the individual has no prior experience, an unknown. The most famous display of hesitation in the face of this unknown is Hamlet's:

> Who would fardels bear,
> To grunt and sweat under a weary life,
> But that the dread of something after death,
> The undiscovered country, from whose bourn
> No traveller returns, puzzles the will
> And makes us rather bear those ills we have
> Than fly to others that we know not of?
> Thus conscience does make cowards of us all.[82]

Whether one believes in a beatific afterlife or no life after death, no one has prior knowledge of what it is like to be dead.[83] Obviously, those who choose suicide to escape suffering assume that what comes after death will involve less suffering than their current circumstances; otherwise, they would not make such a choice. But, as Philip Devine argues, one cannot rationally choose death, since one lacks adequate information about one of the alternatives between which the choice is to be made: to choose death is to hazard a leap into the wholly unknown.[84] Nevertheless, one might argue that to avoid something because it is unknown is itself a kind of cowardice, and that suicide is the more courageous act, whereas remaining alive because one fears the unknown is the act of the coward.

Death as an unknown aside, we may still question the original Aristotelian assumption that the avoidance of evils is cowardly. Mere avoidance of pain is not cowardice; we normally call someone a coward only when he or she avoids some painful or dangerous action that he or she might reasonably be expected to perform, or when avoiding pain also involves failing to meet a morally required duty. A man who avoids an attacker is not a coward, unless, say, he is a soldier on duty or a wrestler who has volunteered for the sport. To support the claim that suicide is cowardly, one would have also to demonstrate that it involves failing to do a duty that the individual can reasonably be expected to perform. Unless, as Kant claimed, this duty is to be understood as a general duty simply to continue to live (in which case we must press for further justification of such a claim), the duties the coward avoids must be particular duties, including those to himself, to other persons, and to society in general. Among these might be the duties to preserve one's health, to support one's children, to contribute useful work to society. But in many kinds of suicide undertaken to avoid painful physical conditions or social circumstances, it may be increasingly implausible to speak of such continuing duties, since these are precisely the cases in which the individual cannot continue to function in ways that would satisfy such duties. Unless there is a general duty to live, to show that the suicide of a person who has advanced and debilitating cancer is cowardly, we must show that she is defaulting upon some obligation or duty she ought to perform for herself, her family, or society. But it is just that, in cases of advanced and debilitating cancer, which is particularly hard to do.

Of course, this reply does not answer the position taken by St. Thomas, that suicide is wrong because it is an "inability to bear penal afflictions." Thomas' position is similar to the Orphic doctrine enunciated by Plato: the body is the prison-house of the soul, and one ought not attempt to escape until one's sentence has been served. But Thomas' position invites consideration of a general issue in social and political philosophy: does someone who has been sentenced to "penal afflictions," whether simple incarceration or various forms of physical hardship and torture, have a moral *obligation* to submit to them, and would it be cowardly (rather than prudent) to escape them if one could? We are tempted to answer both in terms of the justice of the sentence (the innocent convict has no obligation to remain; the guilty one does) and in terms of the severity of the punishment (the guilty convict is obligated to submit to confinement, but not to torture). This would suggest that suicide is impermissible only if the "sentence" to life is just and the severity of the afflictions is not great. But again, these may not be the situations in which suicide is most earnestly considered.

The Value of Suffering. In the Christian tradition the argument that suicide is the coward's way of avoiding suffering has taken on an additional element. The basis of this argument is evident as early as St. Paul's assertion that "we welcome our sufferings" (Romans 5:3): this is the notion that there is some positive value in suffering itself. The full-scale argument with respect to suicide is first made explicit by Mme. de Staël at the beginning of the nineteenth century. "Suffering is a blessing," she writes in her long essay "Reflections on Suicide," (written to refute her own libertarian treatise "On the Influence of the Passions," composed many years earlier); "it is a privilege to be able to suffer."[85]

Her argument, briefly stated, is this: it is true that life often presents us with painful circumstances, and we may be inclined to consider suicide as a way of avoiding this suffering. But for the true Christian, suffering is to be *welcomed,* not avoided. For the true Christian, mere happiness is not the goal of life; rather, the true Christian seeks the attainment of blessedness, moral elevation, and eternal life. But the way to salvation is *through* suffering: one must therefore submit oneself willingly to suffering, reenacting the life of Christ, and triumph in one's faith despite one's suffering. To commit suicide in order to avoid suffering would be to fail to see it as the means to grace. As the contemporary Catholic writer Joseph Sullivan says, "It is rather the mark of a good and holy God that he permits so many of his children to undergo that suffering here on earth. Suffering is almost the greatest gift of God's love."[86]

For the Christian, then, suffering is not a phenomenon to be excused or explained away. Rather, for the Christian, suffering—both one's own and that personified in Christ—is real, important, and in the end redemptive: it is the way to the beatific world beyond death.

But this emphasis on the value and centrality of suffering—even of the innocent—is open to a serious objection. If suffering is of value, it would seem to follow that, rather than work to reduce suffering among one's fellows and in the world at large, one ought to impose on them as much suffering as possible. But this, of course, is a wholly repugnant conclusion. We do regard suffering as an evil; it is something that it is our duty to eradicate, not to foster. W. R. Matthews, former dean of St. Paul's, points out that we would revolt "against a person who complacently regarded the suffering of someone else as a 'blessing in disguise' and refused to do anything about it on those grounds."[87] We use anesthetics where they are medically appropriate, whereas if we believed all suffering to be of value, we should hesitate to do so.[88] We engage in charitable works to ease or end suffering where we can.

On the other hand, we are familiar with the attitudes of popular culture toward suffering, and in particular with the folk saying that suffering "will make a better person of you." The popular notion that physical or mental pain may be strengthening and character-building is quite conspicuous in cultural truisms about a variety of areas, from sports to the painful process of emotional maturation. We tend to believe that those who have suffered most—survivors of death camps, for instance—are elevated to a plane not achieved by those who have led untroubled lives. Although at first glance, then, the contention that suffering is valuable may seem to be false and even scandalous, some support for this view may be found in popular ideas, and it appears that the issue here is not confined to religous questions alone.

This dispute may center in part on an empirical question: what are the effects of suffering—physical or mental—on the character of an individual? But combined with this question is that of whether the effects of suffering on an individual are ones we should *value*. For instance, John MacQuarrie, stating a contemporary Anglican position, claims that at least some suffering has a "morally educative character."[89] Teilhard de Chardin gives a religious view of what we might call the purifying and perfecting effects of suffering on society as a whole:

> Without Christ, suffering and sin would be the earth's "slagheap." The waste-products of the world's activities would pile up into a mountain of laborious effort, efforts that failed, efforts that had been "suppressed." Through the virtue of the cross this great mass of debris has become a store of treasure: man has understood

that the most effective means of progress is to make use of suffering, ghastly and revolting though it be.[90]

MacQuarrie suggests that the capacity of an individual for "depth of sympathy" and "love" is a product of suffering, and that the individual who has not known suffering would be incapable of these fundamental human attitudes.[91] Flexibility, humility, self-reliance, and a host of other virtues are also sometimes named as the products of suffering. Whether or not we have empirical evidence to confirm such claims, it cannot be denied that this notion is a strong component of contemporary popular belief.

But one may ask whether *all* suffering can be of morally educative character, and whether all suffering "regenerates the soul." Some contemporary thinkers who deal with this issue distinguish, though not always explicitly, between "productive" or "constructive" suffering and that which is unproductive or even destructive. Many writers on euthanasia hold that suffering of the destructive variety may be legitimately avoided by (voluntary) euthanasia, since such suffering can have "no beneficial result."[92] Presumably, suicide to avoid this sort of suffering would be permitted. On the other hand, it would be cowardly or morally wrong for an individual to kill him- or herself in order to avoid suffering if that suffering could be "regenerative," on the grounds that even though it may mean undergoing considerable pain, the individual has a moral duty to grow and develop where he or she can. The only suffering that one may without cowardice avoid by suicide is that from which no conceivable benefit can come.

If one accepts the premise that suffering is sometimes of value, but recognizes the distinction between constructive and destructive suffering, there will still be problems. It may not be possible for either an observer or the individual who is suffering to tell in advance whether future suffering will be of the constructive or destructive sort. This is particularly difficult in circumstances where the suffering can be expected to be long-term or permanent and comparatively severe, that is, in just the cases where suicide might most likely be considered. Those who are religiously convinced, however, are likely to reject this sort of distinction, since on the central Christian model *all* suffering of the innocent—even that which appears entirely fruitless—can lead to ultimate spiritual reward.

The Religious Invitation to Suicide

The theologically based arguments we have been considering are generally advanced to demonstrate the moral impermissibility of suicide, and although they do not always succeed, it has been widely assumed that the religious arguments are uniformly directed against suicide. But some theologies, particularly Christianity, lend themselves to arguments in favor of suicide; it is these that we now wish to examine. For the most part, these considerations have not been stated explicitly anywhere in historical or contemporary religious literature, and certainly not as explicit arguments in favor of suicide; nevertheless, they are crucial to a full understanding of the religious view of suicide.

Suicide as Reunion with the Deceased

Most Western, as well as some Eastern, theologies promise that life after death will involve reunion with one's already deceased relatives, lovers, associates, and friends. In classical Greek culture, this promise was recognized as a strong motivation for suicide; in the *Phaedo,* for instance, Plato remarks: "Surely there are many who have chosen of their own free will to follow dead lovers and wives and sons to the next world, in the hope of seeing and meeting there the persons whom they loved."[93] The promise of reunion with the dead is an equally strong motivation in many other cultures as well. In *junshi,* one of the three traditional forms of Japanese suicide, a subordinate kills himself upon the death of his master or lord in order to follow him into the next world; the act is viewed as one of ultimate loyalty.[94] In the now virtually abolished Hindu custom of *suttee* (also said to have been practiced in very early Greece and the Nordic countries), the newly widowed wife throws herself upon her husband's funeral pyre. The primary motivation may be the feeling that life has no point without the husband, but voluntary *suttee* is also viewed in part as an act of loyalty on the wife's part in following her husband into the next world.[95] Christian theology, too, tends to promise reunion with loved ones in the afterlife, though exact description of the kind of personal intercourse expected in the afterlife varies considerably among different denominations.

Even if one believes in this kind of afterlife activity, it still does not generate a case in favor of suicide if one's ties and obligations to persons still alive are as strong as to those in the next world. However, if the individual who is the object of one's primary personal loyalty dies, the case may be reversed; it is precisely this that occurs in *junshi* and in *suttee*. Some suicides for love are of the same order: Homer regards it as a mark of Andromache's great nobility that she was willing to sacrifice her own life to join the dead Hector. A variation of this theme occurs in the classic Japanese suicide form known as *shinju* (or *aitaishi*), where lovers who are not permitted union in this world kill themselves together—usually by drowning, tied together by a rope—in order to bring about their union in the next.

Such considerations, of course, do not form an explicit theological argument in favor of suicide in any religious tradition. But they do, I think, show the way in which a theology that offers personal reunion in an afterlife tends, however subtly, to invite suicide.

Suicide as Release of the Soul

A similar, though perhaps more abstract, invitation to suicide occurs in those theologies that view death as the moment of release of the soul. We've already seen that Plato, drawing on Pythagorean and Orphic teachings, conceives of life as a condition of penal imprisonment of the soul within the body. As long as the soul remains imprisoned within the body, it is subject to the body's limitations, and is dependent for knowledge upon the body's sensory faculties: sight, hearing, touch, and so forth. But the senses are untrustworthy and misleading, according to Plato; knowledge gained through them can never be certain. It is only when the soul is freed from these limitations imposed by the body that true knowledge can be attained. Socrates says:

"We are in fact convinced that if we are ever to have pure knowledge of anything, we must get rid of the body and contemplate things by themselves with the soul by itself. It seems, to judge from the argument, that the wisdom which we desire and upon which we profess to have set our hearts will be attainable only when we are dead, and not in our lifetime."[96] To get rid of the body is to die. But if one's goal can be attained only in death, the question arises—and it was an acute one for Socrates—why not hasten that death by suicide?[97]

Plato attempts to resolve the conflict by arguing that suicide is not permitted unless one is compelled to do so by intolerable disgrace or unavoidable calamity, or is ordered to execute oneself by the state.[98] Suicide in sheer eagerness to rid oneself of the troublesome body, or in impatience to reach the afterlife, is condemned. (Plato's restrictions apparently failed to convince the young Greek philosopher Cleombrotus, who, after reading the *Phaedo*'s account of the liberation of the soul in death, threw himself from the city wall into the sea.[99]) While Christian theology does not accept the Platonic metaphysics or epistemology, it does preserve the notion of death as a separation of the soul from the body (though a resurrected form of that body may later be restored). This basic dichotomy, between a world in which the soul is conjoined to a body and an afterworld in which it is not, supplies one of the root views of Christianity. The more flamboyant forms of Christianity might put it this way: in this carnal, corrupt world, the soul is shackled to the lusts of an insatiate body; in contrast, the next world promises luminous, clarified existence, in which the soul, cleansed and purified of its contaminating association with the body, is finally free. While this view is not orthodox, and may conflict with other basic views common to Christianity, particularly those that celebrate the fruitfulness of the world and the goodness of its creator's work, it may be quite a strong leaning, particularly in monastic and popular belief.

Again, this attitude does not give rise to a formal argument in favor of suicide, but it does, as does the notion of personal reunion with loved ones in an afterlife, subtly recommend it.

Suicide as Self-Sacrifice

A third religiously based inducement toward bringing about one's own death, particularly evident in Christianity and in Buddhism, is the importance given to self-sacrifice in the interests of other persons or groups. Self-sacrifice for others may take a variety of forms; so strongly is it emphasized in these two cultures that it is sometimes held laudable even when its object appears insignificant. Mahayana Buddhism, for example, preserves the story of the future Sakyamuni, who sacrificed his body to feed a starving tigress,[100] though in both traditions self-sacrifice is usually practiced for the protection or benefit of other human beings, not animals. Self-sacrifice for the spiritual benefit of another person, Catholicism has traditionally taught, is highly praiseworthy. Christ and Buddha, in their respective traditions, are exemplary of self-sacrifice, and in each tradition the believer is encouraged to emulate them. Self-sacrifice for others also occurs in situations that are not specifically religious; perhaps the best-known of these in recent Western experience is the self-sacrifice of Captain Oates, an ailing member of an antarctic exploration party under Admiral Scott, who walked out into a blizzard to die rather than slow the progress and thus imperil the safety of the rest of the party.[101] Acts of self-sacrifice occur often in military, rescue, and a variety of other secular situations.

Christianity has strongly encouraged self-sacrifice, though it has continued to forbid suicide. Traditionally, it has distinguished between these two forms of self-killing by employing the principle of *double effect,* according to which the primary intention under which an act is performed is to be distinguished from secondary, foreseen but unintended consequences, and the moral status of a given action is judged by its primary intent. According to the principle of double effect, an action is permitted if (1) the action itself is morally good or neutral; (2) the evil effect is not directly intended, although perhaps foreseen; (3) the good effect follows directly from the action and not from the foreseen evil effect; and (4) there is grave reason for allowing the evil to occur.[102] Under this doctrine, it is permitted (to use the traditional examples) for a physician to enter a plague-infected area to treat victims, or a priest to enter a minefield in order to bring the sacraments to a dying soldier, even though both the physician and the priest may die; such cases will generally be called "self-sacrifice" or "heroism," and the term "suicide" is not used. In each case the primary intention is to bring aid to the needy, though in each case the agent also foresees the possibility of death. It would not be permitted, however, to kill oneself in order to provide donor organs for a dying relative; here the act performed, termed "suicide," is regarded as in itself evil, and is not permissible regardless of the good consequences that may flow from it.

In recent years there has been considerable debate, particularly among non-Catholic writers, as to whether the principle of double effect in fact effectively distinguishes between morally good and morally evil actions, not only in cases of self-killing and exposure to death, but in other areas such as abortion.[103] There is no doubt that the principle has been applied in some very strained ways. A particularly glaring example is the traditional justification of suicide by women to protect their virginity: it has been said that if a virgin leaps to her death from a building to escape an attacker, no evil act is involved, since she merely "wished the jump, and put up with the fall."[104] Robert Martin concedes that the principle of double effect distinguishes effectively between kinds of cases we tend to consider permissible and those we do not, but argues that the principle itself is unsatisfactory. He says that although the principle holds that no morally praiseworthy action involves the accomplishment of a worthy goal by means that are intrinsically evil, nevertheless, in punishment we routinely subject persons to suffering in order to bring about repentance or rehabilitation.[105]

One might want to challenge the assumption that suicide is intrinsically evil; thus, it would not need to be excused by the principle of double effect. Alternatively, one might want to point out that the distinction between self-sacrifice and suicide under the principle of double effect depends on the motivation for a given act. Much contemporary psychology suggests, however, that the true motive for a given action is not always evident, either to the agent who performs the action or to outside observers. For instance, although one may believe him- or herself to be submitting to death in order to prove the strength of his or her religious faith or bring aid to another, his or her real (although not fully conscious) reasons for doing so may be quite different. As soon as we admit the possiblity of actions that are performed under intentions not apparent or acknowledged by the agent, the distinction drawn between martyrdom and suicide is blurred. This would apply to any moral theory that considers intentions, but is particularly important in evaluating a highly stressful, often ambivalent act such as suicide.

Emile Durkheim, Richard Brandt, and many other recent and contemporary writers define "suicide" without reference to the intentions under which the death-producing act is performed; it is sufficient, according to such definitions, that the individual know that the act he or she is performing will directly or indirectly bring about his or her death. Durkheim introduces this view:

> The soldier facing certain death to save his regiment does not wish to die, and yet is he not as much the author of his own death as the manufacturer or merchant who kills himself to avoid bankruptcy? This holds true for the martyr dying for his faith, the mother sacrificing herself for her child, etc. Whether death is accepted merely as an unfortunate consequence, but inevitable given the purpose, or is actually itself sought and desired, in either case the person renounces existence, and the various methods of doing so can be only varieties of a single class.[106]

This may seem to be merely a trick of redefinition, but it underscores the crucial point here: it allows us to see the way in which Christianity has actively encouraged its believers to choose death. Christianity does not call such choices suicide, but, rather, heroism and self-sacrifice; nevertheless, death is part of what is knowingly chosen, and Christianity celebrates that choice.

Suicide as Martyrdom and the Avoidance of Sin

One of the strongest pulls toward self-imposed death originates in the early Christian church's celebration of those who suffer, accept, or willingly embrace a violent and painful death at the hands of religious persecutors; it would be difficult to overestimate the importance of these persecutions in shaping the eventual Christian view of suicide. Martyrdom was prevalent in the early years of the church; although reliable data is not available, contemporary estimates of the total number of victims in the years from the onset of persecution under Nero in A.D. 64 until the conversion of Constantine in 313 range from 10,000 to 100,000. The frequency of martyrdom may be strongly overestimated by some of the more fervent writers, but these accounts, even if exaggerated, have been influential in shaping Christianity's attitudes toward suicide. For instance, Eusebius writes:

> Why should I now make mention by name of the rest or number the multitude of the men or picture the various sufferings of the wonderful martyrs, sometimes slaughtered with the axe, as happened to those in Arabia, sometimes having their legs broken, as fell to the lot of those in Cappadocia, and on some occasions being raised on high by the feet with heads down and, when a slow fire was lit underneath them, choking to death by the smoke sent out from the burning wood, as was visited upon them in Mesopotamia, sometimes having their noses and ears and hands mutilated, and the other limbs and parts of the body cut to pieces, as took place in Alexandria?

> Why should we rekindle the memory of those in Antioch who were roasted on hot
> grates, not unto death but with a view to a lingering punishment, and of others who
> let their right hand down into the very fire sooner than touch the abominable
> sacrifice? Some of these, avoiding their trial, before they were captured and had
> come into the hands of the plotters, threw themselves down from high buildings,
> considering death as booty taken from the wickedness of evil men.[107]

Whatever the actual extent of martyrdom, it is clear that the Christians played an
active role in the persecutions. Martyrdom was heavily encouraged. Confessors—
those subjected to imprisonment and torture—attracted widespread support among
the Christian community; they were frequently brought food and other articles while
in prison and were the focus of extensive prayer. Some early Christian writers
condemned the practice of offering support to jailed confessors, claiming that it
undermined the hardships that these individuals had elected; nevertheless, these
practices continued, and the confessors became the Christ-like heroes of their com-
munities. This served, of course, to increase the eagerness of others for a similar
role. The theological writers of the third century began to assert that those who
actually died for the faith—not merely confessors, but martyrs proper—were as-
sured of immediate salvation. They believed that the baptism of blood could completely remit sin, and thus render the sufferer worthy of immediate admission to
paradise. This, too, served to encourage willing subjection to the persecutions.

There was yet another ingredient in the early Christian enthusiasm for death that
invited not merely submission to persecution but an active role in one's own death.
The body was often regarded as the locus of sin. This is not a new idea; it occurs in
many Eastern cultures, though it probably enters Christianity through Greek culture.
Plato, as we have seen, described the body's demands for food, drink, sex, and other
physical pleasures as an obstacle to the soul's achievement of genuine knowledge;
his view of the body as impediment or obstacle was adopted by many early Christian
thinkers. In St. Paul, it is transformed into the notion that the body is an impediment
to true spiritual life.

> For those who live according to the flesh set their minds on the things of the flesh,
> but those who live according to the spirit set their minds on the things of the spirit.
> To set the mind on the flesh is death, but to set the mind on the spirit is life and
> death. For the mind that is set on the flesh is hostile to God; it does not submit to
> God's law; indeed, it cannot; and those who are in the flesh cannot please God.[108]

But if the body inevitably leads one to sin, and if sin in unavoidable as long as one is
in the body, then it is clear that one's chances of leading a sinless life improve if one
can be released from that body. Thus, release from the body is desired not only for
its own sake, but for an additional reason. To die and thereby to avoid this sinful
world altogether is one's best hope of salvation. We see here the characteristic
Christian contempt for this-world existence: what one longs for is not an extension of
one's sinful existence in this corrupt world, but attainment of the blessed life beyond. Suicide, then, is clearly the reasonable and religious choice: by killing oneself
to avoid the sins that one will inevitably commit in this world, one secures one's
hopes of heaven. Death is not an evil; it is merely a gateway, as it were, to the world
beyond, and it is in one's best interests to pass through that gate as soon as possible.

These beliefs invite suicide in very specific circumstances: for maximum effectiveness, one is to end one's life immediately after confession and absolution, at that moment when one has been forgiven for all previous sin, and before any new misdeeds can be committed. St. Augustine sees clearly what the practical consequences of this religious reasoning would be; ironically, he says:

> . . . we reach the point when people are to be encouraged to kill themselves for preference, immediately they have received forgiveness of all sins by washing in the waters of holy regeneration. For that would be the time to forestall all future sins—the moment when all past sins have been erased. If self-inflicted death is permitted, surely this is the best possible moment for it! When a person has been thus set free why should be expose himself again to all the perils of this life, when it is so easily allowed him to avoid them by dong away with himself?[109]

This attitude, together with the growing enthusiasm for martyrdom, made voluntary death a crucial issue for the early church: could one *seek* death or martyrdom, whether to prove one's faith or to avoid sin, in order to achieve salvation? Some early writers actively encouraged the seeking of martyrdom: Tertullian, for instance, applauds a group of North African Christians for voluntarily surrendering themselves to the Roman governor, and counsels confessors and prospective martyrs: ". . . if you have missed some of the enjoyments of life, remember it is the way of business to suffer some losses in order to make larger profits."[110] Valerian, similarly, exhorts his readers to martyrdom on the basis of the same trade-off analogy: "The wise man will hasten eagerly to martyrdom, since he sees that giving up present life is part of the gaining of [eternal] life."[111]

Some writers did take a stand against self-initiated martyrdom; Gregory of Nazianzus, for instance, says that it is "mere rashness to seek death, though cowardly to refuse it."[112] But many applauded voluntary death, especially as a means of preserving one's virtue and faith. Of particular importance was the issue of whether Christian women whose virginity or chastity was threatened (like St. Pelagia, mentioned earlier) might kill themselves in order to avoid violation. While some thought not, Tertullian, Eusebius, and Jerome approved. Eusebius narrates as an example of Christian virtue the following story:

> And a certain holy and marvelous person in virtue of soul, but a woman in body, and otherwise celebrated among all those at Antioch for wealth and birth and good repute, who had brought up two unmarried daughters in the precepts of religion, pre-eminent for beauty and bloom of body, when the great envy that was stirred up over them endeavored in every way to track them to where they were concealed, then on learning that they were staying in a foreign country deliberately called them to Antioch and they presently fell within the trap of the soldiers, on seeing herself and her daughters in difficulty, and giving consideration to the terrible things that will arise from human beings, and the most terrible and unbearable of all, threat of fornication, exhorting both herself and her girls that they should not submit to listening to this even with the tips of their ears, but saying that the surrendering of their souls to the slavery of demons was worse than all deaths and every destruction, submitted that taking refuge with the Lord was the one release from all these troubles, and then when they had agreed with her opinion and had arranged their garments suitably about their bodies, as they came to the very middle of their

journey, they requested of the guards a little time for retirement, and cast themselves in a river that was flowing by.[113]

Numerous other virgin martyrs were venerated for making similar choices.

Not only did the martyr cults flourish, but sects of Christians and deviant Christians openly advocating self-initiated death arose. The Donatists, Augustine
writes,[114] "seek to frighten us with their acts of self-destruction"; the Circumcellions, a still more extreme group within Donatism, openly advocated and practiced
suicide in the effort to achieve martyrdom. They were immediately labeled heretics,
but that apparently did not diminish their zeal. They have been described in this way:

> Warned by a dream or revelation that his time was at hand, a Circumcellion would
> go forth and stop a traveller, or better still, more reminiscent of the heroic age of
> Christianity, a magistrate. The unfortunate would be given the choice of killing or
> being killed. Others would rush in on a pagan festival and offer themselves for
> human sacrifice. These became martyrs automatically . . . The alternative was
> mass suicide. Crowds would fling themselves over precipices or drown in the
> Chotts, or even burn themselves alive . . .[115]

Self-elected death as a way of avoiding inevitable sin, as a way of preserving oneself
from sexual violation, and as a way of achieving the immediate salvation of a martyr
was epidemic in the Christian community, most particularly in North Africa. It took
place individually, but also in group or mass suicides, some of quite large scale. It
was against this situation that Augustine took the stand that has become the central
statement of Christianity on the issue of suicide: suicide is prohibited by the commandment "Thou shalt not kill," and except when expressly commanded by God,
wholly and seriously wrong. So great a sin is suicide, that no other sin—whether
fornication, injury to another, or apostasy—may be avoided by it; no salvation can
be attained by this means.

Although there is little reason to think that Augustine's position is authentically
Christian,[116] and although it clearly was a response to pressing practical circumstances, it nevertheless rapidly took hold and within an extremely short time had
become universally accepted as fundamental Christian law.

Martyrdom, like self-sacrifice, it may be argued, is not the same as suicide, and
the early Christian encouragement of martyrdom should not be interpreted as an
enticement toward suicide itself. But there is clear historical evidence that the early
church's call to martyrdom was in fact interpreted as an invitation to deliberate self-
killing by many (for example, the Circumcellions); it was the early church's enormous enthusiasm for martyrdom that obligated Augustine to formulate his position
against suicide. Of course, the fact that Augustine's condemnation of suicide was
necessitated by historical circumstances does not entail that it is wrong.[117]

Suicide and the Attainment of the Highest Spiritual State

Finally, in what is perhaps the most powerful of the Christian inducements to
suicide, self-willed departure from this life may be viewed as a way of attaining the
highest spiritual state, usually termed salvation or union with God. This notion is
extremely strong in a number of Eastern religious traditions as well. For instance,

the Hindu *Saiva Puranas* advocate suicide by fire or by falling from a mountain cliff, in order to obtain a post-death existence of unalloyed sensual pleasure;[118] the Dharmasutras expressly state that the world of *Brahman* is obtained by self-immolation in fire.[119] Jain thought includes a complex doctrine of the liberation of self by means of ritual death, voluntarily pursued, according to which release from the world of illusion and the eternal cycle of rebirth is said to be attainable by various means, including drowning, self-immolation, starvation, self-dismemberment, or falling from a cliff, often at specific holy sites.[120] Although these religious traditions also contain prohibitions of suicide, and although in particular the Buddha appears to have been opposed to suicide, religious suicide in order to attain the highest religious state has been widely recommended and practiced in Hinduism and Buddhism.

In Christianity, an explicit longing for death in order to achieve the highest spiritual condition is expressed by a great many thinkers; it is also a powerful element in the motivation for martyrdom. John Donne, as has been mentioned, claims that we all have a religiously fortified "natural desire of dying," and he confesses to his own "sickly inclination" to commit suicide.[121] St. Paul had revealed his own desire for death in his letter to the Philippians: "I am torn two ways: what I should like is to depart and be with Christ; that is better by far; but for your [the Church's] sake there is greater need for me to stay on in the body."[122] Where the desire for death is strongest, it is also held most praiseworthy. It is seen as a triumph over the pleasures of the flesh and entanglements of this world, and as devout commitment to the ultimate spiritual experience of the next. The sheer immediacy of one's need for union with God is a sign of the highest spiritual elevation, and it is the individual who has achieved the greatest degree of spiritual enlightment who prays most earnestly for death. As the Christian mystic Angela of Foligno confesses, after experiencing a vision of God:

> So I was left with the certainty that it was God who had spoken with me; and because of this sweetness and the grief of his departure did I cry aloud, desiring to die. And seeing that I did not die, the grief of being separated from Him was so great that all the joints of my limbs did fall asunder . . .
>
> I longed for death that I might attain unto that delight of which I now felt something, and because of this did I wish to depart from this world. Life was a greater grief unto me than had been the deaths of my mother and my children, more heavy than any other grief of which I can bethink me.[123]

The lure exerted by the promise of reunion with the deceased, release of the soul, the rewards of martyrdom, and the attainment of the highest spiritual states, including union with God, all occur in Christianity. Indeed, this sort of lure occurs in any theology that deems earthly life inferior to an afterlife. Thus, the question of the permissibility of suicide arises, though often only inchoately, for any sincere believer in a religious tradition of this sort, whether that individual's present life is a happy one or filled with suffering. Religious suicide is not always a matter of despair; it is often a matter of zeal. The general problem presented by the promise of a better afterlife may be strongest in Christianity, since the afterlife of spiritual bliss depicted by Christianity is a particularly powerful attraction.

The religious invitation to suicide is strong in other cultures, too, but instead of prohibiting suicide entirely, most other religious cultures have continued to permit some religiously motivated suicide. Usually, however, religious suicide is channeled into controlled institutional practices. Putative examples include the ritual deaths of African tribal kings, whose fixed term of office was terminated in compulsory but willingly performed self execution,[124] and the Brahmin practice of retiring into the forest to complete one's life in ascetic rituals culminating in death.[125] However, these religiously based practices serve to regulate not only religiously motivated suicide but also suicides for a variety of other reasons, including ill health, grief, social or political disgrace, and old age. In India, for instance, it was common for persons afflicted with leprosy or other incurable diseases to bury or drown themselves with appropriate religious ceremony;[126] this practice was believed to make them acceptable to the deities, but also served to facilitate both sanitation and humane self-euthanasia among the incurably ill. The ill also practiced self-immolation, believing that this purification guaranteed transmigration into a healthy body.[127] *Suttee,* widely practiced, was the institutional form of suicide associated with bereavement and the potential economic dependence of women. Japanese *seppuku,* the method of punishment frequently required of wrongdoers from the nobility and military classes,[128] was associated with social or political disgrace. In Hindu culture, as in Eskimo, Arab, American Indian, and a great variety of other cultures, the aged committed suicide, sometimes directly and sometimes by acquiescence to abandonment when they were no longer capable of governing a family or contributing to its economic welfare.[129] By and large, widespread efforts to prevent institutionally governed suicides of these sorts developed only after the intrusion of Western, Christian-based culture into these societies.

Christianity, however, has not developed institutional practices regulating suicide, either in cases of religious motivation, or where occasioned by illness, old age, bereavement, economic scarcity, or other practical calamity. Of course, institutional suicide is not entirely unknown in Western, Christian-based culture: for instance, until recently it was expected that the captain would "go down with his ship." Among Prussian army officers of the nineteenth century, suicide was expected of those unable to pay their gambling debts. There are also reports from seventeenth-century Brittany of a religious practice known as the "Holy Stone," whereby, at the request of the victim, the priest would bring down a large stone upon the head of someone suffering from a painful and incurable disease.[130] These practices have been of extremely limited scope, however. By and large, institutional suicide, other than that associated with self-sacrifice and martyrdom, has been unknown in the Christian West. Thus, the issue of whether or not suicide is permissible in the kinds of personal and social circumstances frequently governed by institutional suicide in other cultures has remained acute in Christianity, and is made more acute by the fact that the central, scriptural texts and early history of Christianity do not contain any explicit prohibition of suicide.

I think this is why we find so many of the religious arguments against suicide unconvincing, even if one accepts the theological premises on which they rest. One is struck by their heuristic character and the shallowness of the surface analogies upon which many of them rest. One also sees that these arguments do not account for many of the circumstances in which the question of suicide is most likely to arise.

Arthur Schopenhauer, observing that there is no prohibition or positive disapproval of suicide in the scriptures of the Judaeo-Christian tradition, remarks that therefore ". . . religious teachers are forced to base their condemnation of suicide on philosophical grounds of their own invention. These are so very bad that writers of this kind endeavor to make up for the weakness of their arguments by the strong terms in which they express their abhorrence of the practice . . ."[131] Schopenhauer also remarks that if there were any moral arguments against suicide, "they lie very deep and are not touched by ordinary ethics";[132] one might say that if there are any effective religious arguments against suicide, they, too, are deep, and have not yet been touched by the sort of argument traditionally offered within Christian religion.

We have considered in this chapter the central religious arguments against suicide; a great number of others have been advanced as well. Suicide, some Epicureans and Stoics claimed, was wrong because it involved the destruction of the divine spark or soul. Plotinus held that suicide was a perturbation or pollution of the soul, since its separation from the body was the product of passion.[133] The Council of Arles (A.D. 542) pronounced suicide to be "diabolically inspired"; this view was echoed by Martin Luther, who held suicide to be a work of the devil.[134] Blackstone, commenting on eighteenth-century English law, remarked that the suicide "rushes into God's presence uninvited."[135] In addition to the arguments already considered here, Thomas Aquinas also saw suicide as a "deliberate choice of evil," and a violation of the charity one owed oneself.[136] Because death is "the wages of sin," it has been argued, it is something we ought not deliberately bring about;[137] death is a punishment, and should not be self-inflicted. Suicide is a failure of trust, say others. And it has often been said that God has "appointed" or "fixed" or "allotted" a duration of time that each individual shall spend on earth, so that to commit suicide is to tamper with this plan. Some of these arguments may overlap with those we've already examined; none of them, I think, will survive analysis any more successfully than those already examined, and it is tempting to discard them all as expedients necessary to counteract the strong lure of the tacit Christian invitation to suicide. Nevertheless, the reader is invited to examine these arguments himself, or to add still others to the list; there may be a deeper, more profound religious argument against suicide we have not yet reached. Or the reader may prefer to adopt the attitude of the seventeenth-century cardinal, John De Lugo, who recognized the arguments to be weak and nevertheless asserts their conclusion to be true: "For though its [suicide's] turpitude is immediately apparent, it is not easy to find the foundation for this judgment. Hence (a thing that happens in many other questions), the conclusion is more certain than the reasons adduced by various authors for its proof."[138] This is hardly, however, a philosopher's stance.

Notes

1. Judaism's prohibition of suicide appears to develop in response to, or perhaps simultaneously with, that of Christianity. See Fred Rosner, "Suicide in Biblical, Talmudic and Rabbinic Writings," *Tradition: A Journal of Orthodox Thought*, 11, no. 3 (Fall 1970/71): 25–40, for a detailed account of the development of Jewish thought on suicide. Though Rosner

does not compare this development with that of Christianity, the perceptive reader will observe that both traditions exhibit simultaneous increases in the severity of their suicide prohibitions, beginning with Augustine and the Tractates of the Talmud. Islam contains a thoroughgoing prohibition of suicide from its beginning; but this, too, is post-Augustinian. Buddhism contains a very strong principle of respect for life, but is not strictly prohibitive of suicide; it permits suicide when one has reached the highest possible spiritual state. See L. De La Vallée Poussin, "Suicide (Buddhist)," in *The Encyclopaedia of Religion and Ethics,* vol. 12, ed. James Hastings (New York: Charles Scribner's Sons, 1925), 24–26.

2. David Daube, "The Linguistics of Suicide," *Philosophy and Public Affairs* 1, no. 4 (Summer 1972): 387–427.

3. These include Abimelech (Judges 9:54), Samson (Judges 16:30), Saul and his armor-bearer (1 Samuel 31:4, II Samuel 1:6, I Chronicles 10:4), Ahithophel (II Samuel 17:23), Zimri (I Kings 16:18) in the Old Testament; Razis (II Maccabees 14:41) and Ptolemy Macron (II Maccabees 10:13) in the Apocrypha; Judas (Matthew 27:5) and Paul's jailor (an attempted suicide) (Acts 16:27) in the New Testament. See L. D. Hankoff, "Judaic Origins of the Suicide Prohibition," in *Suicide: Theory and Clinical Aspects,* ed. L. D. Hankoff and Bernice Einsidler (Littleton, Mass.: PSG Publishing Co., Inc., 1979), 6 and *passim* for dating and further information on the old Testament suicides, as well as Brian M. Barraclough, "The Bible Suicides," *Acta Psychiatrica Scandinavia* 86 (1992): 34–39. See also the Church [of England] Assembly Board for Social Responsibility's study, *Ought Suicide To Be a Crime? A Discussion of Suicide, Attempted Suicide and the Law* (Westminster: Church Information Office, 1959), 42 and O. Kirn, "Suicide," in *Schaff-Herzog Encyclopaedia of Religious Knowledge,* vol. 11, ed. Samuel Macauley Jackson (Grand Rapids, Mich.: Baker Book House, 1964), 132–133.

4. I Samuel 31:1–6, trans. *New English Bible.* See the analysis of this case by George M. Landes of Union Theological Seminary in his unpublished paper "Some Biblical Perspectives Relating to the Matter of Suicide," p. 1. In II Samuel 1:10, Saul is not portrayed as a suicide.

5. Matthew 27:5; Judas is said to have hanged himself by a halter. In Acts 1:18, however, Peter is quoted as saying that Judas "swelled up" and died.

6. Except perhaps in the case of Sarah (Tobit 3:10, in the Apocrypha). Sarah decides not to hang herself, as she had intended, but instead begs the Lord to let her die. That the Old Testament contains no explicit discussion of the morality of suicide is not in itself surprising; particularly before the prophetic period, the Jews did not approach ethical questions in a philosophically explicit manner.

7. G. Margoliouth, "Suicide (Jewish)," in *The Encyclopaedia of Religion and Ethics,* vol. 12, ed. James Hastings (New York: Charles Scribner's Sons, 1925), 37–38. "The ancient Hebrews were, on the whole, a naive people, joyously fond of life, and not given to tampering with the natural instinct of self-preservation" (p. 37). See also Jacob Hamburger, *Real-Encyclopädie für Bibel and Talmud,* vol. 2 (Leipzig: In Commission von R. F. Koehler, 1886–1892), 1110, on the rarity of suicide among the early Jews.

8. L. D. Hankoff, "Judaic Origins of the Suicide Prohibition," in *Suicide: Theory and Clinical Aspects,* ed. L. D. Hankoff and Bernice Einsidler (Littleton, Mass.: PSG Publishing Co., Inc., 1979), 18. Hankoff grants that the earliest period of Hebrew civilization, up until the Exodus, may have had—like its Egyptian, Greek, and Babylonian neighbors—no prohibition of suicide (p. 5).

9. H. J. Rose, "Suicide (Introductory)," in *Encyclopaedia of Religion and Ethics,* vol. 12, ed. James Hastings (New York: Charles Scribner's Sons, 1925), 24.

10. Flavius Josephus, *The Jewish War,* III 316–391 (London: William Heinemann, New York: G. P. Putnam's Sons, 1927, vol. 2, 664–687), described the events at Jotapata; a similar

mass suicide, that at Masada, is described in *The Jewish War,* VII 320–406 (1928), 3, 594–619.

11. For instance, the argument that we should not "fly from the best of masters," that is, God, is reminiscent of Plato's argument against suicide at *Phaedo* 62B, where Socrates described men as the property of the gods, and argued that "one should not escape from a good master." Tr. Hugh Tredennick, in *Plato: The Collected Dialogues,* ed. Edith Hamilton and Huntington Cairns (Princeton, N.J.: Princeton University Press, 1961).

12. *Semakhot,* chap. 2. Chapter 2, Rule 2 also provides a definition of suicide, excluding cases of possible accident or murder. "A willful suicide is one who calls out: 'Look, I am going to the top of the roof or to the top of the tree, and I will throw myself down that I may die.' When people see him go up to the top of the tree or roof and fall down and die, then he is considered to have committed suicide willfully. A person found strangled or hanging from a tree or lying dead on a sword is presumed not to have committed suicide intentionally and none of the funeral rites are withheld from him." See Fred Rosner, "Suicide in Biblical, Talmudic, and Rabbinic Writings," 33–34.

13. Louis Zucker, private conversations, University of Utah.

14. Rosner, "Suicide in Biblical, Talmudic and Rabbinic Writings," 39.

15. For an example of *Kiddush Hashem,* see chap. 5 in Margaret Pabst Battin, *Ethical Issues in Suicide* (Englewood Cliffs, N.J.: Prentice-Hall, 1982), on the self-poisonings of the ninety-three maidens of the Beth Jacob School, pp. 166–167.

16. "Thou shalt not kill" is the Fifth Commandment in the Roman Catholic numbering system; it is the Sixth Commandment for Protestants.

17. Augustine's discussion of suicide in *City of God* appears to draw quite heavily from Lactantius' comments in *Divine Institutes* a century earlier (c. 314–317), particularly in its direct arguments against the suicides of Cleombrotus and Cato. However, Lactantius did not rely on the Sixth Commandment as a basis for the prohibition of suicide, but on the Orphic/Platonic argument that "just as we came into this life not of our own accord, so departure from this domicile of the body which was assigned to our protection must be made at the order of the same One who put us into this body, to dwell therein until He should order us to leave." Use of the commandment as the basis for the suicide prohibition appears to be wholly original with Augustine. See Lactantius, *The Divine Institutes,* bk. 3. chap. 18, in *Fathers of the Church,* vol. 49, tr. Sister Mary Francis MacDonald (Washington, D.C.: Catholic University of America Press, 1964), see especially 214.

18. See Joseph Fletcher's discussion of the language of the commandment in his chapter "Euthanasia: Our Right to Die," in *Morals and Medicine* (Princeton, N.J.: Princeton University Press, 1954), 195–196. Also see, on the linguistic basis of this commandment, *The Interpreter's Bible* (New York: Abingdon Press, 1952), 1, 986, and David Daube's thorough account of Hebrew and Greek terms that are used for suicide, in "The Linguistics of Suicide."

19. Augustine, *Concerning the City of God Against the Pagans,* bk. 1, chap. 21, ed. David Knowles, tr. Henry Bettenson (Harmondsworth: Penguin, 1972).

20. Ibid., bk. 1, 21.

21. Ibid., bk. 1, 21.

22. Ibid., bk. 1, 26.

23. Ibid., bk. 1, 26. "We have only a hearsay acquaintance with any man's conscience; we do not claim to judge the secrets of the heart."

24. John Donne, *Biathanatos* (New York: Arno Press, 1977, a photoreprint of the edition of 1647); also *John Donne's Biathanatos: A Modern-Spelling Edition,* Michael Rudick and M. Pabst Battin, eds. (New York: Garland Publishing Co., 1981).

25. Ibid., part 2, distinction 4, sect. 7, lines 3076–3080.

26. Ibid., part 2, distinction 6, sect. 8, lines 3842–3855.

27. J. Eliot Ross, *Ethics from the Standpoint of Scholastic Philosophy* (New York: The Devin-Adair Company, 1938), 143.

28. Joseph V. Sullivan, *Catholic Teaching on the Morality of Euthanasia.* Studies in Sacred Theology (Second Series), no. 22 (Washington, D.C.: Catholic University of America, 1949), 54.

29. T. C. Kane, "Suicide," in *The New Catholic Encyclopaedia* (New York: McGraw-Hill, 1973), 13, 782. It is instructive to compare this account with that of the 1908 edition of the same work; of particular interest is the more recent version's explicit statement that in cases in which it is doubtful whether the person was responsible for his or her act—"and frequently such doubt exists because the person is often mentally deranged"—the doubt is to be decided in his or her favor, and consequently, no ecclesiastical penalties are to be imposed, at least provided no scandal is likely to ensue. In contemporary practice, suicide cases are almost always treated in this way.

30. Donne's *Biathanatos,* Part 3, *passim,* provides a thorough compilation of biblical passages sometimes interpreted as prohibiting suicide, and argues a nonprohibitive interpretation for each of them.

31. Ibid., part 2, distinction 5, sect. 1, lines 5002–5004.

32. Caleb Fleming, *A Dissertation upon the Unnatural Crime of Self-Murder Occasioned by the Many Late Instances of Suicide in this City, etc.* (London: Printed for Edward and Charles Dilly, 1773), 7.

33. Presbyterian Senior Services, The Presbytery of New York City, pastoral letter on euthanasia and suicide, March 9, 1976, p. 3.

34. Landes, "Some Biblical Perspectives Relating to the Matter of Suicide," 3.

35. Thomas Aquinas, *Summa Theologiae,* 2a2ae64.5 (Blackfriars, New York: McGraw-Hill, London: Eyre & Spottiswoode, 1964).

36. Josephus, *The Jewish War,* vol. 3, 374.

37. Immanuel Kant, *Lectures on Ethics,* tr. Louis Infeld (New York: Harper Torchbooks, 1963), 151.

38. John Locke, *The Second Treatise of Government,* chap. 2, par. 6, ed. Thomas P. Peardon (Indianapolis: Bobbs-Merrill, 1952), 5–6.

39. Plato, *Phaedo* 62B-C.

40. Ibid., 62B; my translation.

41. Locke, *Second Treatise of Government,* chap. 2, par. 6.

42. Cicero, *On Old Age,* vol. 7, "Death Has No Sting," tr. Michael Grant (Baltimore: Penguin Books, 1960), 242.

43. Kant, *Lectures on Ethics,* 154.

44. Johannes Robeck, *Exercitatio philosophica de . . . morte voluntaria. . . .* J. N. Funccius, ed., Rintelii, 1736. See also Henry Romilly Fedden, *Suicide: A Social and Historical Study* (London: Peter Davies, 1978), 210–211.

45. R. F. Holland, "Suicide," in *Talk of God,* Royal Institute of Philosophy Lectures, vol. 2, 1967–1968 (London: Macmillan, 1969), reprinted in James Rachels, ed., *Moral Problems* (New York: Harper & Row, 1971, 1975), 388–400; see 397.

46. Cf. Eike-Henner W. Kluge, *The Practice of Death* (New Haven: Yale University Press, 1975): "A gift we cannot reject is not a *gift.* It also follows that if retribution were to be visited upon us because of such a rejection, mistreatment, or destruction of the gift from God, we should have no alternative but to conclude that it would be the individual who visited the retribution and not we ourselves that would be morally guilty. In fact, the very threat to visit such retribution would be immoral, for it would be a calculated threat or actual attempt to interfere with our liberty" (pp. 124–125).

47. Cicero read the ambiguous *phroura* as "guardpost" rather than "prison"; Plato's (Orphic) argument had been that man is in a kind of prison and ought not escape; Cicero rendered this as the claim that man is stationed at a guardpost, and ought not run away. See M. Pabst Battin "Philosophers' Death and Intolerable Life: Plato on Suicide" (unpublished manuscript, University of Utah), footnote 19, and discussions by such commentators as Burnet, Hackforth, Bluck, and Gallop *ad loc.*

48. P. R. Baelz, "Voluntary Euthanasia: Some Theological Reflections," *Theology*, 75 (May 1972): 238–251; reprinted in slightly excerpted form as "Suicide: Some Theological Reflections," in *Suicide: The Philosophical Issues*, ed. M. Pabst Battin and David Mayo (New York: St. Martin's, 1980), 71–83. Baelz does not hold that all suicides are necessarily acts of ultimate despair.

49. It is not easy to identify who actually held the view Hume is attacking; Tom Beauchamp argues that Hume is replying to Aquinas, but Hume's argument is surely a misconstrual of Aquinas' views. Nevertheless, Hume's attack has given this view a conspicuous place in the later history of the discussion of suicide, hence its consideration here. See David Hume, "On Suicide," in *The Philosophical Works of David Hume*, vol. 4 (Edinburgh: Printed for Adam Black and William Tait, and Charles Tait, 1826), 556–567; also, David Hume, *Of the Standard of Taste and Other Essays*, ed. John Lenz (Indianapolis: Bobbs-Merrill, 1965); Tom L. Beauchamp, "An Analysis of Hume's Essay 'On Suicide,'" *The Review of Metaphysics*, 30, no. 1 (September 1976): 73–95.

50. Hume. "On Suicide," 561.

51. Ibid., 562.

52. Ibid., 562.

53. Ibid., 562.

54. Aquinas, *Summa Theologiae*, 2a2ae64.5.

55. Sir Wiliam Blackstone, "Public Wrongs," bk. 4, "Of Homicide," chap. 14, in *Commentaries on the Laws of England*, 18th ed., ed. Archer Ryland (London: Sweet, Pheney, Maxwell, Stevens & Sons, 1829), 188–190.

56. The metaphorical sense in which suicide and other acts held to be sinful are said to cause the "death of the soul" is usually understood as equivalent to the "loss of eternal (heavenly) life"; it means not that the soul ceases to exist, but that it is consigned to permanent damnation.

57. Donne, *Biathanatos*, part 2, distinction 4, sect. 4, lines 2968–2970.

58. Hume, "On Suicide," 563.

59. Baelz, "Voluntary Euthanasia: Some Theological Reflections," 247.

60. Aquinas, *Summa Theologiae*, 2a2ae64.5.

61. Robert Burton, "Prognosticks of Melancholy," part 1, sect. 4, member 1, in *The Anatomy of Melancholy*, ed. Floyd Dell and Paul Jordan-Smith (New York: Farrar & Rinehart, 1927), 374.

62. Josephus, *The Jewish War*, vol. 3, 369–370.

63. Aquinas, *Summa Theologiae*, 2a2ae64.5.

64. Walter Marsden, *The Lemming Year* (Toronto: Clarke, Irwin, 1964), 134–136 cited in Bernice Einsidler and L. D. Hankoff, "Self-Injury in Animals," in *Suicide: Theory and Clinical Practice*, 131–139. This paper cites much of the literature on suicide-like behavior in various animal species. See also Donne, *Biathanatos*, part 1, distinction 2, sect. 2, for seventeenth-century claims concerning pelicans and bees.

65. Einsidler and Hankoff, "Self-Injury in Animals," 133–134 and *passim*.

66. See S. R. Steinmetz, "Suicide among Primitive Peoples," *American Anthropologist*, 7, no. 1 (1894): 53–60; Edward Westermarck, *The Origin and Development of the Moral Ideas* (London: Macmillan and Co., 1908), especially vol. 2, chap. 35, "Suicide"; Fedden,

Suicide, and Ruth Cavan, *Suicide* (New York: Russell and Russell, 1965), for surveys of suicide in preliterate and non-Western cultures. Cavan writes, reflecting what is probably the prevailing consensus, "Suicides for personal motives are reported from so many sources that it must be assumed that they occur in all except the most isolated groups with extremely simple cultures" (p. 64), and she observes that institutionalized suicide, including *suttee,* self-punishment, self-senicide, and "running amok," is found in widely varied societies in all parts of the world. However, the consensus also holds that suicide rates in most small-scale societies are relatively low. See also Jean La Fontaine, "Anthropology," in *A Handbook for the Study of Suicide,* ed. Seymour Perlin (London, Toronto, New York: Oxford University Press, 1975), 77–91. For a perceptive analysis of the way data in such sources as the Human Relations Area Files have been influenced by the interests of anthropologists who gather them, and a conjecture that this seriously distorts findings concerning suicide, see Jean Baechler, *Suicides,* tr. Barry Cooper (New York: Basic Books, 1975), 38–42.

67. Donne, *Biathanatos,* part 2, distinction 3, sect. 1, lines 2710–2715.

68. See Sigmund Freud, *Mourning and Melancholia,* in *The Standard Edition of the Complete Works of Sigmund Freud,* ed. and tr. James Strachey (London: The Hogarth Press, 1915), 14, 250–252; also chap. 5 of *The Ego and the Id,* and the last pages of "The Economic Problem of Masochism."

69. Edward O. Wilson's *Sociobiology: The New Synthesis* (Cambridge, Mass.: Harvard University Press, 1975), is the central statement of this thesis; his newer *On Human Nature* (Cambridge, Mass.: Harvard University Press, 1978) examines claims concerning altruism in animals and human beings.

70. For an early allusion to this point, see Donne, *Biathanatos,* part 1, distinction 2, sect. 2, lines 1689–1697.

71. Austin Fagothey, S. J., "Natural Law," chap. 11, in *Right and Reason* (St. Louis: C. V. Mosby Co., 1953), 152.

72. A number of critics maintain that Saint-Preux's arguments defending suicide, rather than Lord Bomston's against it, represent Rousseau's actual views, and this is probably the case; nevertheless, the arguments voiced by Bomston in this novel remain an excellent statement of the natural-law view. The discussion between Saint-Preux and Bomston is contained in letters 114 and 115 of *Julie, or the New Heloise;* however, these letters have been severely abridged in the only widely available English translation. The quotations used here are from pp. 166–190 of *Eloisa, or, A Series of Original Letters.* (London: Printed for C. Bathurst, 1795).

73. Ibid., 182.

74. Ibid., 190.

75. Henry Davis, S. J., *Moral and Pastoral Theology,* vol. 2 (London: Sheed and Ward, 1936), 114.

76. Aristotle, *Nicomachean Ethics* 116a, tr. W. D. Ross, in *The Basic Works of Aristotle,* tr. Richard McKeon (New York: Random House, 1941).

77. Augustine, *City of God,* bk. 1, chap. 22, 33.

78. Aquinas, *Summa Theologiae,* 2a2ae64.5.

79. See Augustine's discussion of the suicides of Cato and Regulus at *City of God,* bk. 1, chaps. 23–24; Augustine says that Regulus is a "nobler example of fortitude" than Cato, although Christians supply much nobler instances.

80. An account of Wallace Proctor's suicide, as aided by his close friend Morgan Sibbett, is available in *The New York Times,* Dec. 11, 1977; in the Public Broadcasting System's "All Things Considered" for Friday, Dec. 2, 1977; and in Berkeley Rice, "Death by Design: A Case in Point," *Psychology Today,* January 1978, 71.

81. Paul-Louis Landsberg, "The Moral Problem of Suicide," in *The Experience of Death and The Moral Problem of Suicide*, tr. Cynthia Rowland (New York: Philosophical Library, 1953; original French edition 1951), 68. Landsberg himself once planned suicide, but changed his mind after a religious experience while captured by the Nazis.

82. Shakespeare, *Hamlet*, act III, sc. 1, lines 76–83. (Baltimore: Penguin, 1970), 89–90.

83. There have, of course, always been claims about those "returned from the dead," fueled by Raymond A. Moody, Jr.'s *Life After Life* (New York: Mockingbird Books, 1975; Bantam, 1976), but scientifically verifiable accounts of what it is like to be dead are nowhere available, and the life-after-life reports describe only experiences occurring within a very few minutes after clinical "death," not, so to speak, death on a long-term basis.

84. Philip Devine, *The Ethics of Homicide* (New York: Cornell University Press, 1979), 24–28; reprinted as "On Choosing Death" in *Suicide: The Philosophical Issues*, ed. Battin and Mayo, 138–143.

85. Mme. de Staël-Holstein [Anne Louise Germaine (Necker), the baroness Staël-Holstein], "Reflections on Suicide," in *The Constitution of Man, Considered in Relation to External Objects*, ed. George Combe, "Alexandrian Edition" [not in other editions] (Columbus: J. and H. Miller, 18–?), 99–112 of second half of volume. The earlier work is *A Treatise on the Influence of the Passions upon the Happiness of Individuals and of Nations*, tr. K. Staël-Holstein (London: George Cawthorne, 1798).

86. Sullivan, *Catholic Teaching on the Morality of Euthanasia*, see especially 73–76, "The Catholic Philosophy of Suffering." See also Léon Meynard, *Le Suicide: Étude morale et métaphysique* (Paris: P.U.F., 1966), 105.

87. W. R. Matthews, "Voluntary Euthanasia: The Ethical Aspect," in *Euthanasia and the Right to Death*, ed. A. B. Downing (London: Peter Owen, 1969), 25–29, citation, 26.

88. Fletcher, *Morals and Medicine*, points out in chap. 1 that anesthetics, especially in childbirth, in fact were opposed on these grounds when first introduced.

89. John MacQuarrie, "Suffering," in *Dictionary of Christian Ethics* (Philadelphia, Pa.: The Westminster Press, 1967), 335.

90. Pierre Teilhard de Chardin, *Writings in Time of War*, tr. Rene Hague (New York: Harper & Row, 1968), 67–68.

91. MacQuarrie, *Dictionary of Christian Ethics*, 335.

92. Matthews, "Voluntary Euthanasia: The Ethical Aspect," 26.

93. Plato, *Phaedo* 68A, 50.

94. According to Tasuku Harada's entry, "Suicide (Japanese)," in *The Encyclopaedia of Religion and Ethics*, vol. 12, 35–37, in ancient Japanese society *junshi* was an act of loyalty required by custom, until the emperor Juinin (29 B.C.–70 A.D.) ordered the substitution of clay images for the bodies of attendants and animals. The custom was revived during the feudal period in Japan and forbidden again in 1744; however, occasional modern examples still occur, such as the suicide by *hara-kiri* of General Nogi and his wife at the time of the funeral of the emperor Meiji in September 1921. For a classification of types of suicide in Japanese culture, see Mamoru Iga and Kichinosuke Tatai, "Characteristics of Suicides and Attitudes Toward Suicide in Japan," in *Suicide in Different Cultures*, ed. Norman L. Farberow (Baltimore: University Park Press, 1975), 255–280.

95. See Upendra Thakur, *The History of Suicide in India* (Delhi: Munshi Ram Manohar Lal, 1963), for a discussion of many types of suicide in Indian culture, and A. Venkoba Rao, "Suicide in India," in *Suicide in Different Cultures*, 231–238, especially 233 ff. on *suttee*. In Hinduism, the "next world" referred to is not the next incarnation, but Hinduism's dimly defined interval between this incarnation and the next. Of course, *suttee* can be explained on other grounds; as Venkoba Rao points out (p. 233), in at least some areas *suttee* was a matter

of law intended to prevent the wife from poisoning her husband, since if the poisoning were successful she would be required to die with him.

96. Plato, *Phaedo* 66E, 49.

97. This issue is discussed in Battin, "Philosopers' Death and Intolerable Life: Plato on Suicide."

98. Plato, *Laws* IX, 873C, 1473.

99. Cicero, *Tusculan Disputations* I, 34, 84, quoting Callimachus. The story of Cleombrotus is also discussed by Augustine in *City of God,* bk. 1, chap. 22.

100. De La Vallée Poussin, "Suicide (Buddhist)," in *The Encyclopaedia of Religion and Ethics.* The reference cited is to the *Jatakamala,* bk. i.

101. For a brief account of Captain Oates' self-sacrifice, see Holland, "Suicide," 394. Holland quotes from vol. 1, 462 of *Scott's Last Expedition* (London, 1935).

102. An accessible statement and useful discussion of the principle of double effect in bioethical contexts may be found in Tom L. Beauchamp and James F. Childress, *Principles of Biomedical Ethics* (New York: Oxford University Press, 1979), 102–105. Their footnote 10, on p. 131, provides further references to the literature on double effect.

103. See especially Philippa Foot, "The Problem of Abortion and the Doctrine of the Double Effect," *Oxford Review* no. 5 (1967), reprinted in James Rachels, *Moral Problems,* 59–70.

104. Davis, *Moral and Pastoral Theology,* 2, 116.

105. Robert Martin, "Suicide and Self-Sacrifice," in *Suicide: The Philosophical Issues,* ed. Battin and Mayo, 48–68.

106. Emile Durkheim, *Suicide: A Study in Sociology,* tr. John A. Spaulding and George Simpson (New York: Free Press, 1951).

107. Eusebius, *Ecclesiastical History,* bk. 8, chap. 12, tr. Roy J. Deferrari (New York: Fathers of the Church, Inc., 1955), 29, 184–185.

108. Romans 8:5–8.

109. Augustine, *City of God,* bk. 1, 27.

110. Tertullian, Letter "To the Martyrs," in *Disciplinary, Moral and Ascetical Works,* vol. 40, tr. Rudolph Arbesmann (New York: Fathers of the Church, Inc., 1959), 20.

111. Valerian, Homily 15, "The Excellence of Martyrdom," in *Saint Peter Chrysologus, Selected Sermons, and Saint Valerian, Homilies,* vol. 17, tr. George E. Ganss (New York: Fathers of the Church, 1953), 397–403; quotation, 398.

112. Gregory of Nazianzus, *Orationes* xlii, 5, 6, cited by Maurice H. Hassatt, "Martyr," in *Catholic Encyclopaedia* (New York: The Gilmary Society; Robert Appleton Co., 1910, The Encyclopaedia Press, 1913), 9, 736–740.

113. Eusebius, *Ecclesiastical History,* chap. 12, 185–186.

114. Augustine, Letter 204, to Dulcitius, in *Letters,* vol. 5, tr. Sister Wilfrid Parsons (New York: Fathers of the Church, Inc., 1956), 5, 3.

115. W. C. Frend, *The Donatist Church* (Oxford, Clarendon, 1952), 175.

116. See A. Bayet, *Le Suicide et la Morale* (Paris: Alcan, 1922). See also the strong objection to my view and the argument pursued here in Darrell W. Amundsen, "Suicide and Early Christian Values," in *Suicide and Euthanasia: Historical and Contemporary Themes,* ed. Baruch A. Brody (Dordrecht: Kluwer Academic Publishers, 1989), especially 141.

117. Baelz, "Voluntary Euthanasia," 240.

118. See Thakur, *The History of Suicide in India,* in the section on "Religious Suicides," 77–111, for this and other examples of Hindu, Buddhist, and Jain religious suicide.

119. A. Berriedale Keith, "Suicide (Hindu)," in *The Encyclopaedia of Religion and Ethics,* vol. 12, 33–35.

120. Thakur, *History of Suicide in India,* 79. Also see Rao, "Suicide in India," 231–232;

S. Settar, *Pursuing Death: Philosophy and Practice of Voluntary Termination of Life* (Dharwad: Institute of Indian Art History, Karnatak University, 1990).

121. Donne, *Biathanatos,* preface.

122. Philippians 1:23.

123. Angela of Foligno, "Of the Many Visions and Consolations Received by the Blessed Angela of Foligno," treatise 3, in *The Book of Divine Consolation of the Blessed Angela of Foligno,* tr. Mary G. Steegman (New York: Cooper Square Publishers, 1966), 167–168.

124. Fedden, *Suicide,* 23, describes such practices on the Malabar coast, based on accounts in James Frazer's *The Dying God;* these accounts have been challenged.

125. Rao, "Suicide in India," 232.

126. Thakur, *History of Suicide in India,* 78.

127. Ibid., 78.

128. Harada, "Suicide (Japanese)," 35–37. See also Iga and Tatai, "Characteristics of Suicides and Attitudes towards Suicide in Japan."

129. Simone de Beauvoir's *The Coming of Age,* tr. Patrick O'Brian (New York: G. P. Putnam's Sons, 1972) provides a readable survey of senicide and self-senicide practices in a wide variety of cultures; see especially part 1, chap. 2: "The Ethnological Data."

130. Fletcher, *Morals and Medicine,* 180.

131. Arthur Schopenhauer, "On Suicide," in *Studies in Pessimism,* in *Complete Essays of Schopenhauer,* tr. T. Bailey Saunders (New York: Wiley Book Co., 1942), 25.

132. Schopenhauer, *Foundation of Morals,* sec./par. 5.

133. Plotinus, *Enneads,* tr. A. H. Armstrong (Cambridge: Harvard University Press, 1966), Ennead I, ix, 322–325.

134. Martin Luther, *The Table Talk or Familiar Discourse of Martin Luther,* tr. William Hazlitt (London: David Bogue, 1848), DLXXXIX, 254. The saying attributed to Luther is: "It is very certain that, as to all persons who have hanged themselves, or killed themselves in any other way, 'tis the devil who has put the cord round their necks, or the knife to their throats."

135. Blackstone, *Commentaries on the Laws of England,* bk. 4, 189.

136. Aquinas, *Summa Theologiae,* 2a2ae64.5.

137. Church Assembly Board, *Ought Suicide To Be a Crime?,* 26, discusses this view but does not adopt it.

138. John De Lugo, *De Justitia et Jure,* disp. 10, sec. 1, 2. (Lugduni: Sumpt. Lavrentii Arnaud, & Petri Borde, 1670), 237.

12

Assisted Suicide: Can We Learn from Germany?

As the United States' public discussion of euthanasia and assisted suicide grows increasingly volatile, our interest in the Netherlands—the only country that openly permits the practice of euthanasia—has grown enormously. How do they do it? we ask. What drugs do they use? How many cases of euthanasia are performed in a year? Is there abuse? In asking these questions, and in listening to the legions of bioethicists and reporters and concerned physicians who have been to the Netherlands to scrutinize this practice, we are in effect regarding the Netherlands as a kind of natural laboratory for our own possible experiments in right-to-die legislation. Should we legalize euthanasia, as was on the ballot in the state of Washington in 1991 and in California in 1992? Let us look to the Netherlands, we say.[1] Of course, examining euthanasia in the Netherlands has led to considerable controversy about just what is to be observed there—some claim there is virtually no abuse, others insist abuse is widespread[2]—and about the degree to which the things we learn can be translated to the United States, given differences in law, health-care systems and other social factors,[3] but all parties seem to agree that whatever is happening in Holland, it has important lessons for us.

However, voluntary active euthanasia is not the only form of aid-in-dying on the ballot in the United States. Washington's Initiative 119 and California's Proposition 161 would also have legalized physician-assisted suicide. Yet although the Netherlands also now tolerates physician-assisted suicide under the same legal device that it tolerates euthanasia, the rates of practice are quite different: while about 1.8 percent of all deaths in the Netherlands are the result of euthanasia, only about 0.3 percent involve physician-assisted suicide.[4] It is euthanasia in the Netherlands that has attracted the world's notice; assisted suicide has played only a very minor supporting role.

Yet in the United States, there seems to be nearly as much—or perhaps more—public sympathy for assisted suicide as for active euthanasia. In a *Boston Globe/Harvard* survey taken in October 1991, 54 percent of a national sample of 1,311 adults said that if they had an illness with no hope of recovery and were suffering a great deal of physical pain, they would or probably would consider asking their doctor to

From *The Hastings Center Report* (March–April 1992): 44–51. Copyright © 1992 by the Hastings Center.

administer lethal drugs or a lethal injection; and 53 percent said that in the same circumstances they would or probably would ask their doctor to prescribe a lethal drug that they could decide to take later on; a Roper poll of the West Coast put these figures at 54 percent and 60 percent, respectively.[5] The opposition to Initiative 119 and Proposition 161 focused almost exclusively on the dangers of euthanasia, not assisted suicide: prevent "medical homicide," was the cry,[6] but little was said about restricting a patient's freedom to choose suicide—which, in Washington and California, as in almost all other states, is not illegal. Given chaotic health-care financing in the United States, preferring assisted suicide to active euthanasia is not, I think, an unrealistic position—at least until there has been thorough health care reform. Because the United States is so sensitive (as it should be) to the risks of abuse, and because permitting assisted suicide would require a less dramatic change in the law, I think that the United States will come to accept assisted suicide in the relatively near future, officially as well as tacitly, but is likely to resist legalizing active euthanasia for a longer time.

But if this is so, then there is something ironic about turning only to the Netherlands for insight into issues of aid-in-dying: the Netherlands evidently prefers euthanasia to assisted suicide. What lessons can we learn from a country that sees things the other way around? Germany openly permits the practice of assisted suicide, but rejects euthanasia. Thus, in a sense it is the obverse of the Netherlands; hence, despite many other differences, the lessons to be learned here should be at least equally, or perhaps more, instructive for us.

That the Germans view aid-in-dying issues differently from the Dutch is of little surprise, given their quite opposite histories in World War II. In the minds of most Germans, the very term *euthanasia* is associated with the Nazis, and, in general, it is understood as involuntary killing on potentially political rather than medical grounds. Rejection of euthanasia may also be associated with distrust of physicians in an authoritarian medical climate. To be sure, since the mid-1980s there has been some renewed discussion among bioethicists of voluntary active euthanasia, but recently even the very discussion of it has been vigorously combatted by a coalition of protest groups. They claim that even to speak of euthanasia is to legitimize it; speeches have been silenced and entire conferences driven out of the country to prevent the raising of this issue.[7] For a complex set of reasons, however, attitudes toward assisted suicide are conceptually different from attitudes toward euthanasia, and unlike in the United States and Holland, assisted suicide is not regarded simply as a variant of euthanasia that differs primarily in who delivers the fatal dose.

The situation with respect to assisted suicide in Germany is marked by two important features. For one thing, the practice is both legal and partly institutionalized; it occurs on what may be a much larger scale and in different ways than in Holland, and of course occurs in a way not currently possible in the United States. Second, the practice of assisted suicide in Germany is embedded in a distinctive cultural climate, especially concerning the background conception of suicide; its features can best be made evident by looking at linguistic differences between German and English. Not only do patients with terminal illnesses have different options concerning suicide in Germany than they do in the United States; they are also able to talk differently about it and presumably think differently about it as well. The two main parts of this chapter will address these two principal concerns.

The Character of German Medicine

At least in what was formerly West Germany, medicine is technologically advanced, and, under a complex national health insurance system, provides a high level of care to virtually all inhabitants. Like the United States, Germany has entered the most advanced stage of what is known as the epidemiological transition, and the majority of deaths no longer occur, as they did in earlier historical periods and still do in the third world, as the result of parasitic or infectious disease, but as the result of advanced deteriorative disease late in life—cancer, heart and other deteriorative organ failure, stroke, neurological diseases, and so on. Like American medicine, German medicine has the capacity to "prolong" the lives of dying patients by means of respiratory, nutritional, and other support, but by no means always does so: a substantial proportion of expected deaths are "negotiated," the result of artful giving up. As in the United States, in Germany it is also often held appropriate to withhold or withdraw treatment from patients in the late stages of terminal illness, when survival is unlikely and treatment seems only to prolong dying. In these respects, American and German medicine are similar.

However, German medicine is often said to be quite authoritarian. Although empirical data have yet to be published, a large study currently in progress at the University of Göttingen is exploring a number of hypotheses that are often said to characterize medical decision-making.[8] These center on the claim that decision-making remains largely in the hands of the physician; although consent by the patient is legally required, and, indeed, consent forms for major procedures are routinely signed, neither patient understanding nor patient consent are emphasized. In circumstances in which the patient faces oncoming death, according to the hypotheses of the Göttingen study, it is the physician who makes decisions about the initiation or withdrawal of life-sustaining therapy. In these decisions, the evaluations and views of nurses and other caregivers play a considerable role, and consent typically is sought from the patient's relatives; however, in most cases the patient, who is often no longer competent, is not included in decision-making. Living wills are rarely used; the durable power of attorney became a legal possibility January 1, 1992, but is so far unused. Do-not-resuscitate (DNR) orders are rarely put in written form; for the most part they are made in agreement with the family but without discussion with the patient. Where they are written at all, DNR orders are only very briefly documented and supported. The wishes of a competent patient are considered, but only if they are very clearly expressed, if they are firmly supported by relatives, and if the conditions for patient decisions—namely, adequate information and explanation—have been met. However, this is the exception, not the rule. For the most part, there is no such thing as physician support of patient decision-making. In general, decisions about life-sustaining therapy are made by the physician, not the patient, and are consented to by the family. If the physician favors initiating intensive measures and the patient or family do not, the physician's preference usually prevails, and although explicit

disagreement is rare, where a lucid patient expresses the wish to decline life-prolonging measures, this wish may well be ignored. The only case, according to the
hypotheses of this study, in which patient or family preferences appear to prevail
over those of the physician is when the physician opposes initiating intensive measures, but the patient or family demand them.

It is in this medical climate that Germany's distinctive practices concerning
suicide in end-of-life situations have begun to develop. For the most part, patients
"in the system" of hospital care do not demand or achieve self-determination in
matters of dying. However, taking advantage of the legal situation in Germany with
respect to suicide, there has developed a substantial movement to avoid such situations altogether. It is led by a large, independent, nongovernmental, and nonmedical
organization, the Deutsche Gesellschaft für humanes Sterben (DGHS), or German
Society for Humane Dying, which has actively supported suicide or assisted suicide
as a way of achieving a painless, self-determined death.

Suicide and Euthanasia under German Law

The existence of the DGHS is made possible by a distinctive feature of German law,
a feature in which German law differs from that of England, the United States, the
Netherlands, and most of Europe. During the Middle Ages, in most of Europe
suicide was a felony punishable by desecration of the corpse, burial at a crossroads,
forfeiture of the decedent's estate to the crown, and, in some instances, execution if
the suicide attempt was not fatal. Suicide was not decriminalized in England and
Wales until 1961, primarily for the purpose of permitting medical and psychiatric
treatment without criminal onus for those who had attempted suicide. In contrast,
suicide was decriminalized in Germany by Frederick the Great in 1751. Assisting
suicide is not a crime in Germany either, provided that the person about to commit suicide is *tatherrschaftsfähig,* that is, capable of exercising control over his or
her actions, and also that he or she acts out of *freiverantwortliche Wille,* or freely
responsible choice.[9] Thus, although assisting the suicide of a disturbed, depressed,
or demented person or a person coerced by external forces would not be permitted
under German law, aiding an informed, voluntary suicide, including what we might
be tempted to call a "rational suicide," is legal. However, killing upon request—the
act involved in euthanasia—is illegal under German law.

To be sure, the details of German law on these points have been receiving
extended discussion, especially with respect to the apparent conflict between the fact
that assisted suicide is not illegal but that there may be a duty to rescue a suicide in
progress. Like U.S. law, German law imposes an obligation to rescue upon specific
parties standing in certain professional or personal relationships to other persons;
this is the basis of the physician's legal duty to rescue his or her patient. Thus, as one
widely prevalent interpretation of the legal situation holds, although the physician is
not prohibited from giving a lethal drug to a patient, once that patient has taken the
drug and becomes unconscious, the physician incurs a duty to resuscitate him or
her.[10]

These provisions of German law—all currently highly controversial—have the effect of curtailing the role of German physicians in suicide, and tend to insulate the patient from physician aid. Thus, German law reinforces a posture that might also seem to be a product of fear of euthanasia and suspicion of authoritarian physicians: in Germany, taking death into one's own hands in these contexts is an individual, private matter, to be conducted outside the medical establishment and largely without its help. This is not to say that the provisions of German law are the product of studied judicial deliberation or current political consensus; they are often viewed as an artifact of earlier times. In any case, although it apparently would not be illegal for physicians to assist in the initiation of their patients' suicides, as a matter of practice they do not do so. There is some move to suggest that the obligation to rescue extends beyond the physician to a spouse, friend, or any person with knowledge of a suicide in progress, but this is currently an extremely controversial issue in German law.

That neither suicide nor assisted suicide are illegal under German law does not mean that there can be no attempts to prevent suicide. Indeed, Germany has an active organization for suicide prevention, the Deutsche Gesellschaft für Suizidprävention (the German Society for Suicide Prevention), which directs its attention in particular to recognizing suicidal tendencies in disturbed, depressed, or demented persons—that is, persons who cannot be said to be in control of their actions and who are not exhibiting freely responsible choice. Since, of course, it is not always possible to determine in advance whether a given person's suicide might count as in control or not in control, or as the product or not the product of freely responsible choice, in practice Germany's suicide prevention efforts look very much like those elsewhere, and are generally directed across the board at preventing suicide. [11]

It is in this climate, then—a climate in which there are active programs of suicide prevention, in which suicide and assisted suicide are not illegal, and in which terminal patients have little control within the medical establishment—that the German Society for Humane Dying, the DGHS, has developed. It is not much known in the rest of the world, among other reasons, because it has not joined the World Federation of Right-To-Die Societies. This is in part a function of its very different attitudes about the relationship of suicide and euthanasia, explained by the profound mistrust Germans have of euthanasia: the DGHS insists that euthanasia cannot be legalized without *prior* legalization of assisted suicide;[12] the World Federation and the national right-to-die organizations that are its members support the immediate legalization of euthanasia and assisted suicide as well, as would have been the case with the state of Washington's Initiative 119 and California's Proposition 161. In part because the Dutch, American, and most other national right-to-die societies, including the Hemlock Society in the United States, see the issue of euthanasia in a way quite opposite from the DGHS, there is little love lost between them, and even in Germany the DGHS remains a highly controversial organization. Nevertheless, the DGHS is a major, functioning organization, and its activities are important to understand for those discussing end-of-life issues in the United States and other parts of the world.

The German Society for Humane Dying

Founded in 1980 to facilitate suicide for those who are terminally ill as a way of avoiding the medicalization of the end of life, by early 1993 the DGHS had grown to some fifty-five thousand members, and had been adding new members at the rate of one thousand per month. Many of its members are already elderly or already terminally ill. After a person has been a member of the organization for at least a year, he or she may request a copy of DGHS's booklet *Menschenwürdiges und selbstverantwortliches Sterben,* or "Dignified and Responsible Death," which is not commercially available. The DGHS does not charge for this booklet. The booklet itself includes a statement of the conditions under which it is obtainable—including the requirement that the member has not received medical or psychotherapeutic treatment for depression or other psychiatric illness during the last two years. Each copy is numbered; the member is urged to keep track of it, not to give it to third parties, and not to make public its contents in any other way. The booklet is to be returned to DGHS after the member's death. The DGHS reports approximately two thousand to three thousand suicides per year among its members, though this remains a small fraction—at most 0.5 percent—of Germany's annual mortality.[13]

The specific advice provided in the DGHS's booklet contains, among other things, a list of ten drugs available by prescription in Germany, mostly barbiturates and chloroquines, together with the specific dosages necessary for producing a painless, nonviolent death. In addition to the drugs that will produce death, the booklet lists companion drugs for preventing vomiting and for inducing sedation. It also lists drugs available without prescription in other European countries (some just a few hours' drive from parts of Germany), including France, Italy, Spain, Portugal, and Greece. DGHS recommends that the member approach a physician for a prescription for the drug of choice, asking, for example, for a barbiturate to help with sleeping or chloroquine for protection against malaria on a trip to India. Where this deception is difficult or impossible, the DGHS may also arrange for someone to obtain drugs from a country where they are available without prescription. In unusual cases, it will also provide what it calls *Sterbebegleitung* or "accompaniment in dying": this is provided by a companion who will remain with the person during the time that is required for the lethal drug to take full effect, often as much as ten to twelve hours or longer. However, the DGHS now urges that family members or friends, rather than DGHS staff or members, provide "accompaniment," and has recently inaugurated an "Akademie der Sterbebegleitung" or Academy of Accompaniment in Dying to train such persons in what to expect and how to be supportive.

DGHS also supports refusal of treatment, where that is what the patient wishes, and in general attempts to protect a broad range of patients' rights. It provides members with a series of forms, including copies of Germany's version of the living will and durable power of attorney. In the format provided by the DGHS, both of these forms not only stipulate health-care choices or persons empowered to make them on behalf of a no-longer-competent patient, they also include provisions authorizing the DGHS to take legal action against any person or organization (that is, any physician or hospital) that refuses to honor the patient's antecedently stipulated wishes. For those who choose suicide as a way of bringing their lives to an end, the

DGHS also provides a form intended to provide clear evidence both of the considered nature of that choice and to dispel any suspicion of foul play. The form—printed on a single sheet of distinctive pink paper—is to be signed once when the person joins the DGHS, asserting that he or she is a member of the organization and that he or she wishes to exercise the right to determine the time of his or her death; the same form is to be signed again at the time of the suicide—presumably, at least a year later—and left beside the body.

DGHS also relies heavily on its network of regional bureaus to encourage and facilitate feedback. Because assisting suicide is not illegal in Germany, there is no legal risk for an individual in soliciting information about suicide or in that person's family reporting back information about methods of suicide attempted or used. DGHS attempts to keep very careful track of its members' experiences with the information it provides, and uses this feedback to revise and update its drug recommendations. To facilitate this, the drug information provided in its booklet is printed on a separate sheet inserted in a slip pocket inside the back cover, and this list of current recommendations is revised and updated on a monthly basis. DGHS thus claims to be able to do what is much riskier in countries where assisting suicide is illegal: to make extensive use of feedback about actual methods of suicide. In mid-1991, when *Final Exit*, by the Hemlock Society's president, Derek Humphry, hit the top of *The New York Times* how-to bestseller list,[14] DGHS president Hans Henning Atrott complained that the American book's information wasn't fully reliable: it was based, Atrott claimed, on published toxicological information, or information about which drug doses *might* prove sufficiently toxic to cause death, and not on empirical information about which drug doses would be *certain* to cause death. Because of the quite different legal situation in Germany, DGHS is able to collect reports about its own members' suicides and thus to adjust its drug recommendations on the basis of actual experience. Humphry replied that he gets just as much information from the forty-seven thousand members of the Hemlock Society, including explicit information about suicide deaths from patients' families, from doctors, and even occasionally from patients whose suicide attempts were not fatal,[15] but it is clear that such information is collected in a very different climate in the United States. Fearing that they would be subpoenaed, the Hemlock Society was forced several years ago to burn first-person reports from a sizeable number of physicians about cases of euthanasia they had performed or suicide in which they had assisted.

Early in 1993, the DGHS was struck by scandal. As a result of undercover investigations by the police, it emerged that the DGHS founder and president, Hans Henning Atrott, was selling cyanide for exhorbitant sums, personally pocketing the profit. (DGHS literature does not list cyanide among the drugs it recommends for suicide.) Atrott was arrested on charges of tax evasion and eighty-eight counts of violating the drug dispensing laws, though since assisted suicide is not illegal in Germany and all his clients (perhaps with one exception) had been competent and acting voluntarily, no charges were brought against him on these grounds. *Der Spiegel*, the approximate German equivalent of *Time*, devoted a long cover story to the scandal, describing Atrott's operation as "Mafia-like," and some labelled the DGHS a "band of murderers."[16] Some fifteen hundred members resigned from DGHS; the DGHS board fired Atrott. Although the DGHS received an extensive amount of negative publicity, most of the negative comment applied to Atrott's profiteering—not to the principle that assistance in suicide is permissible if the person is competent and capable of freely responsible choice. This remained unchallenged.

Language and the Cultural Acceptance of Suicide

Beyond doubt, the unique legal situation in Germany contributes to the rather different way in which end-of-life issues are often viewed; so too does the rapid growth of an organization such as the DGHS. But there are deeper cultural factors involved, and these are nowhere more evident than in the German language itself.

In current usage, English provides one principal term to denote self-caused death, *suicide*. In contrast to English's primary reliance on a single term, German employs several distinct ones: the traditional terms *Selbstmord* and *Selbsttötung*, the scientific term *Suizid,* and the literary *Freitod*.[17] *Selbstmord* and *Selbsttötung* are the analogues of the English terms *self-murder* (also *self-murther*) and *self-killing,* which were in widespread use in English during the seventeenth and eighteenth centuries; in English these terms were eventually supplanted by the Latin construct *suicide* and have virtually disappeared from contemporary use. The German terms both remain current. The German *Selbstmord,* the term most frequently used in ordinary spoken and written discourse, carries extremely negative connotations, no doubt associated with its literal meaning "self-murder," including the implication of moral wrong. In partial contrast, *Selbsttötung,* literally "self-killing," has connotations that are comparatively neutral in their factual quality but still decidedly negative, just as *killing* is neutral in English compared to *murder* but is still decidedly negative. *Selbsttötung* is used primarily in bureaucratic and legal contexts. The German term *Suizid,* the Latinate construct linguistically analogous to the English term *suicide,* also literally means "self-killing" but is comparatively neutral in its moral connotations; instead, it conveys an implication of psychiatric pathology, and is the technical term characteristically used by clinicians and researchers. While these terms are primarily found in their conversational, bureaucratic, and clinical applications, respectively, they are also sometimes used interchangeably.

German's fourth term for self-caused death, however, is quite another matter. *Freitod* (literally "free death" or "voluntary death") is a positive term, free from connotations of either moral wrongness or pathology; it also avoids the drabness of bureaucratic facticity. It is associated with voluntary individual choice and the expression of basic, strongly held personal values or ideals, especially those running counter to conventional societal norms, and suggests the triumph of personal integrity in the face of threat or shame. *Freitod* has an archaic flavor, often associated with Romanticism, and would not generally be used in ordinary conversation; however, it is readily recognizable to most German speakers. Although the most common term for suicide, *Selbstmord,* and the comparatively uncommon literary one, *Freitod,* both refer to the act of bringing about one's own death, they have very different connotations and describe what are understood to be quite different sorts of acts. *Selbstmord* is taken to involve a generally repugnant, tragic act, generally associated with despair, anger, or depression; *Freitod,* in contrast, is seen as expressing voluntary, idealistic choice. Even the verbs used with the different German terms for suicide reinforce their semantic differences: one "commits" *Selbstmord* (*man begeht Selbstmord*), but one "chooses" *Freitod* (*man wählt den Freitod*). It is not grammatically possible to speak either of "choosing" *Selbstmord* or of "committing" *Freitod*.

To be sure, both English and German also offer a variety of peripheral terms to refer to suicide—for example, English's *self-destruction* and the archaic *self-slaughter*, German's *Selbstentleibung* (literally, "self-disembodiment"), all terms with strong connotations of violence, as well as an assortment of verbal expressions, many of which appear in similar forms in both English and German. In addition to the abstract *sich das Leben nehmen* ("take one's own life"), there are many expressions that make reference to the means of death employed: *sich erhängen* ("hang oneself"), *sich erschießen* ("shoot oneself"), *sich ertränken* ("drown oneself"), and so on. But the central contrast lies between English's current reliance on a single principal term, *suicide,* and German's routine use of several different terms, especially *Selbstmord, Selbsttötung, Suizid,* and *Freitod.* Despite its comparative archaism and infrequent usage, this latter term, *Freitod,* plays an especially significant role and is crucial to understanding the nature of institutionalized assisted suicide practices in contemporary Germany.

The term *Freitod* is often thought by educated Germans to date from the eighteenth century, emerging around the same time that Frederick the Great was decriminalizing suicide. The term seems particularly associated with the *Sturm und Drang* or Storm and Stress movement in German literature, especially the plays of Goethe and Schiller—plays read, of course, by German students during their high school years. Perhaps the most familiar, celebrated example of *Freitod* in German literature would be said to be the death of Goethe's character Werther, the hero of his 1774 novella *The Sorrows of Young Werther:* in this compelling tale, a projection of Goethe's own ill-fated love affair with Charlotte Buff, Werther chooses to end his own life rather than sink from a condition of extraordinary sensitivity and sensibility into the respectable tedium of everyday life.[18]

Curiously, however, etymological sources do not actually trace the word *Freitod* as far back as Goethe; rather, they find that it originates with the title of section 22 of Nietzsche's *Also Sprach Zarathustra* (1883), "Vom Freien Tode" (variously translated "On free death" or "On voluntary death").[19] In this work, Nietzsche developed the notion of *Übermensch* or "superman," a concept later misunderstood and appropriated by National Socialism, and asserted a central teaching of Zarathustra: "Die at the right time." *Meinen Tod lobe ich euch, den freien Tod, der mir kommt, weil ich will,* says Zarathustra ("I commend to you my death, free death, that comes to me because I want it.").[20] The death to be avoided is the "common, withered, patient death" of those who are "like sour apples": their lot is to "wait until the last day of autumn: and at the same time they become ripe, yellow, and shrivelled." The death that Zarathustra preaches is an active, extraordinary, heroic death, an earlier, self-willed death of which the ordinary man is hardly capable.

Perhaps because of the association of Nietzsche's *Übermensch* with Nazism, *Freitod,* with its quite positive connotations, is rarely thought to originate there, and is instead attributed, erroneously, to the pre-Romantic ideal. But the term is not found in either Goethe or Schiller, and indeed the single term, *Freitod,* is not even found in Nietzsche, though it originates from Nietzsche's two-word phrase,[21] first merged into a single term in a letter by his sister. Yet, however problematic its actual origins, the term does have a distinctive, well-recognized sense in contemporary German: although it refers to the act of bringing about one's own death, it does not convey the very negative moral connotations associated with *Selbstmord,* the factual but still negative connotations of *Selbsttötung,* or the pathological ones associated with *Suizid.* On the contrary, the connotations of *Freitod* are wholly positive: achieving this kind of death is an admirable, heroic—if very difficult—thing to do.

There is no analogous term in English. Although there have been recent attempts at coinages in English (e.g., *self-deliverance*) to describe suicide but avoid that term's negative connotations, there is no widely recognized, familiar English term with long historical resonances of the sort that *Freitod* seems to have. The only other English terms for suicide that do not have negative connotations carry either pronounced religious associations or the implication that the suicide serves the interest of some other person or cause: these are terms like *self-sacrifice* and *martyrdom.* The very concept of *Freitod*—a notion without religious, altruistic overtones and without negative moral or psychological implications, but that celebrates the voluntary choice of death as a personal expression of principled idealism—is, in short, linguistically unfamiliar to English speakers. Language is crucial in shaping attitudes about end-of-life practices, and because of the very different lexical resources of English and German, it is clear that English speakers cannot straightforwardly understand the very different German conception of these matters. Even in situations of terminal illness, the very concept of voluntary death resonates differently for the German speaker who conceives of it as *Freitod* than it does for the English speaker who conceives of it as *suicide.* To be sure, not every German speaker is familiar with the term *Freitod,* and some claim that it is synonymous with their language's other terms for suicide,[22] but this is just to say that some speakers may not be sensitive to the full resources of the language.

Thus, while one sees in both Germany and the United States the development of notions of what is often called rational suicide and the conception that this may be a reasonable choice in terminal illness, they occur in very different cultural climates. In an English-speaking country like the United States, in contrast, there is no tradition that recognizes a distinctive sort of suicide, different from immoral or pathological suicide, and no tradition of legal or other protection for it. Not even among the English Romantics is there a literary model quite like Werther, whose death could readily be described as *Freitod.* The sense of the German term *Freitod* is simply not to be found in any single term in English. Furthermore, it could be constructed in English only with comparatively clumsy circumlocutions: "suicide that is self-centered but without the negative connotations of either 'suicide' or 'self-centered' "; "self-deliverance but with long, positive historical resonances," and so on, but these paraphrases would hardly capture the rich connotative field that has developed around the term *Freitod.* This is not to say that German speakers are always actively aware of the history and connotations of *Freitod,* but that the German language provides resources for thinking about, expressing, and experiencing choices about suicide in terminal illness in a way that English does not. It is tempting to say, then, that these choices themselves may be rather different for the German speaker than the English speaker. If so, it is also plausible to suppose that choices of suicide in terminal illness, protected not only by legal but also by linguistic and hence conceptual supports, may be much easier to make in Germany than they are in the United States, where legal, linguistic, and conceptual structures all militate against them. Furthermore, presumably, not only may these choices be easier for the German speaker to make, they may also be easier for family members and other survivors to accept and for the culture as a whole to acknowledge. Of course, there are factors in German culture that militate against suicide as well— religious sanctions, for example; but the picture may nevertheless be rather different from the one we see in the United States.

Indeed, the DGHS deliberately exploits the conception of ending one's life in terminal illness as *Freitod* rather than *Selbstmord*. The distinctive pink form mentioned earlier, to be signed when joining the DGHS and to be signed again at the time of one's final act, does not refer to that act as suicide, but as free death: it is labelled *Freitod-Verfügung*, or "free death directive." On the line just prior to the space for the second signature, the form reads: *Ich habe heute meinen Freitod eingeleitet:* "I have brought about my free death today." This is the form that will be found beside the body. The terms *Selbstmord* and *Suizid* appear nowhere in this document, and the bureaucratic term *Selbsttötung* appears only on the reverse side in the language of quotations from German law about the legal status of suicide.

From Language to Practice

To be sure, many objections can be raised to the conception of suicide that the notion of *Freitod* supports or to its institutionalization in the practices of the DGHS. For example, because the German practice of assisted suicide, as shaped both by law and by linguistic expectation, tends to minimize the role of the physician, it tends as well to minimize the opportunity for whatever evaluation, counseling, and psychiatric consultation the physician might provide. It also leaves to the patient the primary responsibility for deciding whether the physician's diagnosis is accurate and the prognosis realistic, and whether there are other effective methods of treatment or symptom relief. There is little or no role for psychiatrists here, or for any other outside, "objective" evaluation of a patient's mental state. *Freitod* is conceived of as a profoundly individual, private matter, not one subject to external examination, which, in any case, runs counter to commonplace societal norms. This is not to say that every terminally ill person who commits suicide in Germany conceives of this act as *Freitod* or approximates it to the independent, Romantic/Nietzschean model as an expression of one's basic values, but the likelihood of this is, of course, much greater than in the United States, where an analogous conceptual model is not readily available at all.

Some objections are also raised to the portrayal of suicide in terminal illness as *Freitod* rather than as *Selbstmord, Selbsttötung,* or *Suizid.* For example, in a 1977 discussion of issues in voluntary death, the writer Gabriele Wohmann said she did not like to use the term *Freitod* in these discussions because it was "simply too pretty, too seemingly tasteful."[23] Nor do all discussions of the issue trade on emphasizing the opposition between *Selbstmord,* with its highly negative connotations, and *Freitod,* with its positive ones; many of the academic discussions employ the comparatively neutral term *Selbsttötung* instead,[24] and others attempt to cleanse the usual term *Selbstmord* by rejecting its negative connotations.

Questions can also be raised about the fit between the concept of *Freitod* and the assisted suicide practices possible in contemporary Germany. *Freitod* itself is conceived of as an individual, intensely personal, and thus characteristically solitary act. The word itself does not suggest (as is often the case, in contrast, with euthanasia in the Netherlands) that the period of dying is one in which one might expect to be surrounded by a devoted family or close friends, or supported by a trusted authority such as a priest or doctor. Nor does the German term suggest that one would be guided in one's decision by professionals or family members. It is an act in which one insists on choosing a different, individual course contrary to ordinary expectations: it is in this sense that it is "free" death. This has its advantages: almost by definition, *Freitod* cannot be socially "expected," required by policy, advised by counselors, or in any other way the norm, and hence it may be more resistant to abuse. Yet this does raise the issue of what tensions might arise for the person for whom the rhetoric of *Freitod* seems to describe a choice more individualistic and idealistic than he or she is actually making, or, conversely, what tensions might arise for the person for whom accusations of *Selbstmord* from unsympathetic physicians, family, or religious advisors seem to belittle the personal, reflective nature of his or her final choice. While choices of suicide in terminal illness may be easier to make in a linguistically richer culture than in one that is more limited in its resources for describing this choice, such tensions are no doubt very real. After all, DGHS is an organization that offers membership and provides help with suicide, both in giving information and in training family members or others to be present, and hence in this way the person may be accompanied and not alone. Yet, even in the current scandal, the linguistic and cultural model to which it appeals is one of solitary, profoundly individual choice.

What, If Anything, Can We Learn from Germany?

As we observe the increasing ferment in the United States over right-to-die issues, we can, I think, predict that of the two forms of aid-in-dying that are the focus of attention in the United States—active euthanasia and assisted suicide—it is the latter that will more readily find some degree of social acceptance. This might seem to make the German experience with assisted suicide as much or more relevant to us than the Dutch experience with active euthanasia, and to suggest that we should attend to the ways in which not only Dutch but also German culture has faced such issues. Certainly examining other cultures is an important remedy for our often isolationist myopia about social issues; observing a culture that has a far more open, widespread practice of assisted suicide in terminal illness will be enormously instructive for us.

What we discover, however, is that the issue is much more difficult than we thought, and that cross-cultural lessons are harder to draw. For what we see is that we are limited by our own language, and do not have the linguistic resources for understanding the issue in the way members of another culture can. We do not and perhaps cannot fully understand German attitudes toward what *we* call "suicide," and we cannot really comprehend this other way of looking at the issue—even though our cultures, economies, and medical establishments are in many ways very similar. For the German, *Selbstmord, Selbsttötung,* and *Suizid,* those phenomena described in terms with connotations of moral wrongness, bureaucratic factualness, or psychopathology, are, of course, to be prevented, even though the law neither prohibits them nor prohibits assisting them where they are performed by a person who is in control of his or her actions and acting out of freely responsible choice. On the other hand, the German tends to respect *Freitod,* however difficult it may be to say exactly what differentiates this phenomenon from the previous forms of self-caused death, and tends to regard *Freitod* as a matter of right—that is, to assume that one ought not interfere with it and that one always has the right to this choice. Thus, it is at best difficult for us in the United States fully to understand how members of German culture see these matters, and it is also difficult to understand what position the German takes him- or herself to be in when reflecting on the prospect of medical-ization of the end of life and the alternative of an earlier, self-caused death. Even if we could somehow capture the distinctions a German speaker senses among the various terms for self-caused death, we could not bring with them the set of back-ground models and the full range of culturally understood connotations. There is no easy English way to convey both what *Freitod* suggests and at the same time avoid what it does not.

If there are distinctions German speakers make but English speakers do not in referring to what we call suicide, perhaps we English speakers cannot even fully understand our own assumptions and beliefs about these matters. We say we are committed to "preventing suicide," for example, but this may be just to say that we are committed to preventing *Selbstmord, Selbsttötung,* and *Suizid.* Are we also committed to preventing *Freitod,* when we cannot distinguish it from these other forms of self-caused death, or, on the contrary, do we simply lack any reflective, principled view about whether we ought to do so? We cannot easily say whether we ought to prevent it, given our commitment to suicide prevention, because *we cannot even fully conceive of what it is,* and we cannot even say either that it is "a kind of suicide" or that it is not.

That we cannot make this distinction is not to say that we are altogether incapa-ble of making distinctions among accepted, even respected forms of self-caused death and those we reject or consider candidates for prevention. On the contrary, as noted earlier, English speakers readily make the closely related distinction involving altruistically or religiously motivated self-caused death. Typically, English speakers respond with approval, for example, to the jet pilot going down with the plane in order to avoid the crowded schoolyard, but mark the conceptual difference by insisting that "that's not suicide." This is a response analogous to the one German speakers would use to differentiate *Selbstmord* and *Freitod,* but the distinction is not the same one. The distinction between suicide as a moral wrong or psychological aberration and as a religiously or altruistically motivated choice is readily marked off in English, but the distinction between suicide as a moral wrong or psychological aberration and an autonomous choice based in personal ideals and values is not.

Curiously, the same article in *Der Spiegel* that denounced DGHS president Atrott's cyanide profiteering in Germany referred to the thirteen suicides in which

Dr. Jack Kevorkian had at that time assisted with the term *Freitod*,[25] rather than with the usual more negative expressions; this raises the issue of whether readers of German news accounts using this term might see Kevorkian's actions rather differently from readers of accounts in the English-language press.

What practical lessons, then, does this closer examination of assisted-suicide practices in contemporary Germany teach us about the United States, and particularly about the kinds of practices the United States should or should not legally recognize, morally recognize, or otherwise adopt? The central issue, it seems to me, has to do with the role of the physician. What is so striking about the German practice is the comparative absence of the physician from the scene; the question for the United States is not merely whether the physician ought to play the same absent role, but whether the cultural conceptions that might make suicide in terminal illness a possible choice in an English-speaking world argue for or against such a role. In examining both the Netherlands and Germany, we see two strikingly different physician roles: one in which the physician responds to the patient's request for euthanasia and it is *only* the physician (not a nurse, family member, or any other person except the patient him- or herself) who may administer the lethal drug, and in which the physician is expected to remain with the patient (and the patient's family) throughout the time it takes for the drug to produce death; the other in which the physician is not consulted, except perhaps to obtain the drug, and in any case is not present while the drug is ingested or during the period of dying. Determining what ought to be the role of the physician in the United States, if suicide in terminal illness is to be both morally respected and legally protected, is of course a question of certain practical matters—on the one hand, to exclude the physician seems to preclude the possibility of counseling, confirmation of the diagnosis and prognosis in this context, and physician presence and assistance, perhpas even reassurance, at the time of death, while on the other hand, to include the physician seems to bring with it the possibility of paternalism, control, institutional regulation, and potential inflexibility. But it is not only a question of these practicalities, however important they may be. It is also a matter of the fit between persons' conceptions of what they are doing and the structures within which it is possible for them to do it, and this is a much subtler matter indeed.

A remarkable further twist in the fortunes of the German Society for Humane Dying has direct bearing on the fit between what people take themselves to be doing and the structures within which they do it. In May 1993, five months after the jailing of Atrott, the DGHS elected a new president: Dr. Hermann Pohlmeier, a psychiatrist and noted expert on suicide *prevention*. Dr. Pohlmeier, the founder and long-time president of the German Society for Suicide Prevention, had served on the scientific advisory board of DGHS, but at the time of his election he had been a member for only eight days. Pohlmeier clearly announced that he would be working to change the direction and emphasis of the DGHS, encouraging members to express rights of self-determination in dying by refusing unwanted treatment, by making living wills, and by seeking hospice-style care, but not primarily by turning to suicide. On the contrary, Pohlmeier seeks to reverse what he believes has been a tendency to *encourage* suicide. Gone is the brochure describing methods of suicide and the list of recommended drugs, inserted in the slip pocket inside the booklet's back cover; the new view, according to Pohlmeier, is that while "everybody has the right to suicide, he must do it himself and not with the support of others.''[26] He insists that the issue be confined to cases of terminal illness. DGHS efforts to lobby for the legalization of active voluntary euthanasia have been discontinued. The Academies of Accompaniment in Dying still exist, but they are to be forums for discussion, not outlets for a clandestine trade in cyanide, and the size of the DGHS is to be scaled back. There will be increased contact with right-to-die societies in other countries. Like Pohlmeier, the executive officer will be a professional, scientific figure, and henceforth the discussion of aid-in-dying is to be conducted on a factual basis, meeting international scientific standards.

It is extraordinarily difficult to assess the significance of this seemingly quite radical shift. Some may view it as a defensive move in the face of rumors that the German parliament, acting in the wake of the Atrott scandal, will move to make assistance in suicide illegal, though probably not before the next elections, scheduled for the fall of 1994. Others may see it as a simple takeover of a patients'-rights group by the forces of professional suicide prevention. Still others may see it as the appropriate course-correction of a society whose well-intentioned founder had been corrupted by greed. Few have defended Atrott, or asked what is it about dying in contemporary times and within a modern medical system that would lead so many to pay so much for the promise of an instantaneous, painless death? At the moment, it is far too early to tell whether the change of direction in the DGHS represents a genuine change in the attitudes of the Germans generally, whether it is a temporary reaction to a visible occasion of scandal, or whether it is a closer approximation to the attitudes about voluntary death that have characterized German culture all along: ''everyone has the right, but not with the support of others,'' since support belies the individual, intensely personal, characteristically solitary notion of ''free death,'' even though the law actually permits assistance. The precise nature of the relationship between *Freitod* and assisted suicide may be difficult for Germans to capture in practice, and virtually impossible for English speakers to understand.

These are not easy issues to resolve. Worse still, in trying to do so we may find ourselves at an impasse: it is well indeed to look at other cultures for help with our own dilemmas, but doing so also obliges us to recognize our own severe limitations in attempting to resolve them. We may be able to recognize what our problem is: because our language is impoverished in its lexical resources for referring to self-caused death, we are paying the price in increasing social tension over this issue. Yet this insight does not tell us how to resolve our problem. I suspect we will find that while both the Netherlands and Germany can provide profoundly useful lessons (if we are careful to see what they are), neither the Netherlands nor Germany will prove quite the right model for the United States. Instead, we can expect to watch ourselves spend the next decade or two developing distinctive, conceptually and culturally fitting aid-in-dying practices of our own, drawing on but not adopting these other models.

Notes

I'd like to thank Sylvia Sauter and Hans Henning Atrott of the Deutsche Gesellschaft für humanes Sterben for various interviews in Berlin and Hamburg, September 1991 and Hermann Pohlmeier, M.D., for interviews in Göttingen in March 1992. I'd also like to thank Ali Wilson for her assistance under the Undergraduate Research Opportunities Program at the University of Utah.

1. In the Netherlands, euthanasia remains a violation of statutory law, but the physician who adheres to a careful set of guidelines is protected from prosecution under a series of lower and supreme court decisions.

2. Among the most recent works claiming to find evidence of abuse, see Carlos F. Gomez, *Regulating Death: Euthanasia and the Case of the Netherlands* (New York: Free Press, 1991), and John Keown's "On Regulating Death," *Hastings Center Report* 22, no. 2 (March–April 1992): 39–43; both drawing to some extent on the earlier claims of Dutch cardiologist Richard Fenigsen. Such works tend to conflate two issues: whether abuse is actually occurring, and whether there are adequate protections against abuse; within the former category, they also fail to distinguish between procedural abuse (e.g., not following the guidelines) and substantive abuse (killing patients against their will).

3. See my "Seven Caveats Concerning the Discussion of Euthanasia in Holland," *Perspectives in Biology and Medicine* 34, no. 1 (1990): 73–77, incorporated into chap. 6 of this volume.

4. These are the findings of the Remmelink Committee report, the first full-scale empirical study of euthanasia in the Netherlands. A summary of the findings is available in English in P. J. van der Maas, J. J. M. van Delden, L. Pijnenborg, and C. W. N. Looman, "Euthanasia and Other Medical Decisions Concerning the End of Life," *Lancet* 338 (14 September 1991): 669–674.

5. KRC Communications Research, 1991 *Boston Globe*/Harvard Poll; some results published in *Boston Globe*, 3 November 1991; Roper Poll of the West Coast (California, Oregon, Washington), May 1991.

6. The phrase is former Surgeon General Everett Koop's, used in TV spots in Washington on the eve of the election in November 1991.

7. See Peter Singer. "On Being Silenced in Germany," *The New York Review of Books*, August 15, 1991, 36–42, and Bettina Schöne-Seifert and Klaus-Peter Rippe, "Silencing the Singer: Antibioethics in Germany," *Hastings Center Report* 21 no. 6 (1991): 20–27, for accounts of responses to discussion of euthanasia and other topics. Also see the more comprehensive volume, *Zur Debatte über Euthanasie* (On the debate over euthanasia), ed. Rainer Hegselmann and Reinhard Merkel (Frankfurt: Suhrkamp Verlag, 1991), containing much of the discussion as well as responses to it. An example of the opposition is to be found in Christian Stadler, *Sterbehilfe—gestern und heute* (Aid-in-dying: Yesterday and today) (Bonn: Psychiatrie-Verlag, 1991).

8. Personal communication, Karl-Heinz Wehkamp. The study at the University of Göttingen, "Ärztliche Entscheidungen in Konfliktsituationen" (Physician decision-making in situations of conflict), is directed by Hannes Friedrich, Eva Hampel, Klaus Held, Stefan Tilz, Bettina Schöne-Seifert, and Jürgen Wilhelm. The expected completion date is December 1993.

9. See Volker Krey, "Tötung durch Zulassen eines Selbstmordes" (Killing by allowing a suicide to occur), *Strafrecht Besonderer Teil*, vol. 1, 7th ed. (Stuttgart: Verlag W. Kohlhammer, 1972, 1989), 35–37.

10. See Volker Krey, "Euthanasie nach deutschem Strafrecht—Strafrechtliche Probleme der Sterbehilfe für unheilbar Erkrankte" (Euthanasia according to the German criminal law: The problem of aid-in-dying for the terminally ill), in *5. Europäischer Kongress für humanes Sterben* (Augsburg: Deutsche Gesellschaft für humanes Sterben e.V., 1985), 145–150, and also the previously cited work.

11. See, however, Hermann Pohlmeier, *Selbstmord und Selbstmordverhütung* (Suicide and suicide prevention) (Munich: Urban & Schwartzenberg, 1983) for a discussion of suicide

and suicide prevention that also considers the relationship of suicide prevention to issues about freedom to choose suicide; a briefer statement can be found in his editorial, "Suicide and Euthanasia—Special Types of Partner Relationships," *Suicide and Life-Threatening Behavior* 15, no. 2 (1985): 117–123.

12. Personal communication, Hans Hennig Atrott, president, DGHS, January 8, 1992.

13. As Hans Wedler points out in his open letter, strongly objecting to this article ("Offener Brief an Frau Professor Battin," *Suizidprophylaxe* (Suicide Prevention), vol. 14, no. 2, 1992, p. 68), even if these figures were correct, they would represent only 0.5% of the total annual mortality in Germany (700,000), and only 2% of the cancer deaths (170,000).

14. Derek Humphry, *Final Exit: The Practicalities of Self-Deliverance and Assisted Suicide for the Dying* (Eugene, Ore.: The Hemlock Society, 1991).

15. Personal communication, Derek Humphry, president, The National Hemlock Society, February 4, 1992.

16. "Zyankali: 'Letzter Liebesakt' " (Cyanide: "Last Act of Love") *Der Spiegel*, no. 8, February 22, 1993, 90–101.

17. See *Der große Duden: Synonymwörterbuch*, 1964, s.v. *Selbstmord*.

18. Considerable critical discussion has been devoted to the issue of whether Werther's death—depicted as resulting a dozen hours after a self-inflicted gunshot wound to the head, clearly involving considerable suffering, is really intended by Goethe as a pure example of *Freitod*, or whether on the contrary it is a parody of it or warning against it. The publication of *The Sorrows of Young Werther* did lead to a rash of copycat suicides among young men, many of whom were dressed in clothing similar to Werther's—a blue waistcoat and a yellow vest.

19. Friedrich Kluge, *Etymologisches Wörterbuch der deutschen Sprache* (Etymological dictionary of the German language) (Berlin: DeGruyter, 1989), 231. See also Karl Baumann's remarkable dissertation on the development of the terms *Selbstmord* and *Freitod: Selbstmord und Freitod in sprachlicher und geistesgeschichtlicher Beleuchtung* (Suicide and free death as illuminated by linguistic and intellectual history) (Gießen: Dissertationsdruckerei und Verlag Konrad Triltsch, 1934), which includes extensive personal reflections from other linguists and over one hundred responses to a questionnaire about usage of these two terms.

20. Friedrich Nietzsche, *Also Sprach Zarathustra* (Stuttgart: Alfred Kröner Verlag, 1956), 76–79. Translation mine.

21. The first known occurrence of the single word *Freitod* is dated 1906, some twenty-three years after Nietzsche's *Zarathustra*. See Baumann, *Selbstmord und Freitod*, 13.

22. Wedler, "Offener Brief an Frau Professor Battin," p. 69.

23. Gabriele Wohmann, in "Auszüge aus der öffentlichen Podiumsdiskussion 'Freiheit zum Tode?' " (Selections from the public panel discussion 'Freedom for Death?'), with Jean Améry and Gabriele Wohmann, in *Selbstmordverhütung: Anmaßung oder Verpflichtung*, ed. Hermann Pohlmeier (Bonn: Keil Verlag, 1978), 13.

24. See, for example, the widely discussed proposal for revisions in the law on aid-in-dying, *Alternativentwurf eines Gesetzes über Sterbehilfe* (Alternative draft of a law on aid-in-dying), developed by a working group of professors of criminal law and of medicine (Stuttgart: Georg Thieme Verlag, 1986), and the volume of commentary edited by H. Atrott and H. Pohlmeier, *Sterbehilfe in der Gegenwart* (Aid-in-dying in the present) (Regensburg: Roderer Verlag, 1990).

25. "Zyankali," *Der Spiegel*, 95.

26. Hermann Pohlmeier, M.D., personal communication, October 1993; see also "Professor Pohlmeier will ramponiertes Image der DGHS wider aufpolieren" ("Professor Pohlmeier seeks to polish the tarnished image of the DGHS") *Ärzte Zeitung*, May 13, 1993, and Christine Alber-Longère, "Kein Verein von Todesengelh" (No Club of Death-Angels), *Neue Westfälische*, Bielefeld, May 15, 1993.

13

Assisting in Suicide:
Seventeen Questions Physicians and
Mental-Health Professionals Should Ask

How ought a physician or a mental-health professional respond to a request for help
in suicide, when that request comes from a person contemplating suicide because of
a terminal illness, severe permanent disability, or advanced old age? To disregard
the request or to attempt to prevent the suicide is simply to assume that there can be
no such thing as "rational suicide" under these conditions; but standard clinical
practices may not provide adequate ways of responding to such requests either. The
medical and mental-health professions, in their clinical and counseling services,
currently fail to serve a potentially enormous clientele often much in need of help.
Not all terminally ill, permanently disabled, or aging persons consider suicide, but
many, many do, and hence the issue of how to respond to a request for help in what
may be rational suicide in these circumstances is not arcane, but of central social
importance. It is, unfortunately, an area in which neither medicine nor the mental-
health professions currently provide adequate guidance.

Many clinicians recognize the possibility of rational suicide,[1] and some widely
read texts point out this possibility.[2] Some hotline agencies refer callers to sympathetic professionals, and a new, physician-staffed organization in the state of Washington, Compassion in Dying, provides extensive counseling and, if desired, assistance in suicide for the terminally ill. In 1993, the National Association of Social
Workers changed its code of ethics to allow its psychotherapist members to engage
in full, open discussion of assisted suicide with clients considering it. Nevertheless,
most medical, suicide prevention, and mental-health services do not provide for
suicide as a sane, honorable choice in terminal illness, permanent disability, or old
age. Although many physicians and mental-health professionals believe that suicide
can be rational and discussion of rational suicide is widespread, there is no readily
available, institutionally accepted way of responding to requests for help in rational
suicide that does not also directly or indirectly aim at prevention. Furthermore,
suicide hotlines and counseling services—those organizations which often provide

From *Crisis* 12:2 (1991): 73–80. Originally titled "Rational Suicide: How Can We Respond to a Request
for Help?" Reprinted by permission of the publisher.

the first contact with clinical resources for a person contemplating suicide—are often especially ill-equipped for doing so, since they tend to emphasize suicide prevention on an emergency basis rather than open, cooperative, ongoing response to suicide plans. But because suicide hotlines and counseling services are for the most part committed to suicide prevention even when they recognize the possibility of rational suicide, persons considering suicide for reasons of terminal illness, severe disability, or old age cannot readily trust them or even consult them, for fear that an option they see as real and important will be taken away from them. Thus, they cannot make use of the professional help their doctors, psychologists, psychiatrists, or other counselors have to offer in exploring choices of suicide and which might provide them with very real help. As a result, some older, disabled, or dying persons commit suicide when they do not really wish to do so, while others endure the worst indignities of terminal illness, permanent disability, or extreme old age when that is not their choice.

What follows is a list of seventeen considerations a physician, a mental-health professional, or for that matter, a friend, religious advisor, or any other counselor, might want to review with a person contemplating suicide. These considerations, formulated without antecedent bias toward prevention and without interpreting interest in suicide as evidence of mental illness, have the effect of inviting the person to try to assess the rationality or irrationality of such a choice. They presuppose that the person is capable to a substantial degree of rational self-inspection, and they will not work and should not be used with people who are clearly agitated, disoriented, seriously depressed, out of touch with reality, or otherwise mentally ill, and they cannot be used with someone in pain so severe that reflective thought is impossible. These considerations will be most effective if raised in approximately the order listed, either in one or several consecutive sessions, and if flexibility is exercised in formulating, amending, and augmenting them. There is a great deal of overlap among the various points; this is intended to encourage continuing consideration of the most basic issues.

1. *Is the person making a request for help?* Is it really a request for assistance in suicide, either in obtaining the means for suicide or in carrying out the act? Or is it a request for help in deciding whether to commit suicide? Is it a request for help in justifying the suicide to others? Is it a request for help in avoiding a suicide one has already decided to commit? Is it all of these? Does it cloak some other request? Or is it not a request for help at all? (This initial question is of central importance because the answer to it will determine how the subsequent questions are understood, though it is also the question to which a clear, unambigous answer is least likely to be found. During the rest of the interchange, the clinician may want to refer back to this initial question repeatedly, as it becomes clear that the "help" the person seeks variously shifts through all these forms.)

2. *Why is the person consulting a physician or a mental-health professional?* Has the person been referred by another physician? Has the consultation been urged by a family member or friend? Has the person been obliged or forced to see a physician or a mental-health professional, either through involuntary commitment or some other process? Or is the person seeking help of a physician or a mental-health professional because these caregivers have specific training and skills, and if so,

what does the person perceive these to be? Does the person seek reassurance that it is "normal" to have thoughts of suicide in such circumstances? If the person simply wishes to communicate his or her thoughts and intentions, wanting only an opportunity to "talk it out," why has he or she picked a physician or a mental-health professional for this purpose?

3. *What has kept the person from attempting or committing suicide so far?* Why hasn't the person simply pursued suicide on his or her own, for instance, by jumping, shooting, or overdose? Is it fear of death or fear of violent means of death that discourages such action? Fear of afterlife consequences? Or is it the case that the person does not fear suicide, but given advanced illness or the physical limitations of severe disability or old age, simply cannot obtain the means of causing death, such as pills or a gun, or travel to a location such as a bridge or window ledge? Or does the person think the time for suicide is not yet right? Does the person seem to need approval for the act, either from other persons or from the physician or mental-health professional in this consultation? What are the deterrents to suicide so far?

4. *Is the request for help in suicide a request for someone else to decide?* If so, who? The physician or mental-health professional? Family members? The religious advisor? If it is a request for someone else to decide, why is the decision being displaced? Does the person characteristically displace most major decisions onto someone else, or only this one?

5. *How stable is the request?* Is it a solution to the person's problem which he or she has been considering or planning for a long time? Or is it a response to a recent event, such as the death of a spouse or the diagnosis of an additional medical problem? When the person thinks of suicide, does someone else come to mind, for instance, a family member or a public figure, perhaps one who has recently committed suicide? Does the person change his or her mind about suicide a lot? Sometimes? Never?

6. *Is the request consistent with the person's basic values?* Does it reflect the general outlook on moral values the person has in other areas? For example, does the person support self-determination in, say, reproductive matters or political policies, or does he or she have more conservative views about self-determination which would seem at odds with a choice of suicide? If there is a discrepancy, does this mean suicide cannot really be this person's own choice? If the choice of suicide is incompatible with the tenets of a religious group with which the person continues to identify, how does the person come to terms with this?

7. *How far in the future would the suicide take place?* Is the request preemptive or reactive? That is, is it intended to solve a future problem, for instance, the eventual onset of intractable pain or mental deterioration, or to put an end to problems already occurring?[3] If the suicide is seen as occurring in the future, not now, how does the person expect to know when the time for suicide has come? If the suicide is planned for now, is it premature? Could a suicide planned for now be postponed, and if so, for how long?

8. *Are the medical facts cited in the request accurate?* Is the diagnosis accurate? How probable is it? What confirmation of the diagnosis does the person have? What about the prognosis: how secure is it? Has an independent second or third opinion been obtained? Does the person accurately understand treatment options for future

states of a terminal illness, such as pain control in terminal cancer? Has the person been willing to try possible effective treatments? Has the person tried adaptive strategies for coping with disability? Does the person trust his or her doctor? Is the person afraid of abandonment by the doctor as the condition worsens?

9. *How accurate are other nonmedical facts cited in the request?* Does the person accurately understand that although attempting suicide is not itself a violation of the law in most jurisdictions, it may be grounds for involuntary commitment, and that others who assist in an attempt may be subject to criminal penalties? That suicide does not invalidate life insurance coverage, except during the initial one or two years? Does the person know whether injuries sustained in a nonfatal suicide attempt would be covered by health insurance?

10. *Is the suicide plan financially motivated?* Is it intended to avoid catastrophic medical expenses? To avoid excessive home-care expenses? To supply insurance proceeds to a survivor? Is the timing of the projected suicide determined by such considerations?

11. *Has the person considered the effects of his or her suicide on other persons?* Has he or she considered possible emotional trauma to survivors, especially among immediate family? What about the stigma associated with suicide? What about financial and other effects on survivors? What about co-workers, those involved in joint projects, friends, and so on? Or does the person assume that others will be untouched or even relieved at his or her death? Would the person want to try to mitigate the effects of the suicide on others? If so, has the person given any thought to how this could be done? If not, why not? (Clinicians usually recommend against bringing up issues about the effect on others during counseling with suicidal persons. This is in order to avoid triggering hostile reactions toward family members, lovers, or others, and hence reinforcing the motivation for suicide. However, since the kinds of suicides considered here are typically not dyadic in character, such problems are much less likely.)

12. *Does the person fear becoming a burden?* Is the person's assessment of his or her domestic situation realistic? How willing, in fact, are family members to care for the person in terminal illness, permanent disability, or old age? Is he or she being manipulated by family members? How could the person tell? Has there been any frank and open communication between the person and his or her relatives?

13. *What cultural influences are shaping the person's choice?* Are religious beliefs playing a major role, for instance by categorizing suicide as sinful or by promising a negative or positive afterlife? Are cultural prejudices, especially against the handicapped and the aged, contributing to feelings of worthlessness? What other cultural beliefs play a role, for instance, in shaping views about heroism, suffering, the value of life, the nature of death, and so on?

14. *Are the person's affairs in order?* Has he or she set domestic and financial matters straight? Made a will? Made funeral arrangements? Signed a living will or durable power of attorney, should a suicide attempt be incapacitating but not fatal?

15. *Has the person picked a method of committing suicide?* If so, is it a realistic method which the person is likely to be able to accomplish fully? Does the person know what kinds of injuries are likely to result if the attempt is not fatal, including permanent neurological damage from a sublethal overdose? Is the person committed

to one method only, or has he or she considered various different methods? What features of the method chosen makes it suitable for this person? Would another method be more suitable? If the person has not chosen a method, does this reveal ambivalence about committing suicide at all, or only lack of information or resources?

16. *Would the person be willing to tell others about his or her suicide plan?* Would he or she be willing to confide the plan in his or her spouse? Tell the children? Explain to friends or co-workers? Tell the minister, priest, or other religious advisor? Have it publicly known? Or would the person want the suicide kept secret, and if so, why?

17. *Does the person see suicide as the only way out?* Does he or she have any alternative plans for coping with terminal illness, permanent disability, or old age, and if so, how realistic are these plans? If these plans were subjected to the same previous sixteen questions listed here, would the answers be more or less consistent and coherent than those associated with suicide? To which plan is the person most realistically and rationally committed, or is no such commitment evident at all?

To be sure, a list of exploratory questions such as these will be modified in practice, but one thing must remain central: the exploration of a person's request for help cannot begin with an antecedent bias toward prevention, and it cannot begin by assuming that an interest in suicide is de facto evidence of depression or other psychopathology. Rather, the set of questions presented here is intended to explore whether the person's interest in suicide is rational, or whether, like suicide plans in many other human circumstances, it is the product of emotional trauma or mental illness which could be treated and relieved.[4] The results will not only make it clearer to the person involved, assuming that he or she is indeed capable of some degree of rational self-inspection, whether to proceed with the suicide or not, but it will also make clearer to the physician or mental-health professional what his or her own obligations are and what dilemmas they raise. If the person's interest in suicide reveals itself as ill-considered, incoherent, unstable, misinformed, rooted in depression, unrealistic, or otherwise irrational, the professional's clear obligation is to provide whatever further assistance and treatment is needed for controlling suicidal impulses, though open discussion of them may well prove sufficient to put them to rest. On the other hand, if the person's interest in suicide proves to be a rational and rationally held response to his or her situation—autonomous, informed, stable, considerate, uncoerced, and in accord with his or her basic values—then the professional is faced with a dilemma of personal and professional conscience, especially if he or she is a member of a medical or mental-health professional association opposed to suicide or lives in a legal jurisdiction which criminalizes assistance in suicide. Should he or she act in some more positive way to help the person accomplish suicide? I believe so. Of course, the considerations here cannot resolve such dilemmas—after all, they provide topics for discussion, not rules for behavior—nor can they answer certain hard questions: what to do in a case in which the person's contemplation of suicide seems partly rational and partly irrational, or what to do when suicidal ideation seems irrational in character but the person's circumstances are irremediably very, very bad. Nevertheless, this set of considerations can provide a more respectful and humane way physicians and mental-health professionals can respond to persons who, in a society now beginning to consider suicide as a rational and even responsible way of avoiding what they view as the degradations of terminal illness, severe permanent disability, or extreme old age, wish to explore this option with a trained and sympathetic professional. After all, if such persons cannot trust them in the first place, a paramount opportunity for providing help will be lost.

Notes

I'd like to thank Jerry Motto, Lee Ann Hoff, Ad Kerkhof, and, at a later date, Thomas Preston for comments on this paper.

1. Jerome A. Motto, "The Right to Suicide: A Psychiatrist's View," *Suicide and Life-Threatening Behavior,* vol. 2, no. 3 (Fall 1972); Timothy E. Quill, Christine Cassel, and Diane Meier, "Proposed Clinical Criteria for Physician-Assisted Suicide," *New England Journal of Medicine* 327:19 (November 5, 1992), 1380–1383.

2. Lee Ann Hoff, *People in Crisis: Understanding and Helping,* 3d ed. (Redwood City, CA: Addison-Wesley, 1989).

3. C. G. Prado, *The Last Choice: Preemptive Suicide in Advanced Age* (Westport, Conn.: Greenwood Press, 1990).

4. For an excellent example of how to explore a patient's request for assistance in suicide, see Timothy E. Quill, M.D., "Doctor, I Want to Die. Will You Help Me?" *Journal of the American Medical Association* 270:7 (August 18, 1993), 870–873.

14

Suicide: A *Fundamental* Human Right?

Do persons have the right to end their own lives, that is, the right to suicide? Of the philosophical issues concerning suicide, it is perhaps this that is most hotly disputed, and it is this upon which the most diverse claims have been made. Arthur Schopenhauer, for instance, says: ". . . It is quite obvious that there is nothing in the world to which every man has a more unassailable title than to his own life, and person."[1] Ludwig Wittgenstein, in contrast, holds that "If suicide is allowed then everything is allowed. If anything is not allowed then suicide is not allowed. This throws a light on the nature of ethics, for suicide is, so to speak, the elementary sin."[2]

When we are confronted with actual cases, our own views may be equally diverse. Consider, for instance, the real-life case of a woman I shall call Elsie Somerset:

> . . . an 80-year-old woman who had for two years been living in a nursing home. She suffered from glaucoma, which had almost completely blinded her, and from cancer of the colon, for which she was receiving chemotherapy. Her husband was recently dead. To relieve her chronic pain, and perhaps to mitigate the side effects of chemotherapy, she was being given hydromorphone, a morphine-like drug. In order to save up a week's supply of hydromorphone tablets she suffered through 168 hours of uninterrupted pain. Then she swallowed her hoard and went into a coma.
>
> She was rushed to a hospital emergency room and subjected to a variety of procedures to save her life, including the intravenous injection of naloxone, a powerful morphine antagonist. The naloxone worked and she was returned to the nursing home—still suffering from glaucoma and from cancer.[3]

We may be strongly inclined to say that Elsie Somerset had a right to take these pills, and a right to die undisturbed after she had done so. But our intuitions often swing the other way. In St. Paul, some years ago, a fifteen-year-old boy jumped to his death from a bridge, saying that he was doing so because his favorite television program, "Battlestar Galactica," had been canceled.[4] Here we are very much less inclined to say that such people—even if they were able to make a clear-headed choice—have a *right* to end their lives, and certainly not to assistance in so doing.

How then, in the face of these two very different cases, do we resolve the issue of whether there can be said to be a right to suicide?[5]

Suicide and Rights

There are two general strategies that traditionally have been used to attempt to resolve this issue. The first one attempts to show that although there is some general obligation or moral canon that prohibits suicide, certain sympathetic cases can be allowed as exceptions. For instance, Aristotle said that suicide violates one's obligation to the community; one might reply that exceptions should be made in cases where suicide benefits the community.[6] Plato and Augustine claimed that one has a prior obligation to obey the command of God; both acknowledge as exceptions, however, instances (such as Socrates and Samson) in which God directs rather than forbids the ending of one's life.[7] Immanuel Kant held that suicide is forbidden because one has an obligation to respect the humanity in one's own person; he, too, though otherwise strictly impermissive of suicide, recognized at least one exception: the case of Cato.[8] On this first strategy there is no right to suicide, though certain special cases may be permitted as exceptions to an otherwise general rule.

If, however, one finds the arguments for general obligations against suicide unpersuasive (as many contemporary thinkers have), a second strategy for taking account of our divergent intuitions concerning suicide may suggest itself: to grant that an individual may have a prima facie right to suicide, but point out that there are (frequent) circumstances in which this right is overridden. Under this second strategy, suicide is construed as a right in virtue of the individual's general liberty to do as he or she chooses, provided, of course, that his or her choices do not harm the interests or violate the rights of other persons. In other words, suicide, on this second strategy, is construed as a liberty right (of the sort propounded by John Stuart Mill);[9] one then attempts to do justice to one's initial sense that suicide in some cases is not a matter of right by showing that the liberty right to suicide is often overridden on the basis of considerations of its effects on others. The emphasis here is typically placed on the injury suicide causes to others, particularly in emotional and psychological ways, but often in financial and social respects as well. Because, it is argued, suicide can frequently be extremely damaging to the survivors of the individual who takes his or her own life—and clinical studies do show that it can severely distort the lives of spouses, parents, children, and intimate friends[10]—therefore the individual's prima facie liberty right to suicide is often, or almost always, overridden. On this account, suicide ceases to be a right not because of what it does to oneself (since on Mill's notion of liberty rights one may have a right to choose things that harm oneself), but because of what it does to others.

Like the first approach, I think this second strategy for taking account of our divergent intuitions concerning the issues of rights to suicide also fails. First, an account that restricts one's right to end one's life just to cases in which doing so will have no bad consequences for others may seem to oblige us to hold, in consistency, that one is obligated to end one's life in cases where the consequences would be good. Second, it leaves the hard work undone: it provides no settled account of what particular circumstances might override the right to suicide.[11] And third, it provides unequal treatment for individuals whose grounds for suicide may be the same but who differ in their surrounding circumstances or their relationships with others. Of two persons afflicted with an identical terminal illness, for instance, one of them might have a right to suicide and the other not, if one is free from family relationships and the other not, even though the pain and medical degradation—the reasons for the suicide—might be the same. And finally, although this is not fully distinct from the preceding objection, appealing to cases makes it evident that this way of construing rights to suicide really misses the mark: what is wrong with the suicide of the "Battlestar Galactica" youth is not just that his parents will be grieved; and what allows Elsie Somerset her right to end her life is not simply that no one around her cares.[12]

Suicide as a Fundamental Human Right

It may be tempting, at this point, to discard the notion that suicide is a matter of rights altogether, and to look for some alternative way of accounting for our sense that some suicide is permissible whereas other cases are not.[13] But I think this move is hasty. After all, persons have at least two sorts of rights:[14] not only liberty rights of the sort just described, but more basic, fundamental rights, to be accounted for in a wholly different way. I wish to claim that the right to suicide is indeed a right, and a right of the fundamental sort.

These more basic rights, as distinct from the liberty rights one has as a function of one's freedom to do as one chooses, we call natural rights, fundamental rights, or fundamental human rights. They are rights of the sort identified in the classical manifestos: the American Constitution and its Bill of Rights, the French Declaration of the Rights of Man, the Communist Manifesto, and the 1948 U.N. Declaration of Human Rights, among others. The rights listed, of course, vary from one manifesto to another, variously including rights to life, liberty, ownership of property; freedom of assembly, speech, and worship; rights to education, employment, political representation, and medical care. However, although the manifestos vary considerably in their contents, the conception underlying them is similar: they declare that certain universal, general, *fundamental* rights are held by individuals just in virtue of their being human.

I shall suggest, then, as a third strategy for achieving resolution of our conflicting intuitions regarding suicide, that it be construed as a *fundamental human right.* On this view, permissible suicide is not merely an exception to the general rules, nor is it mere exercise of one's liberty right to harm oneself if one wishes. Rather, it is a fundamental human right, on a par with rights to life,[15] to liberty, to freedom of speech and worship, to education, political representation, and the pursuit of happiness. Although I do not have space here to give an account of the claims against others, both for noninterference and for assistance, that a fundamental right to suicide might generate, it is at least clear that if what had appeared to be a liberty right to suicide turns out to be a *fundamental* right, the force of ordinary utilitarian arguments against it will collapse.

Of course, there will seem to be a good deal of evidence against this view. For one thing, the "Battlestar Galactica" case reminds us that we intuitively feel that there are cases in which persons have no right to kill themselves at all, let alone a fundamental right. Second, although listing in a manifesto cannot be taken as a reliable index of whether something is a fundamental right, it is nevertheless a conspicuous fact that a "right to suicide" is listed in none, even among manifestos of the most politically diverse sorts.[16] And finally, the fact that we have starkly differing intuitions about rights to suicide in different sorts of cases suggests that if rights of any sort are involved, they surely are not fundamental ones: if suicide were a fundamental right, we should expect all persons to have it, not just some.

Let us consider, however, the way in which fundamental rights are to be accounted for. Of course, I do not have space here in which to develop a full theory of rights, but I would like to sketch the account that I shall take in this argument as a basic premise. *Individuals have fundamental rights to do certain sorts of things just because doing those things tends to be constitutive of human dignity.*[17] "Human dignity," though it is perhaps difficult to define, is a notion rooted in an ideal conception of human life, human community, and human excellence (I shall have more to say about the concept of human dignity in the course of this chapter). On this view, although we may take ourselves to have a variety of relatively superficial and easily overridden liberty rights, we also understand ourselves to have more fundamental human rights because we conceive them to establish and promote human dignity. The right freely to associate with others we recognize as a fundamental right because we take free association with others to contribute to our dignity. Alcoholism, on the other hand, does not typically conduce to human dignity; hence, although it may still be a liberty right, namely, when it does not harm other persons, it is not a fundamental right.

While this account of rights may at first seem to be an ad hoc device for resolving our conflicts about suicide, I think it may also help explain and resolve some of the more volatile disputes concerning other rights and show why there are no disputes concerning some. It is rarely disputed, for instance, that persons have a right to freedom, since it is very widely assumed that freedom contributes to human dignity. On the other hand, although Lockean liberals defend a fundamental right to private property, Marxists and others in the post-Rousseau tradition deny this right: what is really at issue, beneath this dispute about whether private property is a right, is whether the owning of property contributes to or detracts from human dignity, both for the owner and for others as well.

But although this account of rights succeeds, not just for suicide but for fundamental rights in general, it is the particular case of the right to suicide that makes us notice the central way in which it differs from more conventional accounts. On this account, *because fundamental rights are rooted in human dignity, they are not equally distributed.* This claim may well seem initially counterintuitive and perhaps morally offensive as well; although we are of course accustomed to assume that liberty rights are inequally distributed (since for different individuals different special obligations may override them), we insist that the distribution of fundamental rights is uniform: *all* persons have them, simply in virtue of their being human. But this notion that fundamental rights are equally distributed is an illusion (though I think a necessary and desirable one):[18] it reflects not the uniform nature of fundamental rights, but the fact that the things they guarantee tend to be constitutive of human dignity equally for all persons. Thus, it appears to be analytic of the notion of fundamental human rights that they are equally distributed; it is precisely the case of suicide that shows us they are not. Some persons in some situations, we shall see, have a fundamental right to suicide; others do not. Of course, the right to suicide, if it is one, is not alone among fundamental rights in being unequally distributed (we recognize this by saying that fundamental rights are abridged or overridden by such circumstances as incompetence or grave public need);[19] it is merely more unequally distributed than most. It is this matter of unequal distribution, I think, that has disguised from us the fact that suicide is a fundamental right.

In practice, of course, there are obstacles to this account of rights. To hold that fundamental rights are not equally distributed can very well invite abuse. And to claim that one has fundamental rights only when the things they guarantee are constitutive of human dignity brings with it problems, much like those in the calculi of utilitarian theory, of ascertaining the characteristics and outcome of the exercise of a given right. Nor is human dignity any easier to quantify than happiness or utility. Nevertheless, I think an alternative account of rights must be considered if we are to resolve the issue of suicide. The traditional account of rights will not permit us to see *why* there might be a right to suicide; to claim that we do, or do not, have a right to suicide only adds, along with Schopenhauer and Wittgenstein, to the array of unfounded assertions in this regard. What we need to see is that we have a right to suicide (if and when we do) *because* it can be constitutive of human dignity, and that this basis is the same as that on which we have all other fundamental human rights. Even though it may be very markedly unequally distributed, the right to suicide is not an "exception" or a "special" right, or a right that is to be accounted for in some different way; it is of a piece with the other fundamental human rights we enjoy.

Rights and Dignity

Not all suicide is constitutive of human dignity. If we consider the "Battlestar Galactica" versus Elsie Somerset cases, this may seem quite clear. Surely we can imagine other acts on the part of the youth that would grant more dignity than his furtive leap from the bridge: the futures open to him were varied and numerous, including, no doubt, love, purposeful occupation, social contribution, and the attainment of ideals. The boy's death lacks utility, of course, in that it does not promote happiness or well-being in the agent or in others, but it also lacks that dignity that might redeem this fault. Elsie Somerset's suicide, on the other hand, seems to be quite a different case. If we consider the futures open to her, at age eighty, we see that they are different indeed from those of the youth, and a good deal less numerous. An unfortunately realistic picture of old age suggests that she can expect increasing debility, dependence, financial limitation, loss of communication and affection; increasingly poor self-image; increasing depression, isolation, and, due to her glaucoma and cancer, blindness and pain. There are alternative possible futures, of course: one of them is suicide. Another is that which she no doubt wants: a continuing, pain-free, socially involved, productive, affectionate life. But, given her physical condition and the social conditions of the society in which she lives, this may no longer be possible, and so her options may be reduced to only two: suicide, or the catalog of horrors just described. Suicide, then, may be constitutive of human dignity in at least a negative sense; in Elsie Somerset's case it may leave one less example of human degradation in the world.[20]

This kind of observation invites us to establish a procedure for sorting suicide cases into those in which the act surely cannot be constitutive of human dignity (the "Battlestar Galactica" case), and those in which it is (Elsie Somerset)—the category of those who have no right to suicide (or only an overrideable liberty right),[21] and the category of those whose right is fundamental; this would supply the basis for various practical social policies with respect to such activities as suicide prevention, psychiatric treatment, involuntary commitment, and the like. It may seem intuitively obvious that the first of these categories will include unhappy youths, star-crossed lovers, persons suffering from financial setacks or bereavement or temporary depression; the second category will include the so-called rational suicides: those who are painfully terminally ill or suffer from severe disabilities, incurable diseases, other intolerable medical conditions, or who have other good grounds for suicide. But it is just this sort of intuitive classification of suicides that is most dangerous and is the reason we need to be clear about the basis of any alleged right to suicide. To see this, we must examine the notion of dignity.

In one, originally Kantian, sense, all human beings have dignity, or what we might describe as intrinsic human worth. Dignity in this sense is an ideal, a construct that points to ends to be achieved; we might equate dignity with "worthiness of respect." But there is a second, empirical sense of dignity as well, that corrupt or abused persons may not have. In this second sense, we can distinguish observed characteristics of individuals as involving dignity from those that do not.[22] Just as we can observe whether a person is being treated with respect or "as a person"— that is, with dignity—in such situations as the classroom, in commercial relations, or in a bureaucracy, we can distinguish characteristics of the individual him- or herself that show that he or she achieves dignity as a human being. For instance, we can distinguish between the person who bears pain with dignity and the person who, in fright or panic, does not.[23] The ghastly lessons of the Nazi camps provide examples of human beings who suffered unbelievable mistreatment with dignity; and those— the so-called *Muselmänner,* the "walking skeleton" prisoners who were not only physically but psychically destroyed—who did not.

Working from a large range of observed phenomena, we can then begin to formulate the components of dignity;[24] they are probably jointly sufficient for the application of this term, though they do not all seem to be necessary. These characteristics include, to begin with, autonomy vis-à-vis external events, self-determination, and responsibility for one's acts.[25] Dignity also includes self-awareness and cognizance of one's condition and acts, together with their probable consequences. Dignity usually involves rationality, though this may not always be the case. It can also be said to involve expressiveness, or rather self-expressiveness, an assertion of oneself in the world. It surely also involves self-acceptance and self-respect: an affirmation of who and what one is. We can also suggest what tends to undermine dignity: anonymity, for instance, as in an impersonal institution; alienation of labor, crowding, meaningless and repetitive jobs, segregation, and torture.[26]

But dignity, for all its apparent initial similarity to happiness or other utilitarian desiderata, differs from these conditions of the individual in a crucially important way; it is also a characteristic of the individual in relation to his or her world. This is what in part makes it so difficult to define. And yet I think we can isolate its most important characteristic: one cannot promote one's own *dignity* by destroying the dignity of someone else, though one can certainly promote one's own interests, happiness, or reputation at another's expense. My happiness may cost your happiness, and that may be a price I am nevertheless willing to force you to pay; despite this morally repugnant choice, I may still achieve happiness. But if I try to elevate my dignity by robbing you of yours, I lose my own as well—even though I may nevertheless gain happiness, satisfaction of my interests, and other utilitarian benefits. Thus, the concept of dignity is not wholly empirical, but contains ideal features as well, even though it is not a substantive conception of the good.

To destroy your dignity, of course, is not just to graze your ego or to hurt your feelings, and it is even possible, as the Nazi camps have shown, that I may seriously damage your interests or even kill you without destroying the dignity you have. But where an act of mine would tend to destroy your capacities for such things as autonomy, self-awareness, rationality, self-expressiveness, and self-respect, then we will begin to want to say that I lose my own dignity in doing such an act to you. Dignity, although it is a characteristic inhering primarily in the individual and is not simply a relational property, contains essential reference to the dignity of others where others are involved; no act that undermines the dignity of others can be an act constitutive of one's own human dignity, whatever utility it may produce, for it thus violates that ideal conception of human community in which the notion of dignity is in part rooted. Furthermore, although dignity contains essential reference to the dignity of others wherever others are involved, an act may also be an act of dignity even if it affects oneself alone—provided that it honors that ideal conception of human excellence, whatever its specific content, in which the notion of dignity is also based.

Thus there can be no dignity trade-offs, like the interests or happiness trade-offs that plague utilitarian calculations; the problem of sacrificing the dignity of some for the dignity of others cannot arise. It is in this sense that dignity is both an empirical and an ideal notion, and it may be that the actual acts that contribute to dignity are in fact very few. Nevertheless, I do think it is a conception of dignity of this sort that lies at the basis of our ascriptions of fundamental rights.

But can *suicide* satisfy both the empirical and ideal criteria for dignity, and so be an act to which one has a fundamental right? And does the distinction between apparently irrational suicides and those for which one has good cause reflect that between dignity-constitutive suicides and those that are not?

Distinguishing among Suicides

There are many different kinds of suicide, both in terms of the individual's interior states and the act's effects on others involved, yet they can be divided into two principal groups. On the one hand are the "violent" suicides: desperate, aggressive acts, that display both contempt and hatred for oneself and for others as well. Most common among these perhaps are the "get even" suicides, which show a desire for revenge upon one's enemies or erstwhile loved ones and often a despising of the world as a whole. Animosity, ambivalence, and agitation are the symptoms here.

Others, in contrast, are "nonviolent": of these, some may be described as involving cessation or surcease rather than obliteration or annihilation, often anticipated and planned in a resigned but purposeful way; others, not always distinct from the surcease suicides, are sacrificial in character and focus centrally on the benefits to some other person or cause. The nonviolent suicides are nonviolent both toward oneself and toward others, at least in the clearest cases; they do not seek to punish oneself or to injure or retaliate against others. Very often these nonviolent suicides contain a component of what we might, paradoxically perhaps, call self-preservation, a kind of self-respect: "I am what I have been," they sometimes seem to say, "but cannot be anymore." They are based, as it were, on a self-ideal: a conception of one's own value and worth, beneath which one is not willing to slip. Whether the threat to one's self-ideal is from physical illness and pain, as in euthanatic suicide, or from the destruction of other persons or values upon which one's life is centrally focused, as in self-sacrificial suicide, the import is the same: one chooses death instead of further life, because further life would bring with it a compromise of that dignity without which one cannot consent to live.

This distinction between violent, self-aggressive and nonviolent, self-respecting suicides is an intuitive distinction only; it is a distinction not much recognized in clinical practice, though perhaps only because psychiatric clinicians are very much less likely to confront cases of the self-respecting, nonviolent type.[27] It is important to be clear, in addition, that this distinction is not based on the means involved: some deaths by gunshot or jumping are of the nonviolent kind, whereas some deaths by tranquilizers or gas or even refusal to eat are of the violent sort, involving extreme self-aggression and aggression toward others. Nevertheless, it is possible to characterize generally the kinds of suicide that are common among certain groups and in certain kinds of situations. Violence toward oneself and others characterizes a good deal of youthful suicide, even that associated with depression; it is also found among the old. But nonviolent, surcease suicide is much more common in disability and terminal illness cases, and particularly among the old. Self-death or self-directed death in these latter conditions, of course, we often term voluntary euthanasia or sometimes euthanatic suicide; we frequently attempt to distinguish them both morally and legally from "irrational" suicide in nonterminal conditions, that is, suicide for which one does not have good reason.

In distinguishing between irrational suicide and euthanatic suicide, we do recognize that there are important differences between suicide that precludes indefinitely continuing life and suicide in preference to inevitable death by another more painful or degrading means. But this distinction does *not* precisely coincide with the distinction between those kinds of suicide to which an individual has only liberty rights or no right at all, and those kinds of suicide to which the individual has a fundamental human right, one that cannot be overridden by any particular obligations or claims. This is because some cases of noneuthanatic suicide may be constitutive of human dignity—Cato's death is a case in point—whereas some genuine euthanasia cases may not be acts of human dignity but acts of cowardice and fear—hasty, terrified measures that preclude any final human dignity rather than contribute to it. Some writers opposed to suicide in general would have us believe that all euthanatic suicides are of this latter sort—acts of cowardice and fear; I think this is false, but I think it is equally wrong to assume that all suicide in the face of terminal illness is a rational, composed, self-dignifying affirmation of one's own highest life-ideal.

It may be that as a practical matter the nearest workable policy is acceptance of the notion of rational suicide, and the devising of selective suicide-prevention and psychiatric-treatment measures to discourage suicide of the irrational sort. If this is the only really practical policy for selectively permitting suicides of fundamental right and prohibiting those that are not,[28] I think on moral grounds we ought to adopt it, in preference either to maintaining the traditional universal suicide prohibitions or adopting indiscriminately permissive policies. We should bear in mind, however, that the rational/irrational distinction does not quite mirror the difference we want.

Now we see why the temptation to classify suicides into dignity-constitutive and non-dignity-constitutive cases on the basis of external characteristics is such a dangerous one, particularly if such a classification is to become the basis for various practical policies: the circumstances under which it occurs do not determine the character of the act. There can be suicides of dignity in conditions of despair; there can be suicides without dignity even when the circumstances are such that the individual might have every reason to die.

In his paper "Suicide as Instrument and Expression,"[29] David Wood invents a case: the suicide (by jumping) of an architect who pioneered high-rise apartment buildings and realizes too late what he has done. Is this a suicide of dignity, and so one to which he has a fundamental right, or is it a suicide of the violent, non-dignity-promoting sort, one to which he does not have such a right? We can imagine the case either way: as the final, desperate act of self-loathing and self-contempt, occurring as the confused climax of long years of self-reproach; but we can also imagine it as a considered, courageous statement of principle, a dignified final act transcending one's own defeat. If it is a violent suicide of loathing, we can imagine reminding the man that he has obligations to his family, his friends, his gods, and himself, that is, we can imagine treating it as a liberty right, quickly to be overridden by the claims of others. But if it is a genuine suicide of dignity it is difficult to know what objection we could make, since we must only admire his attainment of a difficult human ideal. That the price of this attainment is high—very high—is perhaps lamentable, but it is not grounds for interfering with his exercise of the right.

What of Schopenhauer and Wittgenstein, and the disparate philosophical views with which we began? Perhaps now we can venture some explanation that, though it is conjectural, may also explain the apparent inconsistency in our own precritical views. When Wittgenstein claims that suicide is "the elementary sin," he is perhaps conceiving (no doubt in an autobiographical way) of cases in which the act is one of self-annihilation and the annihilation of one's social world; it is the ultimate act of disrespect and violence. When Schopenhauer, on the other hand, said that man had no "more unassailable title than to his own life and person," it may be that even though he regards suicide as a moral and metaphysical error, since it results not from cessation but frustration of the will, he is nevertheless appealing to a notion of suicide as what we might consider an act of ultimate dignity: the final act of self-determination and self-affirmation in an immoral, unyielding world. In this way both views are correct, and not after all incompatible: individuals in the cases Wittgenstein has in mind have no right, or, at most, only an overrideable liberty right, to kill themselves, whereas individuals in the cases Schopenhauer sees have a basic, non-overrideable, fundamental human right to end their lives. The only real mistake Schopenhauer and Wittgenstein make is this: they assume that the ''right to suicide'' is a uniform right, held by all individuals or none at all.

Notes

I'd like to thank Bruce Landesman and, at a later date, Govert den Hartogh for comments on this paper.

1. Arthur Schopenhauer, ''On Suicide,'' from *Studies in Pessimism,* in *Complete Essays of Schopenhauer,* tr. T. Bailey Saunders (New York: Wiley Book Co., 1940).

2. Ludwig Wittgenstein, *Notebooks 1914–1916,* ed. G. H. von Wright and G. E. M. Anscombe (Oxford: Basil Blackwell, 1961), 91e. Wittgenstein continues, however, in this final entry of the notebooks: ''And when one investigates it [suicide], it is like investigating mercury vapour in order to comprehend the nature of vapours. Or is even suicide in itself neither good nor evil?''

3. Adapted from Edward M. Brecher, ''Opting for Suicide,'' *The New York Times Magazine,* March 18, 1979, quoting from the October 1978 issue of *Hospital Physician.*

4. *Minneapolis Star and Tribune,* Saturday, August 25, 1979, p. 1A.

5. One may be said to have a right to x, or a right to do x; that to which a person may have a right can be an object, a condition, a state of affairs, or an action. Construing suicide as an action, I shall speak throughout only of the right to (commit [''do'']) suicide, rather than, say the right to the object or condition (death) that suicide brings about.

6. Aristotle, *Nichomachean Ethics* 1138a.

7. Plato, *Phaedo* 61C–62E; Augustine, *City of God,* bk. 1, chaps. 17–27.

8. Immanuel Kant, ''Suicide,'' in *Lectures on Ethics,* tr. Louis Infield (New York: Harper Torchbooks, 1963), 148–154.

9. John Stuart Mill, *On Liberty* (Harmondsworth: Penguin Books, 1982), originally published 1859. It is interesting that Mill does not discuss suicide directly, although it might seem the most crucial case for the application of his views. In *On Liberty* he argues that one may not sell oneself into slavery because this would fail to preserve one's liberty; one might infer from this that Mill would also repudiate suicide on the same grounds. However, one might argue that since after suicide the individual does not exist in an unfree state (but, rather, does not exist at all), Mill provides no basis for an objection to this practice.

10. There is a large sociological and psychological literature on the effects of suicide on those persons surrounding the individual. See, for example, Albert C. Cain, ed., *Survivors of Suicide* (Springfield, Ill.: Charles C. Thomas, 1972), and many more recent works.

11. Of course, this is not a theoretical objection to the liberty rights account of suicide, but it does point out that without further elaboration the account is not a particularly helpful or informative one.

12. Paul-Louis Landsberg, in *The Moral Problem of Suicide,* tr. Cynthia Rowland (New York: Philosophical Library, 1953), 84, puts the point in this way: ''It is purely and simply antipersonalist to try to decide such an intimately personal question as to whether or not I have

the right to kill myself by reference to society. Suppose I die a little sooner or a little later, what has that to do with society, to which, in any case, I belong for so short a space?''

13. See, for example, James Bogen, ''Suicide and Virtue,'' in *Suicide: The Philosophical Issues,* ed. M. Pabst Battin and David Mayo (New York: St. Martin's, 1980), 286, who claims that an adequate treatment of the morality of suicide cannot be made in terms of obligations, rights, and duties.

14. In addition to liberty rights and fundamental rights, we also recognize legal rights. Given, however, the very uneven situation of the law with regard to suicide (in this connection, see the papers of Alan Sullivan and Leslie Francis, in *Suicide,* ed. Battin and Mayo, 229 and 254). I have restricted the scope of this chapter to moral rights alone.

15. Note that a fundamental right to suicide does not preclude an equally fundamental right to life, because both may be constitutive of human dignity. This is so even in euthanasia cases: there may be dignity in an individual's struggling against the inevitable oncoming of decay, medical degradation, and pain; there may equally well be dignity in his or her choosing to avoid these by ending his or her life. In general, one may have fundamental rights to various incompatible actions, as, for instance, one may have fundamental rights to own private property or to join a communal economic group, when either course of action is the kind that can be constitutive of human dignity. Thus, rights are not to be conflated with duties.

16. One might mention ''the right to die'' now being championed by various patients' rights groups; this, however, is usually understood as the right to freedom from unwanted medical treatment, or a ''right to passive euthanasia.'' The scope of a ''right to suicide'' would be considerably broader.

17. This account appears to resemble in some respects that put forward by William T. Blackstone in ''Human Rights and Human Dignity,'' *The Philosophy Forum* 9, nos. 1/2 (March 1971), and perhaps even the counterthesis in the same volume, Herbert Spiegelberg's ''Human Dignity: A Challenge to Contemporary Philosophy.'' It also resembles one component of the account Arnold S. Kaufman defends in ''A Sketch of a Liberal Theory of Fundamental Human Rights,'' *The Monist* 52 (No. 4), though for Kaufman fundamental human rights may be justified either on the basis of dignity or on the basis of maximum utility together with equality. Also relevant in connection with this issue is Michael S. Pritchard's ''Human Dignity and Justice,'' *Ethics* 82 (No. 4, July 1972).

18. The fiction that fundamental rights are universally distributed is both necessary and desirable for the following reasons. The present account of rights (although I believe it to be correct) is hopelessly particularist, in that it holds that an individual has a fundamental right to do just that sort of act, or just that act, which is conducive to human dignity. But it is extremely difficult to predict whether an act of a given kind will in fact contribute to human dignity, and so be an act of the kind to which that individual has a fundamental right. This may vary from one individual to the next, or change for a given individual over a period of time. Furthermore, despite certain empirical earmarks of dignity, it is in principle impossible to diagnose with full reliability whether a given individual does or does not achieve complete human dignity. The best we can say is that *on the whole,* certain types of actions or things— for example, free assembly, free speech, freedom from the quartering of soldiers in one's house, etc., tend to be constitutive of human dignity, whether or not we can in fact make a reliable, confirmable assessment in any given case. Thus we are forced to assume that fundamental rights are universally or at least very widely distributed; this is the ''necessary'' feature. But once we have made this assumption, we must then produce justification for any abridgment of those (alleged) fundamental rights; this is the ''desirable'' part. For example, because we allow ourselves to assume that the right to free assembly is a fundamental right, shared by all human beings, we thus compel ourselves to justify any abridgment of that right. Hence, protection of these rights is made much more likely. If we were to recognize and honor

an individual's fundamental right to, say, free assembly only in cases in which we could establish that the exercise of free assembly would conduce to the dignity of that individual, we would risk abridgments of this right in very, very many cases.

Whether such a fiction is either necessary or desirable in the case of suicide, however, is quite a different question. I think it is intuitively clear that not all persons in all circumstances have a right to suicide, though some persons in some circumstances do: we are not forced to assume that, *on the whole,* suicide is constitutive of human dignity, because we clearly see that it is not. Nor is it clearly desirable to adopt a fiction that, in practice, would place the burden of justification on those who would interfere with a suicide rather than on those who plan suicide for whatever reason.

19. Conventional theories of rights hold that fundamental rights are overridden in circumstances such as incompetence (e.g., the right of a severely retarded person to freedom of travel may be abridged) or requirements of community interest (the felon's right to freedom of travel may also be abridged); on the present account, fundamental rights are never overridden, but in cases such as these simply do not apply. It is silly to insist that the seriously retarded individual has a "fundamental right to freedom of travel" when travel (at least without assistance) can mean nothing but helpless wandering in an unfriendly world, or that the recidivist felon has a right to freedom of his or her person when exercise of that right conduces to anything but human dignity. Since this is so, nonvoluntary institutionalization of such persons does not genuinely represent an abridgment of their fundamental rights, though institutionalization in a cruel environment, or without facilities for special education, etc., might do so.

20. Human degradation in the empirical sense, of course. The dual concept of human dignity suggests that all human beings continue to have dignity in the ideal sense, that is, all human beings remain worthy of respect, regardless of how degrading the conditions and circumstances in which they are forced to live.

21. I cannot attempt here to resolve the issue of whether suicide, in cases in which it does not conduce to dignity and hence is not a fundamental right, is nevertheless a liberty right, or is, rather, no right at all. If it were a liberty right, it would of course be subject to overriding on the basis of a variety of considerations. If it is a fundamental right, it is a liberty right and should be a legal right as well.

22. This dual account of the concept of human dignity is developed in several of the papers mentioned in note 17.

23. See Abraham Edel, "Humanist Ethics and the Meaning of Human Dignity," in *Moral Problems in Contemporary Society: Essays in Humanistic Ethics,* ed. Paul Kurtz (Englewood Cliffs, N.J.: Prentice-Hall, 1969), 234.

24. This is done here, of course, only in a somewhat a priori and very tentative way. But it is the sort of task we might wish philosophers will do.

25. This is the concept of dignity used by B. F. Skinner in *Beyond Freedom and Dignity* (New York: Alfred A. Knopf, 1991), especially in chap. 3, and also the second sense of dignity for Marvin Kohl, "Voluntary Beneficent Euthanasia," in Kohl, ed., *Beneficent Euthanasia* (Buffalo: Prometheus Books, 1975), 133.

26. The list is Spiegelberg's, "Human Dignity," 60.

27. Surcease suicide in terminal illness is almost never reported as suicide, and is not recorded in that way by the coroner or by insurance companies. It is believed, however, that the practice of surcease suicide in terminal illness, often with the assistance of the physician in providing lethal drugs, is fairly common.

28. Criminal prohibitions, of course, would be most plausibly directed against suicides exhibiting violence against others.

29. *Suicide,* ed. Battin and Mayo, 151.

Index

Aaron, H. J., 79 n.25
Abandonment, death by, 59, 191, 244
Abelson, Raziel, 202 n.1
Abortion: comparison with right-to-die issues, 8; as major social issue, 9; morality of, 17
Abuse: criteria for judging, 166–67; legal protections against, 164; objective indices of, 178–80; potential for, 23–24, 48–49, 55, 73–76, 140–41, 163–67; prevention of, 173–80; types of, 167–73
Academy of Accompaniment in Dying ("Akademie der Sterbebegleitung"), 259, 267
Ackerman, Diana, 56 n.8
Adkins, Janet, 5
Advance directives: of Alzheimer's patients, 147–49, 160, 161–62; authorization of euthanasia with, 137; difficulties in executing, 35; discussions with physicians as, 137; and fundamental rights, 193; legal status of, 14, 28 n.28, 33; planning of, 38; pressuring of patients to have, 172; as requirement for termination procedures, 160, 161–62, 175; specification of euthanasia in 147–49; and uniformity of dying, 91
Advertising of termination procedures, prohibition of, 176
Age of death, fixed, 74–75
Age rationing, 14; as allocation over duration of life, 61–62; alteration of morbidity curve through, 68 (fig.), 68–72, 69 (fig); assumption of scarcity behind,

76–77; as competition among interest groups, 61; through denial of treatment, 63–66, 68, 69, 71; through direct-termination procedures, 68–76, 69 (fig.), 77; individual choice in, 74, 75; issues of abuse in, 73–76; maximization of life in, 70–72; minimization of suffering in, 70; principles of justice and, 61–63; public attitudes toward, 72–73; public understanding of, 76; redistributive dividends of, 77; rights under, 73
Aged, the: as candidates for health care rationing, 60 (see also Age rationing); demands upon health care system, 59–60, 64, 79 n.27; morbidity characteristics of, 66–68, 67 (fig.); obligation to end life of, 58–59 (see also Duty to die)
Aldrich, Virgil, 202 n.2
Aleuts, time to die among the, 73
Altruism: and abuse of patients, 48–49, 55; in amimals, 228; characterizing of self-sacrificial acts as suicide, 188; compatibility with self-interest, 42, 56 n.1; conflict between beneficence and, 45, 48; confrontation with actual sacrifice, 53, 57 n.18; costs to altruist, 50; degree of, 42, 56 n.1; genetic basis for, 228–29; manipulation of, 50, 55; moral significance of, 50, 51, 52–53; objects of, 42, 56 n.1; perception of others by, 52, 57 n.15; precluded by organized medicine, 43–49, 92–93; protecting possibility of, 53–55; psychological consequences of, 50–51; and shifting of

Printed in the United Kingdom
by Lightning Source UK Ltd.
133351UK00001B/143/A

THE LEAST